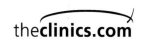

ANESTHESIOLOGY CLINICS

Neurosurgical Anesthesia and Critical Care

GUEST EDITORS
Ansgar M. Brambrink, MD, PhD,
and Jeffrey R. Kirsch, MD

CONSULTING EDITOR
Lee A. Fleisher, MD

September 2007 • Volume 25 • Number 3

SAUNDERS

An Imprint of Elsevier, Inc.
PHILADELPHIA   LONDON   TORONTO   MONTREAL   SYDNEY   TOKYO

W.B. SAUNDERS COMPANY
A Division of Elsevier Inc.

1600 John F. Kennedy Boulevard, Suite 1800 • Philadelphia, Pennsylvania 19103-2899

http://www.theclinics.com

ANESTHESIOLOGY CLINICS	Volume 25, Number 3
September 2007	ISSN 1932-2275
Editor: Rachel Glover	ISBN-13: 978-1-4160-5143-5
	ISBN-10: 1-4160-5143-0

The ideas and opinions expressed in *Anesthesiology Clinics* do not necessarily reflect those of the Publisher. The Publisher does not assume any responsibility for any injury and/or damage to persons or property arising out of or related to any use of the material contained in this periodical. The reader is advised to check the appropriate medical literature and the product information currently provided by the manufacturer of each drug to be administered to verify the dosage, the method and duration of administration, or contraindications. It is the responsibility of the treating physician or other health care professional, relying on independent experience and knowledge of the patient, to determine drug dosages and the best treatment for the patient. Mention of any product in this issue should not be construed as endorsement by the contributors, editors, or the Publisher of the product or manufacturers' claims.

Anesthesiology Clinics (ISSN 1932-2275) is published quarterly by Elsevier Inc., 360 Park Avenue South, New York, NY 10010-1710. Months of issue are March, June, September, and December. Business and Editorial Offices: 1600 John F. Kennedy Blvd., Suite 1800, Philadelphia, PA 19103-2899. Customer Service Office: 6277 Sea Harbor Drive, Orlando, FL 32887-4800. Periodicals postage paid at New York, NY and additional mailing offices. Subscription prices are $101.00 per year (US student/resident), $202.00 per year (US individuals), $246.00 per year (Canadian individuals), $302.00 per year (US institutions), $366.00 per year (Canadian institutions), $134.00 per year (Canadian and foreign student/resident), $263.00 per year (foreign individuals), and $366.00 per year (foreign institutions). To receive student and resident rate, orders must be accompanied by name of affiliated institution, date of term, and the *signature* of program/residency coordinator on institutions letterhead. Orders will be billed at individual rate until proof of status is received. Foreign air speed delivery is included in all *Clinics'* subscription prices. All prices are subject to change without notice. POSTMASTER: Send address changes to *Anesthesiology Clinics*, Elsevier Periodicals Customer Service, 6277 Sea Harbor Drive, Orlando, FL 32887-4800. **Customer Service: 1-800-654-2452** (US). From outside of the US, call **1-407-345-4000**. E-mail: hhspcs@wbsaunders.com.

Anesthesiology Clinics, is also published in Spanish by McGraw-Hill Inter-americana Editores S. A., P.O. Box 5-237, 06500 Mexico D. F., Mexico.

Anesthesiology Clinics, is covered in *Index Medicus, Current Contents/Clinical Medicine, Excerpta Medica, ISI/BIOMED*, and *Chemical Abstracts*.

Printed in the United States of America.

CONSULTING EDITOR

LEE A. FLEISHER, MD, Robert D. Dripps Professor of Medicine; Chair, Anesthesiology and Critical Care, University of Pennsylvania School of Medicine, Philadelphia, Pennsylvania

GUEST EDITORS

ANSGAR M. BRAMBRINK, MD, PhD, Professor of Anesthesiology and Perioperative Medicine and Neurology, Department of Anesthesiology and Perioperative Medicine, Oregon Health and Sciences University, Portland, Oregon

JEFFREY R. KIRSCH, MD, Professor and Chairman, Department of Anesthesiology and Perioperative Medicine, Oregon Health and Sciences University, Portland, Oregon

CONTRIBUTORS

RAFI AVITSIAN, MD, Assistant Professor of Anesthesiology, Cleveland Clinic Lerner College of Medicine of Case Western Reserve University; Staff, Department of General Anesthesiology, Cleveland Clinic, Cleveland, Ohio

AUDRÉE A. BENDO, MD, Professor of Anesthesiology; Vice Chair for Education, Department of Anesthesiology, SUNY Downstate Medical Center, Brooklyn, New York

ANSGAR M. BRAMBRINK, MD, PhD, Professor of Anesthesiology and Perioperative Medicine and Neurology, Department of Anesthesiology and Perioperative Medicine, Oregon Health and Sciences University, Portland, Oregon

J. RICARDO CARHUAPOMA, MD, Assistant Professor, Neurosciences Critical Care Division, Departments of Neurology, Neurosurgery and Anesthesiology and Critical Care Medicine, The Johns Hopkins Hospital, Baltimore, Maryland

DANIEL J. COLE, MD, Professor of Anesthesiology, Deparment of Anesthesiology, Mayo Clinic Hospital, Phoenix, Arizona

EDWARD T. CROSBY, MD, FRCPC, Professor, Department of Anesthesiology, University of Ottawa, The Ottawa Hospital–General Campus, Ottawa, Ontario, Canada

KRISTIN ENGELHARD, MD, Associate Professor of Anesthesiology, Clinic of Anasthesiology, Johannes Gutenberg-University of Mainz, Mainz, Germany

KIRSTIN M. ERICKSON, MD, Assistant Professor of Anesthesiology, Department of Anesthesiology, Mayo Clinic College of Medicine, Rochester, Minnesota

HEIKE GRIES, MD, PhD, Assistant Professor, Department of Anesthesiology and Perioperative Medicine, Oregon Health and Sciences University, Portland, Oregon

LESLIE C. JAMESON, MD, Associate Professor of Anesthesiology, University of Colorado at Denver and Health Sciences Center, Denver, Colorado

DANIEL J. JANIK, MD, Associate Professor of Anesthesiology, University of Colorado at Denver and Health Sciences Center, Denver, Colorado

JEFFREY R. KIRSCH, MD, Professor and Chairman, Department of Anesthesiology and Perioperative Medicine, Oregon Health and Sciences University, Portland, Oregon

W. ANDREW KOFKE, MD, MBA, FCCM, Professor of Anesthesia and Neurosurgery, Department of Anesthesia and Critical Care, University of Pennsylvania, Philadelphia, Pennsylvania

JEFFREY L. KOH, MD, MBA, Professor, Department of Anesthesiology and Perioperative Medicine, Oregon Health and Sciences University; Chief, Division of Pediatric Anesthesia and Pain Management, Doernbecher Children's Hospital, Portland, Oregon

MAREK A. MIRSKI, MD, PhD, Vice Chair, Neurosciences Critical Care Division, Department of Anesthesiology and Critical Care Medicine; Associate Professor, Departments of Neurology, Neurosurgery and Anesthesiology and Critical Care Medicine, The Johns Hopkins Hospital, Baltimore, Maryland

WIBKE MÜLLER-FORELL, MD, Extraordinary Professor of Neuroradiology, Institute of Neuroradiology, Johannes Gutenberg-University of Mainz, Mainz, Germany

NEERAJ S. NAVAL, MD, Assistant Professor, Neurosciences Critical Care Division, Departments of Neurology, Neurosurgery and Anesthesiology and Critical Care Medicine, The Johns Hopkins Hospital, Baltimore, Maryland

JOSE ORTIZ-CARDONA, MD, Clinical Assistant Instructor, Department of Anesthesiology, SUNY Downstate Medical Center, Brooklyn, New York

IRENE ROZET, MD, Assistant Professor, Department of Anesthesiology, University of Washington, Seattle, Washington

ARMIN SCHUBERT, MD, MBA, Professor of Anesthesiology, Cleveland Clinic Lerner College of Medicine of Case Western Reserve University; Staff, Department of General Anesthesiology, Cleveland Clinic, Cleveland, Ohio

TOD B. SLOAN, MD, MBA, PhD, Professor of Anesthesiology, University of Colorado at Denver and Health Sciences Center, Denver, Colorado

MARTIN SMITH, MBBS, FRCA, Consultant in Neuroanaesthesia and Neurocritical Care, Department of Neuroanaesthesia and Neurocritical Care; Honorary Reader in Anaesthesia and Critical Care, The National Hospital for Neurology and Neurosurgery, University College London Hospitals NHS Foundation Trust and Centre for Anaesthesia, University College London, United Kingdom

MICHAEL STIEFEL, MD, PhD, Chief Resident, Department of Neurosurgery, University of Pennsylvania, Philadelphia, Pennsylvania

MONICA S. VAVILALA, MD, Associate Professor, Department of Anesthesiology; Department of Pediatrics; Department of Neurological Surgery, University of Washington, Seattle, Washington

WILLIAM L. YOUNG, MD, Professor and Vice Chair, Department of Anesthesia and Perioperative Care; Professor of Neurological Surgery and Neurology, University of California, San Francisco, San Francisco, California

CONTENTS

> This review outlines the roles of anesthesiologists in the manage-
> ment of patients undergoing invasive endovascular procedures to
> treat vascular diseases, primarily of the central nervous system.
> This practice usually is termed interventional neuroradiology or
> endovascular neurosurgery. The discussion emphasizes periopera-
> tive and anesthetic management strategies to prevent complica-
> tions and minimize their effects if they occur. Planning anesthetic
> and perioperative management is predicated on understanding
> the goals of the therapeutic intervention and anticipating potential
> problems.

> Neuroimaging is essential in the treatment of cerebral nervous sys-
> tem disorders or in patients in the ICU with deterioration of their
> neurologic function. Leading clinical symptoms are acute neurolo-
> gic deficits with different stages of hemisymptomatology, primary
> or progressing loss of consciousness or vigilance deficit, focal or
> generalized seizures, sometimes combined with an acute

respiratory or circulatory insufficiency. The resulting questions can be summarized in those of intracranial space occupying hemorrhage; acute infarction; and signs for reduced cerebral blood flow, cerebrovascular vasospasm, or intracranial mass. Recent evolutions in imaging have contributed to an increase in diagnostic sensitivity and specificity along with reduced side effects. This article illustrates typical and atypical differential diagnoses, with some emphasis on traumatic brain injury.

Anesthetic Considerations for Intraoperative Management of Cerebrovascular Disease in Neurovascular Surgical Procedures

Rafi Avitsian and Armin Schubert

Despite new surgical methods and interventions a considerable number of patients who undergo neurovascular procedures emergently or electively have substantial mortality, morbidity, and disability. Sound knowledge of pathophysiology of cerebral hypoperfusion, reliable and timely information from monitoring devices, and appropriate choice of therapeutic intervention is essential for successful anesthetic management of these patients. The management of perioperative vasospasm and temporary ischemia during aneurysm clipping require an understanding of cerebral vascular pathophysiology and neuroprotective measures.

Perioperative Management of Pediatric Patients with Craniosynostosis

Jeffrey L. Koh and Heike Gries

Craniosynostosis, premature closures of the skull sutures, results in dysmorphic features if left untreated. Brain growth and cognitive development may also be impacted. Craniosynostosis repair is usually performed in young infants and has its perioperative challenges. This article provides background information about the different forms of craniosynostosis, with an overview of associated anomalies, genetic influences, and their connection with cognitive function. It also discusses the anesthetic considerations for perioperative management, including blood-loss management and strategies to reduce homologous blood transfusions.

Perioperative Care of Patients with Neuromuscular Disease and Dysfunction

Ansgar M. Brambrink and Jeffrey R. Kirsch

A variety of different pathologies result in disease phenotypes that are summarized as neuromuscular diseases because they share commonalty in their clinical consequences for the patient: a progressive weakening of the skeletal muscles. Distinct caution and appropriate changes to the anesthetic plan are advised when care is provided during the perioperative period. The choice of anesthetic technique, anesthetic drugs, and neuromuscular blockade always depends on the type of neuromuscular disease and the surgical procedure planned. A clear diagnosis of the underlying disease and sufficient knowledge and understanding of the pathophysiology are of paramount importance to the practitioner and guide optimal perioperative management of affected patients.

Surgery on the cervical spine runs the gamut from minor interventions done in a minimally invasive fashion on a short-stay or ambulatory basis, to major surgical undertakings of a high-risk, high-threat nature done to stabilize a degraded skeletal structure to preserve and protect neural elements. Planning for optimum airway management and anesthesia care is facilitated by an appreciation of the disease processes that affect the cervical spine and their biomechanical implications and an understanding of the imaging and operative techniques used to evaluate and treat these conditions. This article provides background information and evidence to allow the anesthesia practitioner to develop a conceptual framework within which to develop strategies for care when a patient is presented for surgery on the cervical spine.

A variety of anesthetic methods, with and without airway manipulation, are available to facilitate awake intraoperative examinations and cortical stimulation, which allow more aggressive resection of epileptogenic foci in functionally important brain regions. Careful patient selection and preparation combined with attentive cooperation of the medical team are the foundation for a smooth awake procedure. With improved pharmacologic agents and variety of techniques at the neuroanesthesiologist's disposal, awake craniotomy has become an elegant approach to epileptic focus resection in functional cortex.

Transcranial perfusion monitoring provides early warning of impending brain ischemia and may be used to guide management of cerebral perfusion and oxygenation. The monitoring options include measurement of intracranial and cerebral perfusion pressures, assessment of cerebral blood flow, and assessment of the adequacy of perfusion by measurement of cerebral oxygenation and brain tissue biochemistry. Some monitoring techniques are well established, whereas others are relatively new to the clinical arena and their indications are still being evaluated. Currently available monitoring techniques are reviewed and their appropriateness and application to the perioperative period is discussed.

Monitoring and Intraoperative Management of Elevated Intracranial Pressure and Decompressive Craniectomy
W. Andrew Kofke and Michael Stiefel

There are numerous clinical scenarios wherein a critically ill patient may present with neurologic dysfunction. In a general sense these scenarios often involve ischemia, trauma, or neuroexcitation. Each of these may include a period of decreased cerebral perfusion pressure, usually due to elevated intracranial pressure (ICP), eventually compromising cerebral blood flow sufficiently to produce permanent neuronal loss, infarction, and possibly brain death. Elevated ICP is thus a common pathway for neural demise and it may arise from a variety of causes, many of which may result in a neurosurgical procedure intended to ameliorate the impact or etiology of elevated ICP.

Electrophysiologic Monitoring in Neurosurgery
Leslie C. Jameson, Daniel J. Janik, and Tod B. Sloan

Electrophysiologic techniques have become common in the neurosurgical operating room. This article reviews the methods used for mapping neural structures or monitoring during surgery. Mapping methods allow identification of target structures for surgery, or for identifying structures to allow avoidance or plot safe pathways to deeper structures. Monitoring methods allow for surgery on nearby structures to warn of encroachment, thereby reducing unwanted injury.

Risks and Benefits of Patient Positioning During Neurosurgical Care
Irene Rozet and Monica S. Vavilala

Positioning of the surgical patient is an important part of anesthesia care and attention to the physical and physiologic consequences of positioning can help prevent serious adverse events and complications. The general principles of patient positioning of the anesthetized and awake neurosurgical patient are discussed in this article.

FORTHCOMING ISSUES

RECENT ISSUES

ELSEVIER
SAUNDERS

Anesthesiology Clin
25 (2007) xiii–xiv

ANESTHESIOLOGY
CLINICS

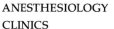

Foreword

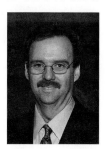

Lee A. Fleisher, MD
Consulting Editor

The twenty-first century has been described by many as the era of neuroscience. There has been an explosion in new imaging modalities and methods to treat neurologic disease. Many contemporary treatments are performed by neurosurgeons and by interventional radiologists. Neuroanesthesiologists have had to adapt to changing requirements for the provision of anesthesia to patients undergoing this vast array of diagnostic and therapeutic procedures. The current issue of the *Anesthesiology Clinics* has approached these changes in the field and has collected a series of state-of-the-art reviews that will benefit all anesthesiologists.

We are fortunate in having two outstanding neuroanesthesiologists from the Oregon Health Sciences University as guest editors for this issue. Jeffrey Kirsh, MD, is currently Professor and Chair of Anesthesiology and Peri-operative Medicine. He has been an active researcher and clinician in both intra-operative neuroanesthesia and in the neuro critical care unit and is a former President of the Society of Neuroanesthesia and Critical Care. He has written more than 90 original articles and has edited five books. He has been funded extensively by the National Institutes of Health to study stroke and brain injury. Ansgar Brambrink, MD, PhD, is Associate Professor of Anesthesiology and Perioperative Medicine and Director of Faculty Development. His research interests include the pathophysiology of cerebral ischemia and

1932-2275/07/$ - see front matter © 2007 Elsevier Inc. All rights reserved.
doi:10.1016/j.anclin.2007.05.012   *anesthesiology.theclinics.com*

reperfusion and poststroke repair and functional recovery. They have invited an outstanding group of international experts to participate in this issue.

Lee A. Fleisher, MD
Anesthesiology and Critical Care
University of Pennsylvania
6 Dulles, 3400 Spruce Street
Philadelphia, PA 19104, USA

E-mail address: fleishel@uphs.upenn.edu

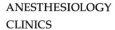

ANESTHESIOLOGY
CLINICS

Anesthesiology Clin
25 (2007) xv–xvii

Preface

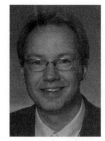 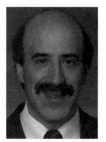

Ansgar M. Brambrink, MD, PhD   Jeffrey R. Kirsch, MD

Guest Editors

Perioperative care for patients who have central nervous system diseases is evolving rapidly as increasing numbers of operative interventional techniques and strategies are developed. Neuroanesthesiologists treat patients throughout the perioperative period, including during diagnostic procedures and interventional radiology procedures.

We believe that the anesthesia provider should have a clear understanding of (1) the disease process, including pathophysiology, specific diagnostics, and treatment options, (2) the concepts and relevant details of the available neurosurgical interventions and techniques, and (3) the necessary means to provide safe and comfortable anesthesia and perioperative care for these patients.

Numerous excellent review articles have been published in recent years on distinct aspects of neurosurgical anesthesia. In June 2002 Dr. Patricia H. Petrozza edited an outstanding volume entitled "Neurosurgical Anesthesia" for *Anesthesiology Clinics of North America.*

Our goal as guest editors of this volume was to provide an update of the key topics in neurosurgical anesthesiology and perioperative care. In addition, we identified several areas of practice for which only limited aggregate information was easily available for review by practicing anesthesiology clinicians. We also have provided reviews on several common problems of the daily practice that had not been examined comprehensively for several years in the accessible body of literature.

We have been fortunate that several international leaders in the fields agreed to contribute to this project. As the key article of this volume we

1932-2275/07/$ - see front matter © 2007 Elsevier Inc. All rights reserved.
doi:10.1016/j.anclin.2007.05.011   *anesthesiology.theclinics.com*

feature a comprehensive review of the state-of-art anesthetic practice for interventional radiology procedures (Dr. Young, San Francisco, CA). This article is paired with an outstanding educational article about diagnostic techniques of the neuroradiologist together with an introduction to the differential interpretation of representative images. Drs. Müeller-Forell and Engelhard (University Hospital, Mainz, Germany) have provided numerous original images to illustrate their topic, which is addressed specifically to the anesthesia provider. In addition, comprehensive updates are provided for the management of patients who have cerebrovascular disease (Drs. Avitsian and Schubert, Cleveland, OH), craniosynostosis (Drs. Koh and Gries, Portland, OR), and neuromuscular disease (Drs. Brambrink and Kirsch, Portland, OR).

Another focus was current developments in specific techniques and concepts pertaining to the intraoperative management in neuroanesthesia. Among those we chose airway management of spine-injured patients (Dr. Crosby, Ottawa, Canada), techniques for awake craniotomy (Drs. Erickson and Cole, Scottsdale, AZ), and monitoring of cerebral perfusion (Dr. Smith, London, UK) and of intracranial pressure including treatment in critical situations (Drs. Kofke and Stiefel, Philadelphia, PA), as well as electrophysiologic monitoring (Drs. Jameson, Janik and Sloan, Denver, CO) and patient positioning during neurosurgical operations (Drs. Rozet and Vavilala, Seattle, WA).

Finally, the issue addresses the often less well appreciated but nevertheless critical challenges during the postoperative period. Drs. Ortiz and Bendo (Brooklyn, NY) summarize the current suggestions for postoperative pain management after neurosurgery, and Drs. Carhuapoma, Naval, and Mirski (Baltimore, MD) review current controversies in neurocritical care.

We are convinced that clinicians in both private practice and academic medicine will benefit from these outstanding review articles. We hope that all clinicians who provide care for patients in the perioperative period enjoy the new 2007 issue on neurosurgical anesthesia, and we are convinced that the information provided may help neuroanesthesiologists further improve the safety and comfort of patients who must undergo these risky procedures.

Ansgar M. Brambrink, MD, PhD
Department of Anesthesiology and Perioperative Medicine
Oregon Health and Science University
3181 S.W. Sam Jackson Park Rd.
Mail Code UHS-2
Portland, Oregon 97239, USA

E-mail address: brambrin@ohsu.edu

Jeffrey R. Kirsch, MD
Department of Anesthesiology and Perioperative Medicine
Oregon Health and Science University
3181 S.W. Sam Jackson Park Rd.
Mail Code UHS-2
Portland, Oregon 97239, USA

E-mail address: kirschje@ohsu.edu

ELSEVIER
SAUNDERS

Anesthesiology Clin
25 (2007) xix

ANESTHESIOLOGY
CLINICS

Dedication

To our families:
Robin, Jodi, Alan, and Ricki (JK); and Petra, Jan, Phillip, Helen, and Lucas (AB).
Thank you for your patience, love, and understanding.

Ansgar M. Brambrink, MD, PhD, and Jeffrey R. Kirsch, MD

1932-2275/07/$ - see front matter © 2007 Elsevier Inc. All rights reserved.
doi:10.1016/j.anclin.2007.06.005 *anesthesiology.theclinics.com*

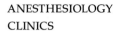
ANESTHESIOLOGY
CLINICS

Anesthesiology Clin
25 (2007) 391–412

Anesthesia for Endovascular Neurosurgery and Interventional Neuroradiology

William L. Young, MD

Department of Anesthesia and Perioperative Care, University of California,
San Francisco, 1001 Potrero Avenue, Room 3C-38, San Francisco, CA 94110, USA

This review outlines the roles of anesthesiologists in the management of patients undergoing invasive endovascular procedures to treat vascular diseases, primarily of the central nervous system. This practice usually is termed interventional neuroradiology (INR) or endovascular neurosurgery. A variety of other names are encountered, highlighting an unsettled and rapidly evolving state of affairs regarding training and practice guidelines. The discussion emphasizes perioperative and anesthetic management strategies to prevent complications and minimize their effects if they occur. There are several fundamental management principles of affording "protection" from injury. Planning anesthetic and perioperative management is predicated on understanding the goals of the therapeutic intervention and anticipating potential problems.

INR is established firmly in the management of cerebrovascular disease, most notably the management of intracranial aneurysm [1], because there is level 1 evidence for aneurysm coiling offering advantages over surgical clipping.

There are several anesthetic concerns that are particularly important for INR procedures, including (1) maintaining immobility during procedures to facilitate imaging, (2) rapid recovery from anesthesia at the end of procedures to facilitate neurologic examination and monitoring or to provide for intermittent evaluation of neurologic function during procedures, (3) managing anticoagulation, (4) treating and managing sudden, unexpected, procedure-specific complications during procedures (eg, hemorrhage or vascular occlusion) which may involve manipulating systemic or regional blood pressures, (5) guiding the medical management of critical care patients

---

E-mail address: ccr@anesthesia.ucsf.edu

doi:10.1016/j.anclin.2007.05.010   *anesthesiology.theclinics.com*

during transport to and from the radiology suites, and (6) self-protection issues related to radiation safety (Table 1) [2,3].

Preoperative planning and patient preparation

Baseline blood pressure and cardiovascular reserve should be assessed carefully. This almost axiomatic statement is important for several reasons. Blood pressure manipulation commonly is required and treatment-related perturbations should be anticipated. Therefore, a clear sense of "where the patient lives" needs to be established. Keep in mind that "autoregulation" as presented in textbooks is a description of a population; individual patients likely will vary considerably, a concept based on the historical observations that underlie modern notions of autoregulatory behavior [4,5]. Stated another way, looking at the usual autoregulation curve, bear in mind that each point on that curve has a 95% CI associated with it—in X and Y directions.

For procedures involving the intracranial, intraspinal, or circle of Willis vasculator, beat-to-beat blood pressure monitoring is suggested, considering

Table 1
Interventional neuroradiologic procedures and primary anesthetic considerations

Procedure	Possible anesthetic considerations
Therapeutic embolization of vascular malformation	
Intracranial AVMs	Deliberate hypotension, postprocedure NPPB
Dural AVM	Existence of venous hypertension; deliberate hypercapnia
Extracranial AVMs	Deliberate hypercapnia
Carotid cavernous fistula	Deliberate hypercapnia, post-procedure NPPB
Cerebral aneurysms	Aneurysmal rupture, blood pressure control[a]
Ethanol sclerotherapy of AVMs or venous malformations	Brain swelling airway swelling, hypoxemia, hypoglycemia, intoxication from ethanol, cardiorespiratory arrest
Balloon A&S of occlusive cerebrovascular disease	Cerebral ischemia, deliberate hypertension, concomitant coronary artery disease, bradycadia, hypotension
Balloon angioplasty of cerebral vasospasm secondary to aneurysmal SAH	Cerebral ischemia, blood pressure control[a]
Therapeutic carotid occlusion for giant aneurysms and skull base tumors	Cerebral ischemia, blood pressure control[a]
Thrombolysis of acute thromboembolic stroke	Post-procedure ICH (NPPB), concomitant coronary artery disease, blood pressure control[a]
Intra-arterial chemotherapy of head and neck tumors	Airway swelling, intracranial hypertension
Embolization for epistaxis	Airway control

[a] Blood pressure control refers to deliberate hypo- or hypertension.

the rapid time constants in this setting for changes in systemic or cerebral hemodynamics. In those cases where intra-arterial catheters are used, the concordance between blood pressure cuff and intra-arterial readings needs to be considered; preoperative blood pressure range likely is known through blood pressure cuff values.

Preoperative calcium channel blockers for prophylaxis for cerebral ischemia may be used and can affect hemodynamic management. In addition, these agents or transdermal nitroglycerin sometimes is used to lessen the incidence of catheter-induced vasospasm.

For cases managed with an unsecured airway, routine evaluation of the potential ease of laryngoscopy in an emergent situation should take into account that direct access to the airway may be limited by table or room logistics. Recent pterional craniotomy sometimes can result in impaired tempomandicular joint mobility.

For intravenous (IV) sedation cases, careful padding of pressure points and working with patients to obtain final comfortable positioning may assist in the patients' ability to tolerate a long period of lying supine and motionless, decreasing the requirement for sedation, anxiolysis, and analgesia. The possibility of pregnancy in female patients and a history of adverse reactions to radiographic contrast agents should be explored.

Secure IV access should be available with adequate extension tubing to allow drug and fluid administration at maximal distance from the image intensifier during fluoroscopy. Access to IV or arterial catheters can be difficult when patients are draped and arms are restrained at the sides; connections should be secure. Infusions of anticoagulants, primary anesthetics, or vasoactive agents should be through IV ports that are as proximal to patients as possible to minimize infusion dead space.

In addition to standard monitors (per guidelines of the American Society of Anesthesiologists), capnography analysis via the sampling port of nasal cannula is suggested for IV sedation cases. A pulse oximeter probe can be placed on the great toe of the leg that will receive the femoral introducer sheath to provide an early warning of femoral artery obstruction or distal thromboembolism.

For intracranial procedures and postoperative care, beat-to-beat arterial pressure monitoring and blood sampling can be facilitated by placement of an arterial catheter. A side port of the femoral artery introducer sheath can be used, but the sheath usually is removed immediately after the procedure. In patients who require continuous blood pressure monitoring or frequent blood sampling postoperatively, it is convenient to have a separate radial arterial blood pressure catheter in place.

Using a coaxial or triaxial catheter system, arterial pressure at the carotid artery, vertebral artery, and the distal cerebral circulation can be measured. Pressures in these distal catheters usually underestimate systolic pressure and overestimate diastolic pressure; however, mean pressures are reliable. Bladder catheters assist in fluid management and patient comfort. A significant volume of heparinized flush solution and radiographic contrast may be used by an interventional team.

A fundamental knowledge of radiation safety is essential for all staff members working in an INR suite. Radiation safety is a critical part of preoperative planning. It probably is reasonable to assume that the x-ray machine always is on. There are three sources of radiation in INR suites: direct radiation from the x-ray tube, leakage (through a collimator's protective shielding), and scattered (reflected from the patients and the area surrounding the body part to be imaged). The amount of exposure decreases proportionally to the inverse of the square of the distance from the source of radiation (inverse square law). Digital subtraction angiography delivers considerably more radiation than fluoroscopy.

Optimal protection includes use of lead aprons, thyroid shields, and radiation exposure badges. Lead aprons should be evaluated periodically for any cracks in the lead lining that may allow accidental radiation exposure. Movable lead glass screens may provide additional protection for the anesthesia team. Clear communication between the INR and anesthesia teams also is crucial for limiting radiation exposure. With proper precautions, anesthesia teams should be exposed to far less than the annual recommended limit for health care workers [6].

Anesthetic technique

Choice of anesthetic technique

Most centers routinely use general endotracheal anesthesia for complex procedures or those procedures that are of long duration. Choice of anesthetic technique varies among centers with no clear superior method and generally follows the dictates of the well-described considerations for operative neuroanesthesia.

General anesthesia

A primary reason for using general anesthesia is to minimize motion artifacts and to improve the quality of image. Relative normocapnia or modest hypocapnia consistent with the safe conduct of positive pressure ventilation should be maintained unless intracranial pressure (ICP) is a concern. The specific choice of anesthesia may be guided primarily by other cardio- and cerebrovascular considerations. There is no clear superiority of one modern anesthetic over another in terms of pharmacologic protection against neuronal injury. Total IV anesthetic techniques or combinations of inhalational and IV methods may optimize rapid emergence. It is appropriate to avoid using nitrous oxide because of the possibility of introducing air emboli into the cerebral circulation and reports that it worsens outcome after experimental brain injury.

It is important to distinguish two general settings where hyperventilation is used in anesthetic practice. First, it is used to treat intracranial hypertension. Hyperventilation is an important mainstay of the acute management of an intracranial catastrophe to reduce cerebral blood volume acutely (Table 2). The second, far more common, application is to provide brain relaxation after the skull is open with the intent of providing better surgical access and, presumably, a lesser degree of brain retraction for a given surgical approach. The former indication may be critical in crisis management; the latter is not relevant to endovascular procedures. Therefore, $Paco_2$ management should aim at normocapnia or mild hypocapnia to the degree consistent with the safe conduct of positive pressure ventilation. If patients have increased intracranial pressure, prophylactic mild hypocapnia may be indicated during induction and maintenance of general anesthesia.

There are some special circumstances for which induced hypercapnia may be indicated, such as embolization of extracranial vascular malformations that drain into the incranial venous system. In these cases, induction of hypercapnia can promote high venous outflow from the cerebral venous system and help minimize the risk for inadvertent movement of embolic material into the intracranial compartment (discussed later).

Intravenous sedation

IV sedation in aneurysm management is used most often for patients coming for interim follow-up angiography to assess the necessity for retreatment

Table 2
Management of intracranial catastrophes

Initial resuscitation
Communicate with endovascular therapy team
Assess need for assistance; call for assistance
Secure the airway ventilate with 100% O_2
Determine if problem is hemorrhagic or occlusive (see text)
Hemorrhagic: immediate heparin reversal (1-mg protamine for each 100 units of heparin given) and low normal mean arterial pressure
Occlusive: deliberate hypertension, titrated to neurologic examination, angiography, or physiologic imaging studies; or to clinical context
Further resuscitation
Head up 15° in neutral position, if possible
$Paco_2$ manipulation consistent with clinical setting, otherwise normocapnia
Mannitol 0.5 g/kg, rapid IV infusion
Titrate IV agent to electroencephalogram burst suppression
Passive cooling to 33°C–34°C
Consider ventriculostomy for treatment or monitoring of increased ICP
Consider anticonvulsants (eg, phenytoin or phenobarbital)

These are only general recommendations and drug doses that must be adapted to specific clinical situations and in accordance with a patient's pre-existing medical condition. In some cases of asymptomatic or minor vessel puncture or occlusion, less aggressive management may be appropriate.

after primary coiling. If further treatment is indicated, the technique can be converted to a general anesthetic. Goals of anesthetic choice for IV sedation are to alleviate pain, anxiety, and discomfort; provide patient immobility; and allow rapid recovery. There may be discomfort associated with injection of contrast into the cerebral arteries (burning) and with distention or traction on them (headache). A long period of lying also can cause significant discomfort.

A variety of sedation regimens is available, and specific choices are based on the experience of practitioners and the goals of anesthetic management. Common to all IV sedation techniques is the potential for upper airway obstruction. Placement of nasopharyngeal airways may cause troublesome bleeding in anticoagulated patients and generally is avoided.

Dexmedetomidine is a new agent that may have applicability in the setting of INR. It is a potent, selective α_2-agonist with sedative, anxiolytic, and analgesic properties, with recent regulatory approval for sedation. Dexmedetomidine is noteworthy especially for its ability to produce a state of patient tranquility without depressing respiration. There are two caveats to consider, however. First, there still are unclear effects on cerebral perfusion [7]. More importantly, there is a tendency for patients managed with dexmedetomidine to have relatively low blood pressure in the postanesthesia recovery period [8]. Because patients who have aneurysmal subarachnoid hemorrhage (SAH) may be critically dependent on adequate collateral perfusion pressure, use of regimens that may result in blood pressure decreases should be used only with great caution.

There is a phenomenon worth mentioning that is characterized inadequately and, perhaps accordingly, lacks a good terminology. It is well known that patients, even with full recovery of a prior fixed neurologic deficit, may emerge from anesthesia with a re-emergence of a prior fixed deficit [9]. These observations are consistent with functional neuroimaging studies that suggest "rewiring" (an inadequately mechanistic metaphor) occurs to compensate for neurologic injury [10]. Why anesthetics cause a temporary reversal of the repair or compensatory process is unknown. For example, Thal and colleagues [9] showed that small doses of either midazolam or fentanyl induced transient focal motor deterioration in patients who had prior motor deficits. Lazar and colleagues [11] demonstrated with more sophisticated methodology that not only motor but also language and spatial functions can be affected by this process. They extend their observations to include patients who suffered recent transient cerebral ischemic episodes and were neurologically intact with negative diffusion-weighted imaging. Midazolam caused re-emergence of prior focal deficits that had been transient and fully resolved [12].

The point to be made for the purpose of this discussion is that potentially there are important effects of IV sedative agents that may complicate neurologic monitoring, especially if functional testing of endovascular manipulations is desirable.

Anticoagulation

Heparin

Careful management of coagulation is required to prevent thromboembolic complications during and after the procedure. Generally, after a baseline activated clotting time (ACT) is obtained, IV heparin (70 units/kg) is given to a target prolongation of 2 to 3 times of baseline. Then, heparin can be given continuously or as an intermittent bolus with hourly monitoring of ACT. Occasionally, patients may be refractory to attempts to obtain adequate anticoagulation. Switching from bovine to porcine heparin or vice versa should be considered. If antithrombin III deficiency is suspected, administration of fresh frozen plasma may be necessary.

Direct thrombin inhibitors

Heparin-induced thrombocytopenia is a rare but important adverse event for heparin anticoagulation. Development of heparin-dependent antibodies after initial exposure leads to a prothrombotic syndrome. In high-risk patients, direct thrombin inhibitors can be applied, recognizing that there are inherent adverse events, such as anaphylaxis, associated with their use. Direct thrombin inhibitors inhibit free and clot-bound thrombin, and their effect can be monitored by either activated partial thromboplastin time or ACT. Lepirudin and bivalirudin, a synthetic derivative, have half-lives of 40 to 120 minutes and approximately 25 minutes, respectively. Because these drugs undergo renal elimination, dose adjustments may be needed in patients who have renal dysfunction. Argatroban is an alternative agent that undergoes primarily hepatic metabolism. A recent report describes bivalirudin as a potential alternative during INR procedures to heparin for IV anticoagulation and intra-arterial thrombolysis [13].

Antiplatelet agents

Although still controversial in the acute setting [14], antiplatelet agents (aspirin, the glycoprotein IIb/IIIa receptor antagonists, and the thienopyridine derivatives) increasingly are used for cerebrovascular disease management [15,16]. Abciximab (ReoPro) has been used for to treat thromboembolic complications. Activation of the platelet membrane glycoprotein IIb/IIIa leads to fibrinogen binding and is a final common pathway for platelet aggregation. Abciximab, eptifibatide, and tirofiban are glycoprotein IIb/IIIa receptor antagonists. The long duration and potent effect of abciximab also increase the likelihood of major bleeding. The smaller molecule agents, eptifibatide and tirofiban, are competitive blockers and have a shorter half-life of approximately 2 hours. Thienopyridine derivatives (ticlopidine and clopidogrel) bind to the platelet's ADP receptors and alter the receptor permanently; therefore, the duration of action is the life span of the platelet. The addition of clopidogrel to the antiplatelet regimen is used commonly for procedures that require placement of devices, such as stents, coiling, or stent-assisted coiling, primarily in patients who have not had an acute event, such as patients who have an unruptured aneurysm.

Reversal of anticoagulation

At the end of the procedure or at occurrence of hemorrhagic complication, heparin may be reversed with protamine. Because there is no specific antidote for the direct thrombin inhibitors or the antiplatelet agents, the biologic half-life is one of the major considerations in drug choice, and platelet transfusion is a nonspecific therapy should reversal be indicated. There is no accurate test currently available to measure platelet function in patients taking the newer antiplatelet drugs. Desmopressin has been reported to shorten the prolonged bleeding time of individuals taking antiplatelet agents, such as aspirin and ticlopidine. There also are increasing recent reports on using specific clotting factors, including recombinant factor VIIa and factor IX complex, to rescue severe life-threatening bleeding, including intracranial hemorrhage (ICH), uncontrolled by standard transfusion therapy. The safety and efficacy of these coagulation factors remain to be investigated more fully.

Deliberate hypertension

During acute arterial occlusion or vasospasm, the only practical way to increase collateral blood flow may be an augmentation of the collateral perfusion pressure by raising the systemic blood pressure. The circle of Willis is a primary collateral pathway in cerebral circulation. In as many as 21% of otherwise normal subjects, however, the circle may not be complete. There also are secondary collateral channels that bridge adjacent major vascular territories, most importantly for the long circumferential arteries that supply the hemispheric convexities. These pathways are known as the pial-to-pial collateral or leptomeningeal pathways.

The extent to which the blood pressure has to be raised depends on the condition of patients and the nature of the disease. Typically, during deliberate hypertension, the systemic blood pressure is raised by 30% to 40% above the baseline in the absence of some direct outcome measure, such as resolution of ischemic symptoms or imaging evidence of improved perfusion. Phenylephrine usually is the first-line agent for deliberate hypertension and is titrated to achieve the desired level of blood pressure. The EKG and ST segment monitor should be inspected carefully for signs of myocardial ischemia.

The risk for causing hemorrhage into an ischemic area must be weighed against the benefits of improving perfusion, but augmentation of blood pressure in the face of acute cerebral ischemia probably is protective in most settings. There also is a risk for rupturing an aneurysm or arteriovenous malformation (AVM) with induction of hypertension. There are no data that assess the risk for induced hypertension directly, other than older case series that report rupture during anesthetic induction in the range of about 1%, presumably the result of acute hypertension. For AVMs, cautious extrapolation of observations for head-frame application suggests the rarity of AVM rupture from acute blood pressure increases. Szabo and colleagues [17] measured blood pressure changes noninvasively in 56 patients who were conscious and unpremedicated and who were undergoing local anesthetic injection and pin insertion; the maximum mean arterial pressure (MAP) was 118 ± 7 mm Hg, representing an increase of 37% from baseline. They concluded that because none of the 56 patients or any of the more than 1000 patients treated in similar fashion suffered a hemorrhage, moderate arterial hypertension does not cause spontaneous AVM hemorrhage.

Deliberate hypotension

The two primary indications for induced hypotension are (1) to test cerebrovascular reserve in patients undergoing carotid occlusion and (2) to slow flow in a feeding artery of brain AVMs (BAVMs) before glue injection (sometimes termed "flow arrest"). The most important factor in choosing a hypotensive agent is the ability to achieve safely and expeditiously the desired reduction in blood pressure while maintaining patients physiologically stable, and if awake, not interfere with neurologic assessment.

The choice of agent should be determined by the experience of the practitioner, the patient's medical condition, and the goals of the blood pressure reduction in a particular clinical setting. IV adenosine has been used to induce transient cardiac pause and may be a viable method of partial flow arrest [18].

Management of neurologic and procedural crises

A well thought-out plan, coupled with rapid and effective communication between anesthesia and radiology teams, is critical for good outcomes. The primary responsibility of an anesthesia team is to preserve gas exchange and, if indicated, secure the airway. Simultaneous with airway management, the first branch in the decision-making algorithm is for the anesthesiologist to communicate with the INR team and determine whether or not the problem is hemorrhagic or occlusive.

In the setting of vascular occlusion, the goal is to increase distal perfusion by blood pressure augmentation with or without direct thrombolysis. If the problem is hemorrhagic, immediate cessation of heparin and reversal with protamine is indicated. As an emergency reversal dose, protamine can be given (1 mg for each 100 units of initial heparin dosage that resulted in therapeutic anticoagulation). The ACT then can be used to fine-tune the final protamine dose. Complications of protamine administration include hypotension, true anaphylaxis, and pulmonary hypertension. With the advent of new long-acting direct thrombin inhibitors, such as bivalirudin, new strategies for emergent reversal of anticoagulation need to be developed.

Bleeding catastrophes usually are heralded by headache, nausea, vomiting, and vascular pain related to the area of perforation. Sudden loss of consciousness not always is the result of ICH. Seizures, as a result of contrast reaction or transient ischemia, and the resulting postictal state, also can result in an obtunded patient. In patients who are anesthetized or comatose, the sudden onset of bradycardia and hypertension (Cushing response) or an endovascular therapist's diagnosis of extravasation of contrast may be the only clues to a developing hemorrhage. Most cases of vascular rupture can be managed in an angiography suite. The INR team can attempt to seal the rupture site endovascularly and abort the procedure; a ventriculostomy catheter may be placed emergently in an angiography suite. Patients who have suspected rupture require emergent CT scan, but emergent craniotomy usually is not indicated.

Specific procedures

Intracranial aneurysm ablation

The two basic approaches for INR therapy of cerebral aneurysms are occlusion of proximal parent arteries and obliteration of the aneurysmal sac. With the publication of the International Subarachnoid Aneurysm Trial (ISAT) results [19], coil embolization of intracranial aneurysms has become a routine first-choice therapy for many lesions. Patients with unruptured lesions or for whom stent placement is contemplated may be placed on antiplatelet agents preoperatively.

There is great interest in the development of stent-assisted coiling methods. The stent can provide protection of the parent vessel. Stent placement requires a greater degree of instrumentation and manipulation, probably increasing the ever-present intraprocedural risk for parent vessel occlusion, thromboembolism, or vascular rupture.

Anesthetic management should proceed with the usual considerations used in the care of patients who have an intracranial aneurysm [20]. Patients who have aneurysmal SAH often have either increased ICP or decreased intracranial compliance, secondary to the mass of SAH, secondary to parenchymal injury from ischemia, or from hydrocephalus.

Anesthesiologists should be prepared for aneurysmal rupture and acute SAH at all times, from spontaneous rupture of a leaky sac, direct injury of the aneurysm wall by the vascular manipulation, perianeurysmal thrombus formation, or arterial branch occlusion.

If a rupture occurs, anticoagulation must be reversed immediately; a Cushing response (hypertension and bradycardia) may be developed. Cerebral perfusion pressure (CCP) should be maintained at adequate levels. Emergent placement of a ventriculostomy should be considered and an emergent CT scan performed to assess consequences of the perforation or rupture.

Angioplasty of cerebral vasospasm from aneurysmal subarachnoid hemorrhage

Approximately one of four patients who have SAH develop symptomatic vasospasm. Angioplasty, either mechanical (balloon) or pharmacologic (intra-arterial vasodilators), may be used as a treatment [21]. Angioplasty ideally is done in patients who already have had the symptomatic aneurysm surgically clipped and for patients in the early course of symptomatic ischemia to prevent hemorrhagic transformation of an ischemia region.

A balloon catheter is guided under fluoroscopy into the spastic segment and inflated to distend the constricted area mechanically. It also is possible to perform a "pharmacologic" angioplasty by direct intra-arterial infusion. There is the greatest experience with intra-arterial papaverine, but there are potential CNS toxic effects [22]. Other agents, such as calcium channel blockers (nicardipine and verapamil), also are used [23]. Intra-arterial vasodilators may have systemic effects (eg, bradycardia and hypotension).

Patients who come for angioplasty often are critically ill with a variety of challenging comorbidities, including neurocardiac injury, volume overload from "triple-H" (intentional hypertension, hemodilution, and hypervolemia) therapy, hydrocephalus, brain injury from recent craniotomy, and residual effects of the presenting hemorrhage. Procedural complications include arterial rupture, reperfusion hemorrhage, thromboembolism, and arterial dissection.

In patients who have symptomatic vasospasm, it is common to be asked to maintain MAP 30% to 50% above baseline MAP, in an attempt to improve cerebral perfusion. If the aneurysm is unsecured, this target may be tempered. Although phenylephrine is a useful agent, if myocardial dysfunction is present from neurogenic injury, an inotrope may be appropriate. When phenylephrine treatment does not allow reaching the target MAP because of reflex bradycardia, a muscarinic antagonist may be appropriate. Unless clinicians are trying to treat increased ICP, hyperventilation should be avoided.

Carotid test occlusion and therapeutic carotid occlusion

Large or otherwise unclippable aneurysms may be treated partly or completely by proximal vessel occlusion. To assess the consequences of carotid occlusion in anticipation of surgery, patients may be scheduled for a test occlusion, in which cerebrovascular reserve is evaluated in several ways. A multimodal combination of angiographic, clinical, and physiologic tests can be used to arrive at the safest course of action for a given patient's clinical circumstances. The judicious use of deliberate hypotension can increase the sensitivity of the test [24]. The most important factor in choosing a hypotensive agent is the ability to achieve the desired reduction in blood pressure safely and expeditiously, while maintaining patients physiologically stable. The choice of agent should be determined by practitioner experience, patients' medical condition, and the goals of the blood pressure reduction in a particular clinical setting.

Brain arteriovenous malformations

Also called cerebral or pial AVMs, BAVMs typically are large, complex lesions made up of a tangle of abnormal vessels (called the nidus) frequently containing several discrete fistulae served by multiple feeding arteries and draining veins. The goal of the therapeutic embolization is to obliterate as many of the fistulae and their respective feeding arteries as possible. BAVM embolization usually is an adjunct for surgery or radiotherapy.

The cyanoacrylate glues offer relatively "permanent" closure of abnormal vessels. N-butyl cyanoacrylate (NBCA) is a low-viscosity liquid monomer that polymerizes to a solid form on contact with ionic solutions including blood and saline, but not dextrose 5% in water. Passage of glue into a draining vein can result in acute hemorrhage; in smaller patients, pulmonary embolism of glue can be symptomatic. For these reasons, deliberate hypotension may increase safety of glue delivery. There is no compelling reason to choose any particular method to achieve the hypotension. The flow through the fistula is a pressure-dependent phenomenon [25].

A major drawback to NBCA is that it is adhesive, with the potential to inadvertently glue the catheter to the injected polymer. Onyx is a new, nonadhesive liquid embolic agent consisting of ethylene-vinyl alcohol copolymer in a dimethyl sulfoxide solvent that theoretically may decrease overall complication rates [26].

Although less durable, polyvinyl alcohol microsphere embolization also commonly is used. If surgery is planned within days after polyvinyl alcohol embolization, the rate of recanalization is low. Ethanol also is used as an agent but has many untoward effects (discussed later) [27].

For AVM evaluation, some centers use superselective Wada testing before therapeutic embolization to test the eloquence of regions adjacent to a lesion. During this test, a short-acting anesthetic (eg, methohexital) is injected into the right or left internal carotid artery (ICA) to suspend the ipsilateral cerebral hemispheres and test the abilities subserved by the contralateral hemisphere in isolation. It is important to consider using a sedation regimen for such cases that have a minimal impact on cognitive or motor examinations (see previous discussion regarding re-emergence phenomena). The purpose of such testing is to establish treatment risk for individual patients.

Such Wada testing, functional imaging studies, and intrasurgical cortical mapping have shown redistribution of language and memory to unpredictable regions [28,29]. Further, developmental cognitive history in these patients indicates that most have at least some background of learning problems during the school-age years with varying degrees of severity [30], reflecting a time when brain reorganization may be occurring.

Dural arteriovenous malformations

Dural AVM is considered an acquired lesion resulting from venous dural sinus stenosis or occlusion, opening of potential ateriovenous shunts, and subsequent recanalization. Intracranial dural arteriovenous fistulas (DAVF) account for approximately 10% to 15% of all intracranial vascular malformations. Symptoms are variable according to which sinus is involved. Venous hypertension of pial veins is a risk factor for ICH. Dural AVMs may be fed by multiple meningeal vessels, and therefore, multistaged embolization often is necessary. DAVF can induce increased venous pressure markedly and decreased net cerebral perfusion pressure. Therefore, presence of venous hypertension should be factored into management of systemic arterial and cerebral perfusion pressure. This is a critical aspect of DAVF perioperative management. It often is assumed that the venous hypertension induces the angiogeneic phenotype by acting through its causing cerebral ischemia, but newer evidence suggests that venous hypertension may be a direct stimulus for angiogenesis [31]. DAVF are unique in that there are promising animal models of their pathogenesis [32,33], unlike most other hemorrhagic brain diseases.

Galen's veins malformations are a special case of DAVF, discussion of which is beyond the scope of this review [34]. These are relatively uncommon but complicated lesions that are present in infants and require a multidisciplinary approach. Patients may have intractable congestive heart failure, intractable seizures, hydrocephalus, and mental retardation. Several approaches have been attempted, including transarterial and transvenous embolization. In infants who have high-output failure, pre-existing right-to-left shunts, and pulmonary hypertension, a relatively small pulmonary glue embolism can be fatal.

Venous malformations

Craniofacial venous malformations are congenital disorders and, in addition to causing significant cosmetic deformities, may impinge on the upper airway and interfere with swallowing. Many of these lesions are resistant to conventional surgery, cryosurgery, or laser surgery. In this procedure, United States Pharmacopeia grade 95% ethanol opacified with contrast is injected percutaneously into a lesion under fluoroscopic guidance, resulting in a chemical burn to the lesion and eventually shrinking it. Sclerotherapy alone may be adequate treatment or may be combined with surgery [35].

This therapy has several inter-reactions with anesthetic management [2]. Because marked swelling occurs immediately after ethanol injection, the ability of patients to maintain a patent airway postoperatively must be considered carefully [35]. Desaturation on the pulse oximeter frequently is noted after injection. Cardiopulmonary arrest is reported [27]. There are anecdotal reports of cardiac arrest during ethanol sclerotherapy, The predictable intoxication and other side effects of ethanol may be evident after emergence from anesthesia, in particular post emergence agitation in children.

Venous malformations of the face or dural fistulas have the potential to drain into intracerebral veins or sinuses. By increasing the $Paco_2$ to 50 to 60 mm Hg, cerebral venous outflow greatly exceeds extracranial venous outflow, and the pressure gradient favors movement of a sclerosing agent, chemotherapeutic agent, or glue away from vital intracranial drainage pathways. Although actual pressure gradients never have been studied, increased intracranial outflow readily is demonstrable in clinical practice with angiography. Addition of CO_2 gas to the inspired gas mixture is the easiest and safest way to achieve hypercapnia. Airway collapse and atelectasis are prevented by maintaining adequate tidal volume. Hypoventilation may be used, however, if CO_2 gas is not available; in this case, addition of positive end-expiratory pressure may be useful to maintain oxygenation.

Angioplasty and stenting for atherosclerotic lesions

Angioplasty and stenting (A&S) for treatment of atherosclerotic disease involving the cervical and intracranial arteries continue to supplant open surgical management [36,37]. Risk for distal thromboembolism is a major issue in this procedure. Catheter systems using some kind of trapping system distal to the angioplasty balloon are being developed. There are many ongoing trials to compare the usefulness of stenting to carotid endarterectomy (CEA) for extracranial carotid disease. The Stenting and Angioplasty with Protection in Patients at High Risk for Endarterectomy trial, a hybrid randomized controlled trial (RCT)/registry trial [38], suggests noninferiority for outcomes when using A&S in a comparison to CEA. The majority was asymptomatic ICA lesions treated with nitinol stents and used emboli protection. The 30-day stroke, death, and acute myocardial infarction (AMI) rates were 9.8% for CEA versus 4.7% for A&S ($P = .09$). The Endarterectomy Versus Stenting in Patients with Symptomatic Severe Carotid Stenosis Trial [39] studied patients who had symptomatic ICA stenosis greater than 60%. This cohort did not have severe coronary artery disease. The trial was stopped prematurely after 527 patients. The 30-day stroke/death rate was 3.9% for CEA versus 9.6% for A&S; the endpoint of any stroke or death at 6 months was 6.1% versus 11.7%, with no difference in 30-day acute myocardial infarction rates.

Preparation for anesthetic management in patients scheduled for A&S may include placement of transcutaneous pacing leads, in case of severe bradycardia or asystole from carotid body stimulation during angioplasty. IV atropine or glycopyrrolate also may be used in an attempt to mitigate bradycardia, which occurs almost invariably to some degree with inflation of the balloon. This powerful chronotropic response may be difficult or impossible to prevent or control by conventional means. Adverse effects of increasing myocardial oxygen demand need to be considered in antibradycardia interventions.

Potential complications resulting from A&S include vessel occlusion, perforation, dissection, spasm, thromboemboli, occlusion of adjacent vessels, transient ischemic episodes, and stroke. Similar to CEA, there is approximately a 5% risk for symptomatic cerebral hemorrhage or brain swelling after carotid angioplasty [40]. Although the etiology of this syndrome is unknown, it is associated with cerebral hyperperfusion and may be related to poor postoperative blood pressure control.

Thrombolysis of acute thromboembolic stroke

In acute occlusive stroke, it is possible to recanalize the occluded vessel by superselective intra-arterial thrombolytic therapy. Thrombolytic agents can be delivered in high concentration by a microcatheter navigated close to the clot. Neurologic deficits may be reversed without additional risk for secondary hemorrhage if treatment is completed within several hours from the onset of carotid territory ischemia and somewhat longer in vertebrobasilar territory. Intra-arterial thrombolysis currently has "off-label" use. Despite an increased frequency of early symptomatic hemorrhagic complications, treatment with intra-arterial prourokinase within 6 hours of onset of acute ischemic stroke with middle cerebral artery occlusion significantly improved clinical outcome at 90 days [41].

A newer and promising approach is the use of mechanical retrieval devices to physically remove the offending thromboembolic material from the intracranial vessel, as reviewed by Smith and colleagues [42,43]. This device seems efficacious in terms of recanalizing occluded vessels. Whether or not outcome also is affected is less clear.

Intra-arterial chemical thrombolysis and mechanical retrevial have an inherent risk for promoting hemorrhagic transformation, just as in the case of IV thrombolysis. This is an important area for investigation because hemorrhagic transformation—or its threat—has great impact on clinical practice. Chemical thrombolysis with tissue plasminogen activator promotes expression and activity of matrix metalloproteinase (MMP)-9, a key protease for tissue remodeling and involved in various kinds of vascular injury that can damage the neurovascular unit and promote hemorrhage [44]. Chemical thrombolysis with tissue plasminogen activator can increase MMP-9 expression in brain endothelium, acting through the low-density lipoprotein receptor-related protein, and promotes up-regulation after focal cerebral ischemia [45]. Patient MMP-9 plasma levels also are increased after treatment [46].

Details of anesthetic management are reviewed elsewhere [47]. Briefly, there are several challenges in providing hyperacute care of a patient population that generally is elderly and has frequent medical comorbidity, especially if little knowledge of patient history is available before treatment. The choice of IV sedation versus general anesthesia must be considered carefully depending on local practices and the potential for patient agitation versus the ability to monitor neurologic status. Intravascular volume management may be challenging for several reasons. There is a high incidence of systemic hypertension in patients who have severe vascular disease, who may be further hypovolemic because of an acute ictus. This complicates management by requiring MAP to be maintained at supranormal levels because of inadequate collateral perfusion secondary to the acute arterial obstruction. The risk for vessel rupture or clot propogation is omnipresent.

Postoperative management

Endovascular surgery patients pass the immediate postoperative period in a monitored setting to watch for signs of hemodynamic instability or neurologic deterioration. Control of blood pressure may be necessary during transport and postoperative recovery (eg, induced hypertension) if indicated. In particular, patients undergoing treatment of extracranial carotid disease are prone to postprocedural hemodynamic instability, similar to postcarotid endartectomy patients [48].

Abrupt restoration of normal systemic pressure to a chronically hypotensive (ischemic) vascular bed may overwhelm autoregulatory capacity and result in hemorrhage or swelling (normal perfusion pressure breakthrough [NPPB]) [40,49]. The pathophysiology for NPPB is unclear but probably it is not simply a hemodynamic effect. The loss of neurovascular unit integrity probably is related to the pathways involved in postreperfusion hemorrhage in the setting of acute stroke (described previously). In addition, cerebral hyperemia probably is exacerbated if uncontrolled increases in systemic arterial blood pressure occur in the postoperative period. In the absence of collateral perfusion pressure inadequacy, fastidious attention to preventing hypertension is warranted. Complicated cases may go first to CT or some other kind of tomographic imaging; critical care management may need to be extended during transport and imaging. Symptomatic hyperemic complications are moreuncommon than "silent" hyperemic states; and with use of more sensitive MRI, ischemic events are found more common than suspected previously [50].

Future directions

There is accelerating interest and discussion regarding appropriate management of asymptomatic cerebrovascular disease. Anesthesiologists traditionally are not caught on the horns of these management dilemmas— at least directly. Optimal provision of perioperative care and effective resource allocation, however, would benefit from active involvement by all practitioners involved in the management of these patients.

The indications for invasive therapy for unruptured AVMs [51] and aneurysms [52,53] currently are undergoing critical discussion. Although generally it is agreed that ruptured lesions need treatment, the aggregate risks for treating all patients who have unruptured lesions may exceed the potential benefits from protecting against future hemorrhage. For example, A Randomized Trial of Unruptured Brain Arteriovenous Malformations is an international, multicenter, randomized controlled trial to test whether or not functional outcome and the risk for spontaneous AVM rupture at 5 years for best medical therapy is superior to procedural intervention, including embolization, microsurgical resection, or radiosurgery [54]. Similarly, the International Study of Unruptured Intracranial Aneurysms is a longstanding effort to document the natural history and treatment outcomes for unruptured lesions [52,55].

Future research directions for vascular disease of the brain present opportunities for neuroanesthesia, perioperative management, and neurologic critical care. Basic or translational questions include the interaction of angiogenesis and vascular remodeling on pathogenesis and clinical course. There is growing evidence suggesting that some of these lesions undergo active angiogenesis and vascular remodeling in the adult life. This new concept— active angiogenesis and vascular remodeling in intracranial vascular malformations—may open new clinical paradigms in which pharmacologic interventions are proposed to stabilize these abnormal blood vessels and prevent further growth or hemorrhage. Recent research on intracranial vascular malformations has been focusing on identifying roles of angiogenic and antiangiogenic factors in their pathophysiology [56].

Abnormal vascular remodeling mediated by inflammatory cells has been identified as a key pathologic component of various vascular diseases, including abdominal aortic aneurysms, BAVMs, and atherosclerosis [57–60]. This concept may provide a new treatment strategy to use agents to inhibit inflammation or cytokines produced by inflammatory cells, such as MMPs. Based on findings from observational studies that analyzed human intracranial aneurysms and experimental studies that used animal models, an emerging concept suggests that a key component of the pathophysiology of intracranial aneurysms is sustained abnormal vascular remodeling coupled with inflammation [61–63].

Consistent with a background contribution of a ubiquitous process, such as inflammation, aneurysmal disease may be conceived of better as a process rather than an event. For example, the long-term durability of aneurysm treatment often is assumed. There is growing appreciation that the traditional notion of "disease treatment" should not necessarily be construed as a "cure," although it may be in many cases. Although treatment clearly decreases new rupture rates, there is a measurable rebleed rate after treatment (surgery or coiling) [1]. The risk for further hemorrhage continues for up to 30 years after SAH [64]. The Dutch ASTRA group reported follow-up CT angiography on 610 patients 1 to 15 years after surgical clipping of a ruptured aneurysm and found an incidence of 16% of new aneurysms [65]. In 24 patients, aneurysms were present at the site of the previous clipping and in three of these, the postoperative angiogram had shown complete aneurysm occlusion. Taken together with observations that a significant fraction of aneurysms enlarge over time [64–66], aneurysmal disease may be a process characterized by generalized vascular dysfunction rather than a sporadic focal event.

Proinflammatory influence on disease susceptibility [67,68] and clinical course [69,70] seems to apply to AVMs also. Tissue interleukin (IL)-6 expression is associated with IL-6-174G > C genotype and linked to downstream targets involved in angiogenesis and vascular instability [71]. Further, IL-6 induced MMP-3 and MMP-9 expression and activity in the mouse brain and increased proliferation and migration of cerebral endothelial cells. Taken together, such observations are consistent with the hypothesis that inflammatory processes influence angiogenic and proteolytic activity, thus contributing to the pathogenesis of ICH.

In the future, genetic variation has the potential to be developed to help predict new ICH in the natural course after presentation [69,70] or used to risk stratify for postoperative complications [72]. Genetic variation or plasma cytokine assays [73,74] have the potential for development to have an impact multiple aspects of perioperative management.

Summary

Endovascular treatment probably never will replace operative neurosurgery completely, at least for the foreseeable future. It will, however, continue to grow in its "market share" of vascular practice and technical sophistication. Anesthesiologists influence optimal patient outcome in equally important albeit slightly different ways as in traditional neurosurgical practice. Perioperative management that is predicated on understanding the goals and methods of the endovascular intervention, and anticipating potential problems, will optimize patient safety and good outcomes.

Acknowledgments

The author would like to thank the members of the UCSF Brain AVM Study Project and the Center for Cerebrovascular Research (www.avm. ucsf.edu) for the opportunities to learn more about cerebrovascular disease and anesthetic management and John Pile-Spellman, Lawrence Litt, Tomoki Hashimoto, Chanhung Lee, and the Neurovascular Medical Group at UCSF for continued collaboration on this topic.

References

[1] Molyneux AJ, Kerr RS, Yu LM, et al. International subarachnoid aneurysm trial (ISAT) of neurosurgical clipping versus endovascular coiling in 2143 patients with ruptured intracranial aneurysms: a randomised comparison of effects on survival, dependency, seizures, rebleeding, subgroups, and aneurysm occlusion. Lancet 2005;366(9488):809–17.

[2] Young WL, Pile-Spellman J. Anesthetic considerations for interventional neuroradiology (review). Anesthesiology 1994;80(2):427–56.

[3] Young WL, Pile-Spellman J, Hacein-Bey L, et al. Invasive neuroradiologic procedures for cerebrovascular abnormalities: anesthetic considerations. Anesthesiol Clin North America 1997;15(3):631–53.

[4] Strandgaard S, Olesen J, Skinhoj E, et al. Autoregulation of brain circulation in severe arterial hypertension. Br Med J 1973;1(5852):507–10.

[5] Drummond JC. The lower limit of autoregulation: time to revise our thinking? [letter] Anesthesiology 1997;86(6):1431–3.

[6] Centers for Disease Control. Guidelines for protecting the safety and health of health care workers (chapter 5). Available at: http://www.cdc.gov/niosh/hcwold0.html. Accessed June 13, 2007.

[7] Prielipp RC, Wall MH, Tobin JR, et al. Dexmedetomidine-induced sedation in volunteers decreases regional and global cerebral blood flow. Anesth Analg 2002;95(4):1052–9.

[8] Arain SR, Ebert TJ. The efficacy, side effects, and recovery characteristics of dexmedetomidine versus propofol when used for intraoperative sedation. Anesth Analg 2002;95(2): 461–6.

[9] Thal GD, Szabo MD, Lopez-Bresnahan M, et al. Exacerbation or unmasking of focal neurologic deficits by sedatives. Anesthesiology 1996;85(1):21–5 [discussion: 29A–30A].

[10] Chollet F, DiPiero V, Wise RJ, et al. The functional anatomy of motor recovery after stroke in humans: a study with positron emission tomography. Ann Neurol 1991;29(1):63–71.

[11] Lazar RM, Fitzsimmons BF, Marshall RS, et al. Reemergence of stroke deficits with midazolam challenge. Stroke 2002;33(1):283–5.

[12] Lazar RM, Fitzsimmons BF, Marshall RS, et al. Midazolam challenge reinduces neurological deficits after transient ischemic attack. Stroke 2003;34(3):794–6.

[13] Harrigan MR, Levy EI, Bendok BR, et al. Bivalirudin for endovascular intervention in acute ischemic stroke: case report. Neurosurgery 2004;54(1):218–22 [discussion: 222–3].

[14] Ciccone A, Abraha I, Santilli I. Glycoprotein IIb-IIIa inhibitors for acute ischaemic stroke. Cochrane Database Syst Rev 2006;4:CD005208.

[15] Hashimoto T, Gupta DK, Young WL. Interventional neuroradiology–anesthetic considerations. Anesthesiol Clin North America 2002;20(2):347–59, vi.

[16] Fiorella D, Albuquerque FC, Han P, et al. Strategies for the management of intraprocedural thromboembolic complications with abciximab (ReoPro). Neurosurgery 2004;54(5): 1089–97 [discussion: 1097–8].

[17] Szabo MD, Crosby G, Sundaram P, et al. Hypertension does not cause spontaneous hemorrhage of intracranial arteriovenous malformations. Anesthesiology 1989;70(5):761–3.

[18] Hashimoto T, Young WL, Aagaard BD, et al. Adenosine-induced ventricular asystole to induce transient profound systemic hypotension in patients undergoing endovascular therapy. Dose- response characteristics. Anesthesiology 2000;93(4):998–1001.

[19] Molyneux A, Kerr R, Stratton I, et al. International Subarachnoid Aneurysm Trial (ISAT) of neurosurgical clipping versus endovascular coiling in 2143 patients with ruptured intracranial aneurysms: a randomised trial. Lancet 2002;360(9342):1267–74.

[20] Drummond JC, Patel PM. Neurosurgical anesthesia (chapter 53). In: Miller RD, editor. Anesthesia, Vol 2. 6th editionPhiladelphia: Elsevier Churchill Livingston; 2005. p. 2127–73.

[21] Newell DW, Eskridge JM, Mayberg MR, et al. Angioplasty for the treatment of symptomatic vasospasm following subarachnoid hemorrhage. J Neurosurg 1989;71(5 Pt 1): 654–60.

[22] Smith WS, Dowd CF, Johnston SC, et al. Neurotoxicity of intra-arterial papaverine preserved with chlorobutanol used for the treatment of cerebral vasospasm after aneurysmal subarachnoid hemorrhage. Stroke 2004;35(11):2518–22.

[23] Feng L, Fitzsimmons BF, Young WL, et al. Intraarterially administered verapamil as adjunct therapy for cerebral vasospasm: safety and 2-year experience. AJNR Am J Neuroradiol 2002;23(8):1284–90.

[24] Marshall RS, Lazar RM, Pile-Spellman J, et al. Recovery of brain function during induced cerebral hypoperfusion. Brain 2001;124(Pt 6):1208–17.

[25] Gao E, Young WL, Pile-Spellman J, et al. Deliberate systemic hypotension to facilitate endovascular therapy of cerebral arteriovenous malformations: a computer modeling study. Neurosurg Focus 1997;2(6):e3.

[26] van Rooij WJ, Sluzewski M, Beute GN. Brain AVM embolization with onyx. AJNR Am J Neuroradiol 2007;28(1):172–7.

[27] Yakes WF, Rossi P, Odink H. How I do it. Arteriovenous malformation management. Cardiovasc Intervent Radiol 1996;19(2):65–71.

[28] Lazar RM, Marshall RS, Pile-Spellman J, et al. Interhemispheric transfer of language in patients with left frontal cerebral arteriovenous malformation. Neuropsychologia 2000;38(10):1325–32.

[29] Lazar RM, Marshall RS, Pile-Spellman J, et al. Anterior translocation of language in patients with left cerebral arteriovenous malformations. Neurology 1997;49(3):802–8.

[30] Lazar RM, Connaire K, Marshall RS, et al. Developmental deficits in adult patients with arteriovenous malformations. Arch Neurol 1999;56(1):103–6.

[31] Zhu Y, Lawton MT, Du R, et al. Expression of hypoxia-inducible factor-1 and vascular endothelial growth factor in response to venous hypertension. Neurosurgery 2006;59(3):687–96 [discussion: 687–96].

[32] Lawton MT, Jacobowitz R, Spetzler RF. Redefined role of angiogenesis in the pathogenesis of dural arteriovenous malformations. J Neurosurg 1997;87(2):267–74.

[33] Terada T, Higashida RT, Halbach VV, et al. Development of acquired arteriovenous fistulas in rats due to venous hypertension. J Neurosurg 1994;80(5):884–9.

[34] Fullerton HJ, Aminoff AR, Ferriero DM, et al. Neurodevelopmental outcome after endovascular treatment of vein of galen malformations. Neurology 2003;61(10):1386–90.

[35] Lasjaunias P, Berenstein A. Endovascular treatment of the craniofacial lesions. In: Surgical neuroangiography. Vol 2. Heidelberg (Germany): Springer-Verlag; 1987. p. 389–97.

[36] Higashida RT, Meyers PM, Connors JJ 3rd, et al. Intracranial angioplasty & stenting for cerebral atherosclerosis: a position statement of the American society of interventional and therapeutic neuroradiology, society of interventional radiology, and the American society of neuroradiology. AJNR Am J Neuroradiol 2005;26(9):2323–7.

[37] Goodney PP, Schermerhorn ML, Powell RJ. Current status of carotid artery stenting. J Vasc Surg 2006;43(2):406–11.

[38] Yadav JS, Wholey MH, Kuntz RE, et al. Protected carotid-artery stenting versus endarterectomy in high-risk patients. N Engl J Med 2004;351(15):1493–501.

[39] Mas JL, Chatellier G, Beyssen B, et al. Endarterectomy versus stenting in patients with symptomatic severe carotid stenosis. N Engl J Med 2006;355(16):1660–71.

[40] Meyers PM, Higashida RT, Phatouros CC, et al. Cerebral hyperperfusion syndrome after percutaneous transluminal stenting of the craniocervical arteries. Neurosurgery 2000;47(2):335–43 [discussion: 343–5].

[41] Furlan A, Higashida R, Wechsler L, et al. Intra-arterial prourokinase for acute ischemic stroke. The PROACT II study: a randomized controlled trial. Prolyse in acute cerebral thromboembolism. JAMA 1999;282(21):2003–11.

[42] Smith WS. Safety of mechanical thrombectomy and intravenous tissue plasminogen activator in acute ischemic stroke. Results of the multi mechanical embolus removal in cerebral ischemia (MERCI) trial, part I. AJNR Am J Neuroradiol 2006;27(6):1177–82.

[43] Smith WS, Sung G, Starkman S, et al. Safety and efficacy of mechanical embolectomy in acute ischemic stroke: results of the MERCI trial. Stroke 2005;36(7):1432–8.

[44] Wang X, Lee SR, Arai K, et al. Lipoprotein receptor-mediated induction of matrix metalloproteinase by tissue plasminogen activator. Nat Med 2003;9(10):1313–7.

[45] Tsuji K, Aoki T, Tejima E, et al. Tissue plasminogen activator promotes matrix metalloproteinase-9 upregulation after focal cerebral ischemia. Stroke 2005;36(9):1954–9.

[46] Horstmann S, Kalb P, Koziol J, et al. Profiles of matrix metalloproteinases, their inhibitors, and laminin in stroke patients: influence of different therapies. Stroke 2003;34(9): 2165–70.

[47] Lee CZ, Litt L, Hashimoto T, et al. Physiological monitoring and anesthesia considerations of the acute ischemic stroke patient. J Vasc Interv Radiol 2004;15(Suppl 1):S13–9.

[48] Qureshi AI, Luft AR, Sharma M, et al. Frequency and determinants of postprocedural hemodynamic instability after carotid angioplasty and stenting. Stroke 1999;30(10):2086–93.

[49] Young WL, Kader A, Ornstein E, et al. Cerebral hyperemia after arteriovenous malformation resection is related to "breakthrough" complications but not to feeding artery pressure. Columbia university AVM study project. Neurosurgery 1996;38(6):1085–93 [discussion: 1093–5].

[50] Cronqvist M, Wirestam R, Ramgren B, et al. Endovascular treatment of intracerebral arteriovenous malformations: procedural safety, complications, and results evaluated by MR imaging, including diffusion and perfusion imaging. AJNR Am J Neuroradiol 2006;27(1): 162–76.

[51] Stapf C, Mohr JP, Choi JH, et al. Invasive treatment of unruptured brain arteriovenous malformations is experimental therapy. Curr Opin Neurol 2006;19(1):63–8.

[52] Wiebers DO, Whisnant JP, Huston J 3rd, et al. Unruptured intracranial aneurysms: natural history, clinical outcome, and risks of surgical and endovascular treatment. Lancet 2003; 362(9378):103–10.

[53] Wiebers DO. Patients with small, asymptomatic, unruptured intracranial aneurysms and no history of subarachnoid hemorrhage should generally be treated conservatively. Stroke 2005;36(2):408–9.

[54] ClinicalTrials.gov, a service of the U.S. National Institute of Health. A randomized trial of unruptured brain AVMs (ARUBA). Available at: http://clinicaltrials.gov/ct/show/ NCT00389181. Accessed June 13, 2007.

[55] International Study of Unruptured Intracranial Aneurysms Investigators. Unruptured intracranial aneurysms–risk of rupture and risks of surgical intervention. N Engl J Med 1998;339(24):1725–33.

[56] Hashimoto T, Young WL. Roles of angiogenesis and vascular remodeling in brain vascular malformations. Seminars in Cerebrovascular Diseases and Stroke 2004;4(4):217–25.

[57] Hashimoto T, Wen G, Lawton MT, et al. Abnormal expression of matrix metalloproteinases and tissue inhibitors of metalloproteinases in brain arteriovenous malformations. Stroke 2003;34(4):925–31.

[58] Knox JB, Sukhova GK, Whittemore AD, et al. Evidence for altered balance between matrix metalloproteinases and their inhibitors in human aortic diseases. Circulation 1997;95(1): 205–12.

[59] Goodall S, Crowther M, Hemingway DM, et al. Ubiquitous elevation of matrix metalloproteinase-2 expression in the vasculature of patients with abdominal aneurysms. Circulation 2001;104(3):304–9.

[60] Loftus IM, Naylor AR, Goodall S, et al. Increased matrix metalloproteinase-9 activity in unstable carotid plaques. A potential role in acute plaque disruption. Stroke 2000;31(1):40–7.

[61] Chyatte D, Bruno G, Desai S, et al. Inflammation and intracranial aneurysms. Neurosurgery 1999;45(5):1137–46 [discussion: 1146–7].

[62] Frosen J, Piippo A, Paetau A, et al. Remodeling of saccular cerebral artery aneurysm wall is associated with rupture: histological analysis of 24 unruptured and 42 ruptured cases. Stroke 2004;35(10):2287–93.

[63] Hashimoto T, Meng H, Young WL. Intracranial aneurysms: links between inflammation, hemodynamics and vascular remodeling. Neurol Res 2006;28(4):372–80.

[64] Juvela S, Porras M, Poussa K. Natural history of unruptured intracranial aneurysms: probability of and risk factors for aneurysm rupture. J Neurosurg 2000;93(3):379–87.

[65] Wermer MJ, van der Schaaf IC, Velthuis BK, et al. Follow-up screening after subarachnoid haemorrhage: frequency and determinants of new aneurysms and enlargement of existing aneurysms. Brain 2005;128(Pt 10):2421–9.

[66] Mangrum WI, Huston J 3rd, Link MJ, et al. Enlarging vertebrobasilar nonsaccular intracranial aneurysms: frequency, predictors, and clinical outcome of growth. J Neurosurg 2005; 102(1):72–9.

[67] Simon M, Franke D, Ludwig M, et al. Association of a polymorphism of the ACVRL1 gene with sporadic arteriovenous malformations of the central nervous system. J Neurosurg 2006; 104(6):945–9.

[68] Pawlikowska L, Tran MN, Achrol AS, et al. Polymorphisms in transforming growth factor-B-related genes ALK1 and ENG are associated with sporadic brain arteriovenous malformations. Stroke 2005;36(10):2278–80.

[69] Achrol AS, Pawlikowska L, McCulloch CE, et al. Tumor necrosis factor-alpha-238G > a promoter polymorphism is associated with increased risk of new hemorrhage in the natural course of patients with brain arteriovenous malformations. Stroke 2006;37(1):231–4.

[70] Pawlikowska L, Poon KYT, Achrol AS, et al. Apoliprotein E epsilon2 is associated with new hemorrhage risk in brain arteriovenous malformation. Neurosurgery 2006;58(5):838–43 [discussion: 838–43].

[71] Chen Y, Pawlikowska L, Yao JS, et al. Interleukin-6 involvement in brain arteriovenous malformations. Ann Neurol 2006;59(1):72–80.

[72] Achrol AS, Kim H, Pawlikowska L, et al. TNF-alpha polymorphism is associated with intracranial hemorrhage (ICH) after arteriovenous malformation (AVM) treatment [abstract]. Stroke 2007;38(2):597–8.

[73] Castellanos M, Leira R, Serena J, et al. Plasma metalloproteinase-9 concentration predicts hemorrhagic transformation in acute ischemic stroke. Stroke 2003;34(1):40–6.

[74] Tung PP, Olmsted EA, Kopelnik A, et al. Plasma B-type natriuretic peptide levels are associated with early cardiac dysfunction after subarachnoid hemorrhage. Stroke 2005;36(7): 1567–9.

ELSEVIER
SAUNDERS

Anesthesiology Clin
25 (2007) 413–439

ANESTHESIOLOGY
CLINICS

Neuroimaging for the Anesthesiologist

Wibke Müller-Forell, MD[a],*, Kristin Engelhard, MD[b]

[a]Institute of Neuroradiology, Johannes Gutenberg-University of Mainz,
Langenbeckstrasse 1, 55131 Mainz, Germany
[b]Clinic of Anaesthesiology, Johannes Gutenberg-University of Mainz,
Langenbeckstrasse 1, 55131 Mainz, Germany

In all cases of acute loss of consciousness, sometimes combined with acute respiratory or cardiologic insufficiency, and especially in traumatic brain injuries with the question of life-threatening central nervous system involvement, the demand for neuroradiologic imaging is justified. It is beyond the scope of this article to give the physical insight of CT and MRI, but some basic facts should be mentioned.

CT

The basis of CT is the measurement of different absorption values after exposure to X-rays. In the slice of interest, the absorption values of parts of a defined matrix (voxels) are transformed to gray-scale units by specific algorithms. These reconstructions are shown on a display, and all data are sampled in a digital manner. The radiation burden of a CT examination can be ignored in case of emergency with vital danger to the patient.

The absorption value is named after its inventor as the Hounsfield unit (HU) [1]. It varies linearly in proportion to the absorption coefficients and is defined arbitrary: water is defined as 0 HU, air may have -1000 HU, and in bone values of more than +2000 HU are measured. In routine examinations, the absolute values are not as important as the relative density of the adjacent tissue. Isodense tissue is defined for tissue with a density of normal brain parenchyma (especially gray matter), whereas tissue of high absorption of X-rays (eg, bone or a fresh hemorrhage) is called hyperdense, appearing bright. Tissue of water content (eg, edema or necrosis) looks hypodense, appearing gray to black.

Because there is a widespread and quick availability of CT equipment, this imaging method is predestined to emergency cases, especially traumatic

---

* Corresponding author.
E-mail address: mueller-forell@neuroradio.klinik.uni-mainz.de (W. Müller-Forell).

1932-2275/07/$ - see front matter © 2007 Elsevier Inc. All rights reserved.
doi:10.1016/j.anclin.2007.06.003 *anesthesiology.theclinics.com*

lesions. Combined with the newest developments of multislice CT, the ability of secondary reconstructions (including three-dimensional and vessel graphs) in any dimension is available, and questions concerning vascular diseases can be answered in an optimal manner [2].

MRI

MRI is a method to generate cross-sectional images from the interior of the body based on the physical phenomena of nuclear magnetic resonance without using ionizing radiation. Hydrogen nuclei (protons) are abundant in human tissue (as in the hydrogen atoms of water molecules), the reason for medical MRI. Brought into an external static and strong magnetic field, and exposed to an external radiofrequency pulse, the protons move in a defined way, emitting electromagnetic waves. The energy of these waves is measured and represents values, which are attributed to the brightness of the individual picture elements of which the pictures are composed by the application of sophisticated mathematical reconstruction algorithm [3].

Different parameters of the MRI examination with different preparations of the radio frequency impulse, and the time of measurement of the electromagnetic energy, stress the characteristic answers of the different tissue, which are dependent of the narrow and global environment of the protons (T2 and T1 relaxation). The MRI characteristics of tissue are defined by the composition of these different components; the manipulation of the parameters enables the investigator to enhance the differences between the local tissues, resulting in a better inherent contrast. The terms "T1-weighted," "proton density weighted," and "T2-weighted" characterize MRI sequences and images, with specific information [3,4]. T1-weighted images are best for anatomic details. After intravenous application of specific contrast material (gadolinium), the definition of the absence or existence of a blood-brain barrier disruption can be made. T2-weighted images best define tissue characteristics as edema, demyelination, or the different stages of hematoma. The fluid attenuated inversion recovery sequence combines T2-weighted characteristics (of high sensitivity for proton accumulation) with suppression of so-called "free," not tissue-bound water (where cerebrospinal fluid [CSF] looks black), enabling a better differentiation of parenchymal defects or brain edema. Out of numerous sequence techniques used to define specific tissue characteristics some should be mentioned: diffusion-weighted imaging (DWI) characterizes a disruption of brownian motion of molecules, reflecting restricted and facilitated diffusion, respectively, the affected areas showing an increased (bright) or a decreased signal enhancement [5]. Reconstruction of a secondary map of apparent diffusion coefficient (ADC) enables a quantitative and reproducible assessment of the diffusion changes of the affected or normal noneffected brain areas. In combination with the diffusion-weighted images, a differentiation between a vasogenic and toxic brain edema can be made. Diffusion tensor imaging enables the definition of tracts (eg, pyramidal tract) [6] not of much interest in the acute course of emergency, but diffusion tensor imaging becomes increasingly important in identifying biomarkers to the outcome of severe traumatic brain injury, especially in children [7].

Anatomy and corresponding pathophysiologic considerations

The discussion of the anatomy is focused on the most important structures in neuroradiologic emergency imaging, including the brain supplying arteries and draining veins, the basal cisterns, the midline structures, and some landmarks to define acute CSF circulation disturbances.

The region of the basal cisterns (Fig. 1) is an important indicator concerning the threats to the patient. The midbrain with its important nuclei is surrounded by a rather narrowed environment, as it passes the tentorial notch (see Fig. 1A), a small pathway between the rigid dura of the tentorium (Fig. 1B). The interpeduncular, suprasellar, and perimesencephalic (ambient) cisterns are the site of the cisternal way of important cranial nerves (N. III oculomotor nerve, N. IV trochlear nerve, and N. V trigeminal nerve). Additionally, it is the region of the circle of Willis (Fig. 1C), an interconnecting arterial polygon between the branches of the internal carotid arteries by anterior communicating artery, and by posterior communicating arteries the basilar bifurcation with its branches of the posterior cerebral arteries (PCA), enabling a collateralization of the main branches of the leptomeningeal arteries (see Fig. 1C). In only 20% of the cases the circle of Willis is complete, common variants include hypoplasia of one or both posterior communicating arteries, a hypoplastic or absent anterior communicating artery, and "fetal" origin of the PCA from the internal carotid arteries with hypoplastic or absent P1-segment of the corresponding PCA. Parallel to the perimesencephalic course of the PCA (*white arrows* in Fig. 1C) is the course of the basal vein of Rosenthal.

In pathologic conditions several findings indicate the seriousness of the individual disease. A narrowing of the basal cisterns indicates an increase of brain pressure, infratentorial or supratentorial. In case of a unilateral supratentorial space-occupying lesion, this acute tentorial herniation normally is accompanied by an ipsilateral anisocoria and a contralateral hemiparesis. In consequence it might lead to posterior cerebral infarction of the affected PCA (Fig. 2).

The basal ganglia and the internal capsule, together with the insular (sylvian) cistern, the location of the main part of the vessels of the medial cerebral arteries, characterize the region of the foramina of Monro (Figs. 3–5). It is the region where the definition of the so-called "midline structures" can be made, because the anterior and posterior interhemispheric fissure is seen in line with the thin third ventricle. Another midline structure is the (mainly) calcified pineal gland, and the corpus callosum, best seen on a midsagittal view (see Fig. 4). The rectus sinus, fixed in the dura, runs as a vascular midline structure in the roof of the tentorium, the demarcation of the posterior fossa

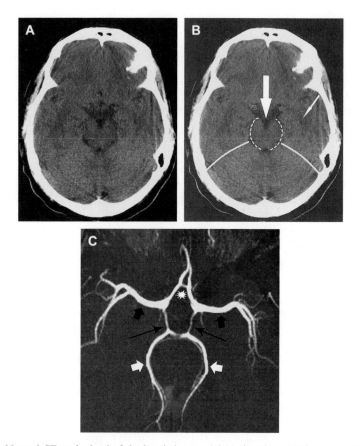

Fig. 1. Normal CT at the level of the basal cisterns. (*A*) Native view. (*B*) Corresponding diagram, indicating the ambient cisterns (*dotted white lines*), the interpeduncular cistern (*thick white arrow*), the normal-sized temporal horn (*thin white arrow*), and the edge of the tentorium at that level (*white lines*), and both internal carotid arteries (ICA) (*small white circles*). (*C*) MR angiography time-of-flight (TOF) of the circle of Willis. The posterior communicating arteries (*thin black arrows*) connect the ICA with the PCA (*thick white arrows*); the anterior communicating artery (Acom; *white star*) connects both anterior cerebral arteries (ACA). The black arrows indicate the medial cerebral arteries (MCA).

from the supratentorial cerebral hemispheres. The configuration of a tent is demonstrated on the coronal view (Fig. 5C), giving an understanding for the different forms of cerebral herniation, a mechanical displacement of brain, CSF, and blood vessels from one cranial compartment to another.

Two types of transtentorial herniation can occur: descending and ascending. By far the most common type is the descending transtentorial herniation, where parts of the temporal lobe (the uncus and parahippocampal gyrus) herniate over the free tentorial margin. In case of unilateral supratentorial mass effect the main symptoms are contralateral hemiparesis, and ipsilateral anisocoria, because of the close vicinity to the pyramidal tract, and

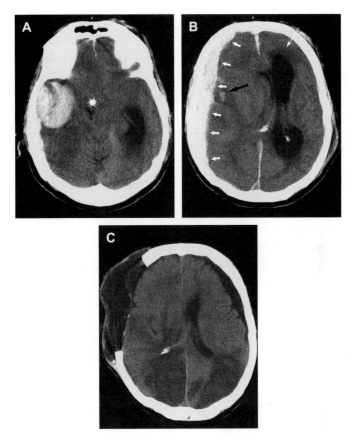

Fig. 2. A 63-year-old man found in coma, after a head trauma of unknown origin, presenting with anisocoria (right OO left). Diagnosis is combined brain injury: subcortical (intracerebral) contusion hematoma and acute subdural hematoma. (*A*) Axial CT at the level of the basal cisterns, demonstrating a space-occupying intracerebral contusion hematoma in the right temporal lobe, leading to an extensive midline shift and transtentorial herniation (the main cause for the anisocoria). Note the dislocation of the right temporal horn (*white star*), the missing basal cisterns, and the enlargement of the left temporal horn, indicating a blockade of the CSF circulation at the level of the foramina of Monro. (*B*) Axial CT at the level of the cella media of the lateral ventricles, demonstrating the entire acute ubdural hematoma (*white arrows*) and another intracerebral contusion hematoma (*black arrow*), and the extensive midline shift. Note the resulting compression of the ipsilateral ventricle and the acute CSF block with elevation of the intraventricular pressure and transventricular CSF leakage (*thin white arrow*). (*C*) Corresponding axial CT 14 days after decompression and evacuation of the acute subdural hematoma: consecutive bilateral infarction of the PCA, caused by transtentorial herniation, and contralateral infarction of a parietal branch of the MCA.

the course of the ocular cranial nerves. In consequence of the compression of the PCA, running in the ambient cistern, an infarction of the corresponding occipital lobe might occur (see Fig. 2C). In cases of severe descending transtentorial herniation all basal cisterns are obliterated, a resulting

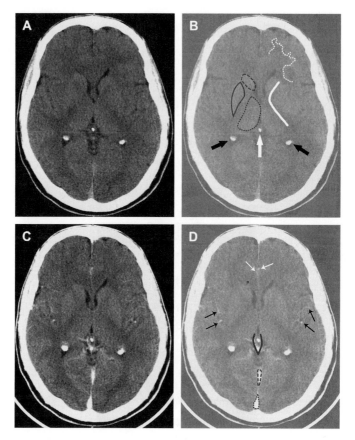

Fig. 3. Normal CT at the level of the basal ganglia and foramen of Monro. (*A*) Native view. (*B*) Corresponding diagram; the pyramidal tract with anterior and posterior leg of the internal capsule (*white line*) divides the head of the caudate nucleus (*dashed black line*) and the lateral basal ganglia (lentiform nucleus) (*black line*) from the thalamus medially (*dotted black line*). Note the slight differences in density, indicating the border of gray and white matter, and the (normal) calcification of choroid plexus (*black arrows*) and pineal gland (*white arrow*). (*C*) Corresponding contrast-enhanced view demonstrating the normal enhancement of the brain, with better delineation of the gray-white matter border, caused by the intensive vascularization of the gray matter. (*D*) Corresponding diagram; note the contrast-enhanced vessels (*small black arrows*) in the insular cistern, the pericallosal arteries (*small white arrow*), the distal internal cerebral veins (*black line*), and parts of the rectus (*dashed line*) and superior sagittal sinus (*dotted line*).

posterior fossa mass effect displaces the cerebellar tonsil inferiorly through the foramen magnum with clinical symptoms of bilateral mydriasis and lost pupillary reflex.

This concurrent tonsillar herniation might also occur in the course of ascending transtentorial herniation. In cases of infratentorial mass effect of any origin, the central cerebellar structures (central lobule, culmen, and superior surface of the cerebellum) are displaced cephalad through the tentorial incisura (Fig. 6). In subfalcine herniation the cingulated gyrus is

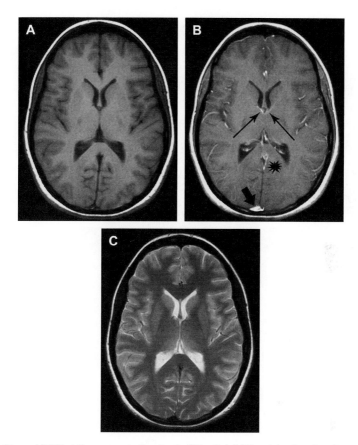

Fig. 4. Normal MRI at the corresponding level of Fig. 2. (*A*) T1-weighted native view; note the better delineation of anatomic details, compared with the corresponding CT. (*B*) Corresponding contrast-enhanced T1-weighted view. The foramina of Monro (*small black arrows*) are indicated by the confluence of the thalamostriate and the pellucid septum veins. The internal cerebral veins converging to the great vein of Galen (*star*), and the superior sagittal sinus (*large black arrow*) are indicated. (*C*) Corresponding T2-weighted view; note the bright signal of CSF in the lateral ventricles and subarachnoid space, and the excellent anatomic details, especially concerning the basal ganglia and gray-white matter border (see corresponding description of Fig. 2B).

displaced across the midline under the inferior free margin of the falx cerebri, with the consequence of infarction of the territory of the anterior cerebral arteries, which run at the inferior border of the falx, or even subependymal veins.

Clinical practice

All patients with loss of consciousness and vigilance deficits may harbor an intracerebral pathology and need neuroradiologic imaging. Many of the

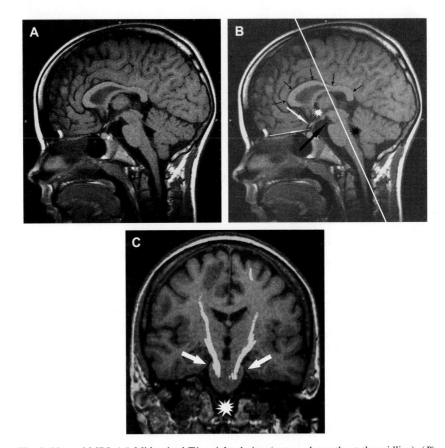

Fig. 5. Normal MRI. (*A*) Midsagittal T1-weighted view (prepared exactly at the midline). (*B*) Corresponding diagram; some midline structures are indicated: the corpus callosum (*thin black arrows*), the third (*white star*) and fourth (*black star*) ventricle, the interpeduncular cistern (*large black arrow*), the chiasm (*thick short white arrow*), and the pituitary stalk (*thin, long white arrow*). The white line indicates the coronal plain of Fig. 4C. (*C*) Coronal T1-weighted view matched with a diffusion tensor imaging, demonstrating the course of the pyramidal tract in close vicinity to the tentorium (*white arrows*); pyramidal decussation is superior to the great foramen (*white star*).

highly endangered patients treated by anesthesiologists are those with traumatic brain injuries.

Cerebral trauma

Traumatic brain injury is an important health problem in western countries, still with a mortality of 20% [8,9]. Primary traumatic craniocerebral lesions include minor or major skull fractures; scalp hematomas; and extra-axial (extracerebral) and intra-axial lesions. The main extra-axial traumatic lesions demanding neurosurgical intervention in emergency are

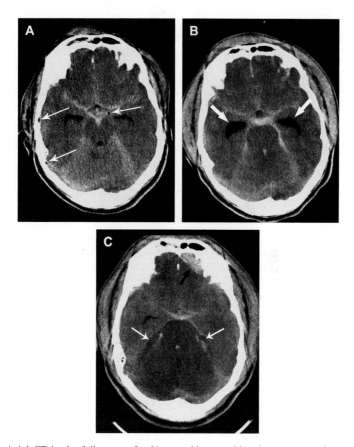

Fig. 6. Axial CT in the follow-up of a 31-year-old man with primary unconsciousness after a fall from a height of more than 6 m, requiring primary intubation and ventilation. Diagnosis is complex brain injury (diffuse axonal injury, traumatic subarachnoid hemorrhage [SAH], multiple skull fractures, multiple extracerebral hematomas) with combined (ascending and descending) transtentorial herniation in the follow-up. (*A*) CT at admission, demonstrating diffuse traumatic SAH in the basal cisterns. Note the accentuation of the temporal horns of the lateral ventricles, and the intracranial air inclusions (*white arrows*), indicating skull fractures. (*B*) The control 5 hours later, indicated because of circulatory instability (corresponding view to Fig. 10A) shows an acute CSF disturbance with widening of the temporal horns of the lateral ventricles (*thick white arrows*), leading to the indication of an open ventricular drainage. (*C*) Another control 16 hours after hospitalization was indicated because of bilateral loss of the pupillary reflex, maximal widening, and increase of intracranial pressure. Note the hypodensity of the entire midbrain, and the cerebellum, bilaterally herniated over the tentorial margin (*white arrows*), and an additional extra-axial hematoma on the left frontal region (*black arrow*).

epidural and subdural hematoma, leading to acute (or slowly progressing) increase of intracranial pressure, and the acute subarachnoid hemorrhage. Intra-axial traumatic lesions include cortical contusions, diffuse axonal injury, deep cerebral and primary brainstem injury, and intraventricular or choroid plexus hemorrhage.

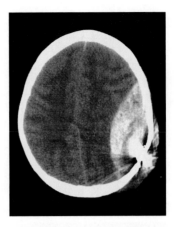

Fig. 7. A 3-year-old boy presenting with inadequate vigilance some hours after cochlear implant of the left ear. Diagnosis is acute epidural hematoma. Axial CT at the level of the centrum semiovale, where the entire dimension of the epidural hematoma is apparent. The etiology was an iatrogenic temporal fracture (not shown) by implantation of the battery.

Twenty-five percent of cases with fatal injuries do not demonstrate a skull fracture, although the incidence of intracranial hematomas in patients who have a skull fracture is much higher than those who do not, but contusions are the main causes for fatal course outcome [10]. There are three types of extracerebral (extra-axial, extrinsic) hemorrhage: (1) epidural hematoma; (2) subdural hematoma; and (3) subarachnoid hemorrhage, the latter in traumatic cases mainly in combination with one of the others.

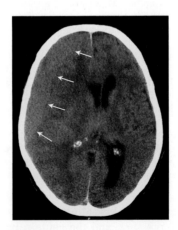

Fig. 8. A 72-year-old woman presenting with syncope and history of progressive headache, disorientation, but without any neurologic deficit. Diagnosis is subacute subdural hematoma. Axial CT showing a relevant midline shift to the left, caused by an isodense extra-axial mass of the right frontal region (*white arrows*).

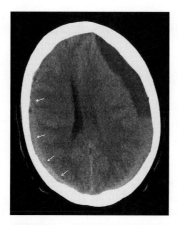

Fig. 9. A 57-year-old man with Marfan syndrome. Some days after thoracoabdominal aortic replacement, caused by aortic dissection, he suffered from acute unconsciousness and anisocoria. Diagnosis is bilateral subdural hematoma of different age. Axial CT with midline shift to the right, caused by a chronic subdural hematoma of the left hemisphere with mixed density and fluid-fluid level. Note the small isodense subacute subdural hematoma of the right hemisphere (*small white arrows*).

Extracerebral lesions

Epidural hematoma. Epidural hematomas are rare (1%–4%), and 10% of these injuries have a fatal outcome, mainly because of delayed referral, diagnosis, or operation. In most cases a skull fracture causes a laceration of a branch of the middle meningeal artery with the consequence of bleeding.

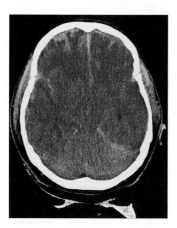

Fig. 10. Axial CT of a 60-year-old male inline-skater who fell down on the road during a race without wearing a helmet. Neurologic state was primary loss of consciousness. Diagnosis is complex brain injury: diffuse traumatic SAH, diffuse brain edema, diffuse shearing injury, and multiple skull fractures (not shown). No differentiation of the basal cisterns caused by diffuse brain swelling. Note the diffuse traumatic SAH in the frontal and temporal sulci, and a small subdural hematoma on the tentorium.

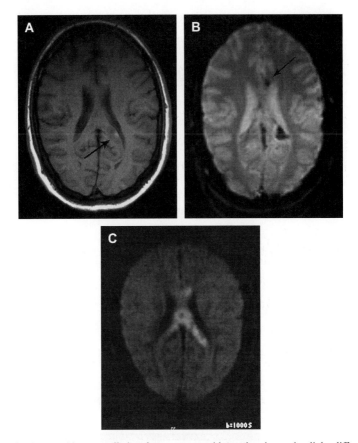

Fig. 11. A 22-year-old man suffering from a car accident, showing only slight diffuse brain edema. After a primary coma he did not awake adequately; CT did not show any structural lesion despite a diffuse, mild brain edema. Diagnosis is diffuse shearing injury. (*A*) T1-weighted image, showing a signal enhancement at the left callosal radiation (*black arrow*), corresponding to an intra-axial hematoma (methemoglobin). (*B*) Corresponding T2*-weighted image, demonstrating the intraaxial hematoma as hypointense area, and another in the anterior corpus callosum (*black arrow*). (*C*) Corresponding diffusion-weighted image. The high signal intensity corresponds to an acute diffusion disturbance, demonstrating the shearing injury of the entire corpus callosum.

Epidural hematomas are located between skull and dura. Because it forcefully strips the dura from the inner table of the skull, which does not cross sutures, it characteristically assumes a focal biconvex or lentiform configuration (Fig. 7). The most common site of epidural hemorrhage is temporoparietal; the posterior fossa or the convexity epidural hematoma are rare.

On CT the typical biconvex extra-axial, mainly hyperdense mass displaces the gray-white matter interface away from the calvarium. In acute epidural hematoma secondary tentorial herniation is very common. In emergency, MRI plays a subordinate role.

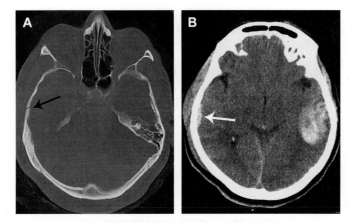

Fig. 12. A 51-year-old female cyclist, hit by a motorbike. Primary loss of consciousness requiring an intubation. Diagnosis is coup-contre-coup lesion with epidural and contusion hematoma. (*A*) Axial CT (bone window) at the level of the upper pyramid demonstrating a right temporal fracture (*black arrow*; site of the coup). (*B*) Axial CT at the level of the basal cisterns, showing a contralateral left intraparenchymatous hematoma (contre coup). Note the upper part of the epidural hematoma on the right (*white arrow*), caused by the temporal fracture.

Subdural hematoma. Traumatic acute subdural hematoma is among the most lethal of all head injuries, with a mortality range from 50% to 85% [11]. Sudden changes in velocity of the head, as it occurs mainly in car accidents, cause stretching and tearing of the bridging cortical veins as they cross the subdural space to drain into an adjacent dural sinus. Subdural hematomas are interposed between the dura and arachnoidea, which may also be torn, leading to a mixture of blood and CSF. The patients with acute trauma may present on admission with low Glasgow Coma Scales; half of them are flaccid or decerebrate [11]. On CT, the main administered primary diagnostic imaging, they typically present as crescent-shaped, homogeneously hyperdense extracerebral hematoma, which spreads diffusely over the affected hemisphere (see Fig. 2B).

Subdural hematoma may present in acute, subacute, or chronic stage, and in some cases, especially in elder patients, a definite history of trauma may be lacking. With time, subdural hematomas undergo clot lysis, organization, and neomembrane formation, delineated by contrast administration, which may demonstrate cortical vessel displacement. On CT subacute subdural hematoma may present as isodense, mainly crescent-shaped (Fig. 8) extra-axial lesion. Recurrent hemorrhage into pre-existing chronic subdural hematoma might present with mixed density or with fluid-fluid levels (Fig. 9), whereas uncomplicated chronic subdural hematoma typically present with low attenuation.

Traumatic subarachnoid hemorrhage. Diffuse traumatic subarachnoidal hemorrhage (see Fig. 6; Fig. 10) is associated with adverse outcome [12].

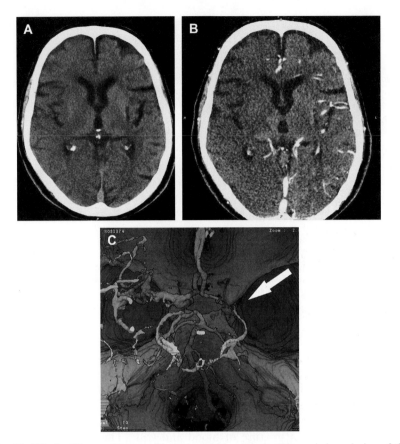

Fig. 13. CT of a 79-year-old man with acute right hemiplegia. Diagnosis is occlusion of the right ICA. (*A*) Axial CT at the level of the basal ganglia, where the right internal capsule is not as well seen as the left. (*B*) Corresponding contrast-enhanced CT, missing not only the branches of the right MCA, but also the capillary contrast enhancement of the entire right hemisphere. (*C*) CT angiography, demonstrating the complete occlusion of the intracranial right ICA (*white arrow*). (Note that the 3D-view is vice verse to the conventional view.)

In most patients traumatic subarachnoid hemorrhage is seen as additional lesion in cases of moderate to severe head trauma. Pseudosubarachnoid hemorrhage is seen in cases of severe, diffuse cerebral edema when the brain becomes very low in attenuation and circulating blood in the cranial vasculature appears unusually hyperdense compared with adjacent structures (Fig. 16).

Intra-axial lesions
Diffuse axonal injury. Diffuse axonal injury ("sharing" injury), together with cortical or subcortical contusions, is the most important cause of significant morbidity in patients with traumatic brain injuries [13]. Typical

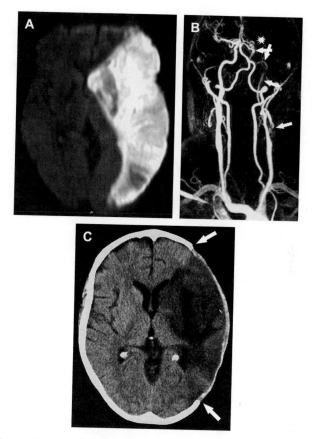

Fig. 14. A 47-year-old man with acute hemiparesis of the right side, progressing to hemiplegia during the next day, combined with fluctuating changes of vigilance, and aphasia. The axial CT (not shown), 3 hours after onset, does not show any significant pathology. Diagnosis is complete infarction of the left MCA caused by dissection and consecutive subtotal occlusion of the left ICA. (*A*) Axial MRI (diffusion-weighted image) at the level of the foramen of Monro, 42 hours after onset, demonstrating the edema in the entire territory of the MCA. (*B*) Contrast-enhanced MR angiography, where only minimal flow is seen in the extracranial and intracranial course of the ICA (*white arrows*), and the absence of any perfusion of the left hemisphere, caused by proximal occlusion of the left MCA (*star*), and no collateral flow of the leptomeningeal vessels. (*C*) Postoperative axial CT after craniectomy (corresponding level to Fig. 14A). The white arrows indicate the borders of the craniectomy. Note the return of the midline structures, despite the complete infarction of the left MCA.

clinical symptoms include loss of consciousness at the moment of impact. Diffuse axonal injury is caused by acute and sudden acceleration or deceleration or rotational forces on the brain. The brain lesions tend to be diffuse, bilateral, and occur in very specific areas: (1) lobar white matter, particularly at the gray-white matter interface; (2) at the corpus callosum; and (3) at the dorsolateral aspect of the brainstem.

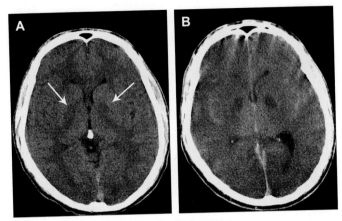

Fig. 15. A 20-year-old man, found in an unconscious state in front of a discotheque. Diagnosis is global hypoxia caused by an overdose of cocaine. (*A*) Axial CT at admission. Note a discrete hypodensity of both globus pallidi (*white arrows*), resembling carbon monoxide intoxication. (*B*) Corresponding, contrast-enhanced view 24 hours later. Note the effacement of the gray and white matter of the insular and temporal region, indicating global ischemia (intravital brain death) beside the better visualization of the damaged globus pallidi.

Initial CT scans are often normal, despite profound clinical impairment. Sometimes only small, subtle hemorrhage in the interpeduncular cistern leads to conclusion of midbrain injury. Diffuse axonal injury is the main indication for MRI in patients with cerebral trauma. Morphologic changes are best

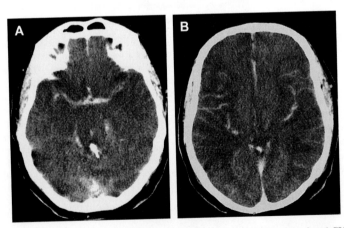

Fig. 16. A 66-year-old man presenting with frozen bilateral pupillary reflex after ACVB-bypass operation in emergency, history of cardiogenic shock 1 week before. Diagnosis is intravital brain death. (*A*) Axial CT at the level of the basal ganglia with indistinct differentiation of gray and white matter, compression of the basal cisterns, and unusual hypodensity of the midbrain. Note that the hyperdensity of the basal cisterns is caused by the slow to minimal flow of the basal vessels, but is not due to an additional SAH. (*B*) At the level of the basal ganglia differentiation (eg, of the internal capsule) is impossible. Note the hyperdensity of the sylvian arteries.

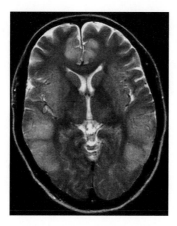

Fig. 17. A 34-year-old woman who presented with progressive unconsciousness after liver transplantation (history of toxic hepatic insufficiency). Diagnosis is metabolic encephalopathy. Axial MRI (T2-weighted), demonstrating symmetric, bilateral cortical and subcortical signal enhancement of frontal, insular, and temporal brain regions.

detected on T2-weighted images with multifocal, hyperintense foci at the gray-white matter interface and corpus callosum, or hemorrhagic lesions (see Fig. 11). Diffusion-weighted images show best the entire extension of the injury, because the disturbance of brownian movement is seen as an area of high signal intensity. Combined with apparent diffusion coefficient maps and diffusion tensor imaging together with spectroscopic measurements of the neuroaxonal damage allow, beside a better inside of the traumatic changes, a correlation with the clinical course and outcome [7,14–16].

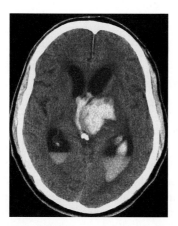

Fig. 18. Axial CT of a 67-year-old woman with history of diabetes and hypertonus, presenting with acute hemiparesis of the right. Diagnosis is spontaneous thalamic hemorrhage with intraventricular involvement.

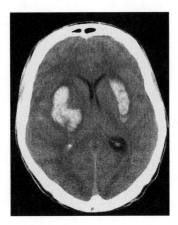

Fig. 19. Axial CT of a 21-year-old man who presented with coma. Diagnosis is spontaneous bilateral hemorrhage of the lateral basal ganglia caused by an overdose of speed.

Cortical contusion. Cortical and subcortical contusions are the second most common primary traumatic neuronal injury; they represent 45% of primary intra-axial traumatic lesions, again induced by differential acceleration-deceleration forces applied to the head. They are less frequently associated with primary loss of consciousness as diffuse axonal injury. Brain contusions are typically superficial foci of punctuate or linear hemorrhages that occur along gyral crests, mainly induced by brain striking on an osseous ridge (or dural fold), or in association with depressed skull fractures. In so-called "coup-contre-coup" lesions, one may find a cortical contusion opposite to the site of the impact (mainly apparent by skull fracture), because of compression of the cortex in continuity to the force direction (Fig. 12) [17].

Stroke

An acute neurologic deficit of different severities is the main symptom in patients presenting with stroke, although the etiology might be diverse. The most frequent and most important etiologies are discussed next.

Cerebral ischemia and infarction
About 85% of all strokes are ischemic. The most common pathway for cerebral artery stroke is an artery-to-artery embolism in patients with severe extracranial internal carotid artery stenosis and atherosclerotic plaque formation. The absence or insufficiency of leptomeningeal collateral circulation leads to neurologic deficit as hemiparesis or hemiplegia (Fig. 13) [18].

Patients with so-called "malignant" middle cerebral artery territory infarctions develop space-occupying brain edema and transtentorial herniation, carrying a mortality of about 80% [19]. Although still discussed

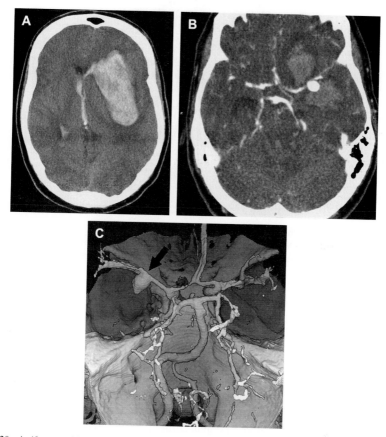

Fig. 20. A 48-year-old man with acute hemiparesis of the right site, rapid development of unconsciousness, leading to intubation and ventilation in emergency. Diagnosis is atypical bleeding of MCA aneurysm. (*A*) Axial CT, showing an extensive insular hemorrhage with an additional intraventricular bleeding (delineation of the midline shift). (*B*) The contrast-enhanced view at the level of the basal cisterns depicts an aneurysm of the left MCA. (*C*) Three-dimensional reconstruction, demonstrating the wide neck of the aneurysm at the left M1-segment, and the so-called "baby-aneurysm" at the dome, the bleeding-site directing to the basal ganglia.

controversial, decompressive hemicraniectomy seems to be a promising therapy (Fig. 14) because it not only saves the life of the individual patient, but can avoid a vegetative state, and even lead to functional independence, especially in younger patients [20–22].

Extracerebral artery dissection is commonly responsible for stroke in young patients. Dissections tear the intima and blood enters the wall of the vessel between the intima and the media, leading the wall to balloon outward and compress the lumen. If stroke results from this condition, it is most often caused by embolus, arising from a thrombus at the tear site,

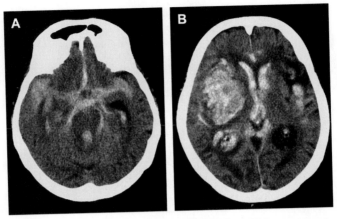

Fig. 21. Axial CT of a 90-year-old man with history marcumar therapy because of atrial fibrillation, presenting in a state of coma. Diagnosis is diffuse intracerebral and SAH. (*A*) CT at the level of the basal cisterns with extensive SAH. (*B*) CT at the level of the cella media of the lateral ventricles, demonstrating a diffuse involvement of the parenchyma with additional intraventricular bleeding. Note the global atrophy, and a postischemic defect of the left frontal operculum.

sweeping up the vessel into the brain (see Fig. 14). Spontaneous artery dissections are rather rare, but known in combination with massive trauma and minor neck injuries, and patients commonly present with pain [18].

Hypoxic-ischemic encephalopathy. Hypoxia, ischemia, and hypoglycemia are conditions with reduced oxygen content of the arterial blood, leading to a compromised supply of oxygen and nutrients to brain tissue. This may result in brain swelling, as water is osmotically drawn into the organelles and cells. Irreparable brain damage with cell death occurs if these hypoxic conditions, including (among others) asphyxia, severe pulmonary failure, or respiratory insufficiency, last too long. Out of several patterns of morphologic post–hypoxic-ischemic damage (including arterial border zone infarctions and cortical laminar necrosis), basal ganglia affection (Fig. 15) and diffuse white matter injury after cardiac arrest may lead to fatal outcome [23]. On imaging diffuse brain swelling and hypodensity of gray and white matter caused by generalized edema is seen (see Figs. 11 and 16). The compromise of the vessels of the circle of Willis should not be misinterpreted as spontaneous subarachnoid hemorrhage, but compression and blood stagnation in the corresponding vessels.

Iatrogenic toxic encephalopathy. Resembling images may be seen in patients with posterior reversible encephalopathy syndrome, an increasing, potentially reversible condition caused by the increase of more aggressive immunosuppression chemotherapy (especially cyclophosphamite) (eg, in patients

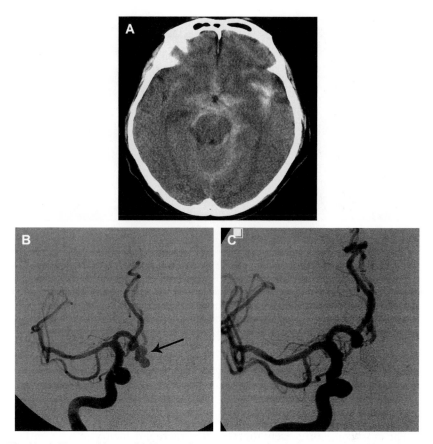

Fig. 22. A 66-year-old man with history of an acute extreme headache, presenting with confusion, drowsiness, but reaction to questions (HUNT and HESS II). Diagnosis is aneurysm of the Acom. Therapy is coiling in general anesthesia. (*A*) Axial CT demonstrating an extent SAH with slight emphasis to the left sylvian fissure. (*B*) Digital subtraction angiography of the right ICA in anteroposterior view depicts a lobulated aneurysm of the Acom (*black arrow*), showing to the left (explaining the preference of the left sylvian fissure, because the rupture nearly always occurs at the dome). (*C*) Corresponding view after coiling of the aneurysm. Note preservation of Acom.

with organ transplants). Clinically, these patients present with altered mental status, headaches, seizures, or cortical blindness (Fig. 17) [24].

Spontaneous intracerebral hemorrhage

Fifteen percent of patients presenting with stroke suffer from spontaneous intracerebral hemorrhage. The most common cause for spontaneous intracerebral hemorrhage is hypertension [25], with the preferred location of the basal ganglia, followed by thalami (Fig. 18), pons, and cerebellar hemispheres. Intracerebral hemorrhages with etiology of amyloid angiopathy, vascular malformation, drug abuse (Fig. 19), cerebral aneurysm (Fig. 20),

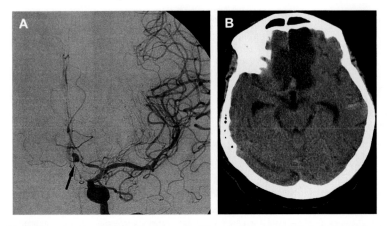

Fig. 23. A 70-year-old woman who presented with unconsciousness, drowsiness, without adequate response (HUNT and HESS III). History of headache and fall 1 week before. A significant increased flow was found in both MCA in Doppler ultrasound. Diagnosis is state of recurrent SAH (primary unrecognized) of an aneurysm of the Acom, complicated by vasospasm. (*A*) Digital subtraction angiography of the left ICA in anteroposterior view, demonstrating a remarkable narrowing of the cerebral vessels, especially the ACA, and an aneurysm of the Acom (*black arrow*). (*B*) Axial CT some days later showing bilateral infarction of the ACA, despite an intraarterial (local) spamolysis with papaverine, and consecutive coiling of the aneurysm.

or iatrogenic drugs (anticoagulants) (Fig. 21), although increasing [26], are less common.

Spontaneous subarachnoid hemorrhage

The most common presentation of an intracranial aneurysm is a nontraumatic subarachnoid hemorrhage and up to 90% of all nontraumatic subarachnoid hemorrhage is caused by rupture of an intracranial aneurysm. Subarachnoid hemorrhage presents on CT with high density of the subarachnoid space (Fig. 22A), filling mainly the basal cisterns and sylvian fissure, because most aneurysms arise from arteries of the circle of Willis. The distribution of the blood in the basal cisterns may lead to localization of the aneurysms. The clinical grading is the Hunt and Hess scale I to V, where patients presenting with grade I are basically asymptomatic or have only minimal headache, whereas patients presenting with grade IV or V demonstrate stupor, hemiparesis, or coma [27], because of the distribution of the bleeding in combination with an increased intracranial pressure caused by acute CSF disturbance or vasospasm (Fig. 23). Because the risk of rebleeding is the most imminent danger [28], diagnosis and therapy (neurosurgical clipping or neuroradiologic coiling) should not be delayed [29].

Cerebral vein and sinus thrombosis

In patients presenting with deterioration of primary unspecific symptoms as headache or seizures, veno-occlusive diseases should be ruled out:

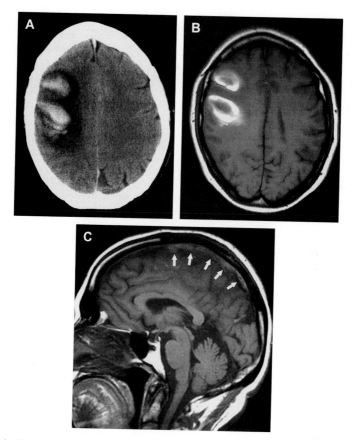

Fig. 24. A 52-year old women who presented with apoplectiform hemiparesis of the left side. Diagnosis is thrombosis of the superior sagittal sinus. (A) Axial CT demonstrating an atypical intracerebral bleeding in the right frontal lobe, suspicious for venous thrombosis. (B) Corresponding T1-weighted view. Note the different signal intensities of the subacute hemorrhage. (C) T1-weighted midsagittal view. The isodense to slightly hyperdense signal of the thrombus in the superior sagittal sinus (white arrows) is apparent.

imaging is critical to the diagnosis of these often underdiagnosed disorders. On CT, atypical intracerebral hemorrhage as a marker of venous congestion (in combination with a hyperdense thrombus in the affected dural sinus) may lead to suspicion of thrombosis of the corresponding sinus. The most commonly effected dural sinus is the superior sagittal sinus (Fig. 24), followed by the transverse sinus [30,31]. The main causes are hormonal disturbances, such as pregnancy and oral contraceptives; dehydration; or infection. In the course of systemic malignancies cerebral venous or sinus thrombosis present as a paraneoplastic syndrome or in combination with chemotherapy [31].

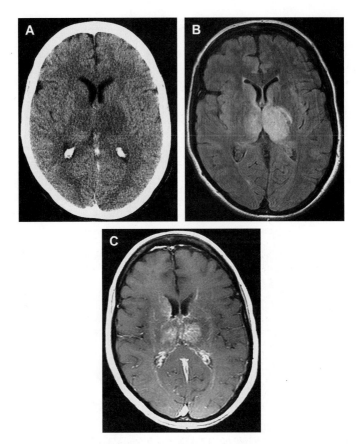

Fig. 25. A 49-year-old woman with progressing headache and loss of vigilance. Diagnosis is thrombosis of internal veins. (*A*) Native CT with hypodensity of both thalami, left more than right. (*B*) Corresponding T2-weighted (FLAIR) MRI demonstrating the edema of both thalami and caudate nuclei head caused by venous congestion. (*C*) Corresponding T1-weighted contrast-enhanced view. Note the widening of the veins of the thalami and basal ganglia, normally not visible (compare with Fig. 5B).

A rather rare condition is deep cerebral vein thrombosis (internal cerebral veins), a disease that might be fatal if misdiagnosed. In case of bilateral edema of the thalami a thrombosis of the internal cerebral veins should always be excluded (Fig. 25).

For the question of cerebral venous thrombosis MRI is the imaging method of choice, not only with morphologic but dynamic venous MR angiography sequences. One should always keep in mind the variable signal characteristics of thrombi at different stages of blood clot, because especially fresh thrombi with isodense signal in T1-weighted images may be overlooked [32].

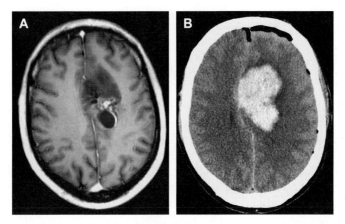

Fig. 26. A 53-year-old man, 1 day after surgery of an intraventricular astrocytoma WHO grade II. After a normal postoperative state (patient was able to walk) he presented with inadequate reactions and changing vigilance but no neurologic deficit. Diagnosis is postoperative complication: space-occupying bleeding. (*A*) Preoperative axial T1-weighted, contrast-enhanced MRI, demonstrating the size of the tumor. (*B*) Corresponding postoperative CT, showing a space-occupying hemorrhage not only in the former tumor bed, but in the cingulated gyrus and the corpus callosum.

Postoperative complications

Attention should be made in the first hours after diverse operative procedures, because even unspecific symptoms might be signs of severe complications (Figs. 26 and 27). That might be the right place to thank the nursing

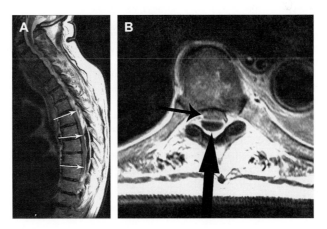

Fig. 27. MRI of a 94-year-old man suffering from urinary retention and progressive paraparesis 1 day after abdominal surgery (because of mesenterial artery occlusion) in peridural anesthesia. Diagnosis is epidural hematoma from D11 to D7. (*A*) Sagittal T2-weighted view of the cervicothoracic spine demonstrating the upper end of the lesion at D4 (*white arrows*); the lower end at D11 was seen on sagittal images of the lumbar spine (not shown). (*B*) Axial T2-weighted view at the level of D7 showing the compromise of the thoracic cord (*thin black arrow*) by the hematoma (*thick black arrow*).

staff, because they are close to patients, and the first who pay attention to any unusual behavior.

Summary

Neurologic disorders can be caused by many different pathologies, such as head trauma, cerebral ischemia, tumors, vessel disorders, intoxication, inflammation, and metabolic diseases. The symptoms of neurologic disorders for all these pathologies are very similar, such as impairment of consciousness, palsy, headache, or seizures. A precise imaging of the brain is necessary. On the basis of the combination of clinical symptoms and CT, angiography, and MRI, most of the diagnoses can be made and a differentiated therapy can be started. This article helps the anesthesiologist to identify most of the causes for neurologic disorders, to decide the optimal approach for each individual patient if he or she has to be operated on, and to choose the right treatment for the patient in the intensive care unit.

References

[1] Hounsfield G. Computerized transverse axial scanning (tomography); part 1: description of the system. Br J Radiol 1973;46:1016–22.
[2] Benvenuti L, Chibbaro S, Carnesecchi S, et al. Automated three-dimensional volume rendering of helical computed tomographic angiography for aneurysms: an advanced application of neuronavigation technology. Neurosurgery 2005;57:69–77.
[3] Wichmann W. Magnetic resonance imaging (MRI). In: Müller-Forell W, editor. Imaging of orbital and visual pathway pathology. Springer Verlag; 2002. p. 18–23.
[4] Wehrli F, McGowan J. The basis of MR contrast. In: Atlas S, editor. Magnetic resonance imaging of the brain and spine. Lippincott-Raven; 1996. p. 29–48.
[5] Mascalchi M, Filippi M, Floris R, et al. Diffusion-weighted MR of the brain: methodology and clinical application. Radiol Med 2005;109:155–97.
[6] Reinges M, Schoth F, Coenen V, et al. Imaging of postthalamic visual fiber tracts by anisotropic diffusion weighted MRI and diffusion tensor imaging: principles and applications. Eur J Radiol 2004;49:91–104.
[7] Wilde E, Chu Z, Bigler E, et al. Diffusion tensor imaging in the corpus callosum in children after moderate to severe traumatic brain injury. J Neurotrauma 2006;23:1412–26.
[8] Rutland-Brown W, Langlois J, Thomas K, et al. Incidence of traumatic brain injury in the united states. J Head Trauma Rehabil 2006;21:544–8.
[9] Boto G, Gomez P, De la Cruz J, et al. Severe head injury and the risk of early death. J Neurol Neurosurg Psychiatry 2006;77:1054–9.
[10] Bullock K, Teasdale G. Surgical management of traumatic intracranial hematomas. In: Vincken P, Bruyn G, editors. Handbook of clinical neurology. New York: Elsevier; 1990. p. 249–50.
[11] Wilberger J, Harris M, Diamond D. Acute subdural hematoma: morbidity, mortality, and operative timings. J Neurosurg 1991;74:212–8.
[12] Armin S, Colohan A, Zhang J. Traumatic subarachnoid hemorrhage: our current understanding and its evolution over the past half century. Neurol Res 2006;28:445–52.
[13] Gentry L. Head trauma. In: Atlas SW, editor. Magnetic resonance imaging of the brain and spine. 3rd edition. Raven Press; 2002. p. 1059–98.

[14] Shanmuganathan K, Gullapalli R, Mirvis S, et al. Whole-brain apparent diffusion coefficient in traumatic brain injury: correlation with Glasgow Coma Scale score. Am J Neuroradiol 2004;25:539–44.

[15] Marmarou A, Signoretti S, Fatouros P, et al. Predominance of cellular edema in traumatic brain swelling in patients with severe head injuries. Neurosurgery 2006;104:720–30.

[16] Marino S, Zei E, Battaglini M, et al. Acute metabolic brain damages following traumatic brain injury and their relevance to clinical severity and outcome. J Neurol Neurosurg Psychiatry 2007;78:501–7.

[17] Jayakumar P, Sastry Kolluri V, Basavakumar D, et al. Prognosis in contre-coup intracranial hematomas–a clinical and radiological study of 63 patients. Acta Neurochir 1991;108:30–3.

[18] Kohorshetz W, Gonzales R. Causes of ischemic stroke. In: Gonzales R, Hirsch J, Koroshetz W, et al, editors. Acute ischemic stroke: imaging and intervention. Springer; 2006. p. 27–40.

[19] Hacke W, Schwab S, Horn M, et al. Malignant middle cerebral artery territory infarction: clinical course and prognostic sign. Arch Neurol 1996;53:309–15.

[20] Harscher S, Reichert R, Terborg C, et al. Outcome after decompressive craniectomy in patients with severe ischemic stroke. Acta Neurochir 2006;148:31–7.

[21] Vahedi K, Hofmeier J, Juettner E, et al. Earlx decompressive surgery in malignant infarction of the middle cerebral artery: a pooled analysis of three randomized controlled trials. Lancet Neurol 2007;6:215–22.

[22] Pillai A, Menon S, Kumar S, et al. Decompressive hemicraniectomy in malignant middle cerebral artery infarction: an analysis of long-term outcome and factors in patient selection. J Neurosurg 2007;106:59–65.

[23] Van der Knaap M, Valk J. Post-hypoxic ischemic damage. In: Van der Knaap M, Valk J, editors. Magnetic resonance imaging in myelination and myelin disorders. Springer; 2005. p. 714–7.

[24] Van der Knaap M, Valk J. Iatrogenic toxic encephalopathies. In: Van der Knaap M, Valk J, editors. Magnetic resonance imaging in myelination and myelin disorders. Springer; 2005. p. 679–89.

[25] Diringer MN. Intracerebral hemorrhage: pathophysiology and management. Crit Care Med 1993;21:1591–603.

[26] Flaherty M, Kissela B, Woo D, et al. The increasing incidence of anticoagulant-associated intracerebral hemorrhage. Neurology 2007;68:116–21.

[27] Cedzich C, Roth A. Neurological and psychosocial outcome after subarachnoid hemorrhage, and the Hunt and Hess scale as a predictor of clinical outcome. Zentralbl Neurochir 2005;66:112–8.

[28] van Gijn J, Kerr R, Rinkel G. Subarachnoid haemorrhage. Lancet 2007;369:306–18.

[29] Mericle R, Reig A, Burry M, et al. Endovascular surgery for proximal posterior inferior cerebellar artery aneurysms: an analysis of Glasgow coma scale by Hunt-Hess grades. Neurosurgery 2006;58:619–25.

[30] Einhäupl K, Masuhr F. Cerebral venous and sinus thrombosis–an update. Eur J Neurol 1994;1:109–26.

[31] Marks M. Cerebral ischemia and infarction. In: Atlas S, editor. Magnetic resonance imaging of the brain and spine. Lippincott Williams & Wilkins; 2002. p. 919–79.

[32] Thulborn K, Atlas S. Intracranial hemorrhage. In: Atlas S, editor. Magnetic resonance imaging of the brain and spine. Lippincott Williams & Wilkins; 1996. p. 265–314.

ELSEVIER
SAUNDERS

ANESTHESIOLOGY
CLINICS

Anesthesiology Clin
25 (2007) 441–463

Anesthetic Considerations for Intraoperative Management of Cerebrovascular Disease in Neurovascular Surgical Procedures

Rafi Avitsian, MD*, Armin Schubert, MD, MBA

Department of General Anesthesiology, Cleveland Clinic, 9500 Euclid Avenue, Cleveland, OH 44195, USA

Improved emergency response systems, especially in major urban areas, have facilitated rapid transport of patients who suffer from subarachnoid hemorrhage (SAH) following a ruptured intracranial aneurysm (IA). New surgical methods and interventions promise a better outcome, but a considerable number of patients who undergo neurovascular procedures emergently or electively have substantial mortality, morbidity, and disability. This article provides a brief description of relevant anatomic, physiologic, and pharmacologic points, followed by a discussion of anesthetic management for IA, arteriovenous malformation (AVM), and extracranial-to-intracranial arterial bypass surgery.

Applicable cerebral anatomy, physiology, and pharmacology

The circle of Willis

Two internal carotid arteries (ICAs) and two vertebral arteries are the four main arteries supplying the brain. The ICAs supply the anterior part of the brain, whereas the vertebral arteries supply the posterior part. These arteries anastomose at the base of the brain to form the circle of Willis, although a perfect functional circle is present in less than 20% of angiographic studies. The ICAs give rise to ophthalmic arteries on their ipsilateral sides. After this branch, the ICAs give rise to the posterior communicating

* Corresponding author.
E-mail address: avitsir@ccf.org (R. Avitsian).

1932-2275/07/$ - see front matter © 2007 Elsevier Inc. All rights reserved.
doi:10.1016/j.anclin.2007.06.002   *anesthesiology.theclinics.com*

artery and then the anterior choroidal artery. In the end the ICAs bifurcate into the anterior cerebral artery and the middle cerebral artery (MCA). Although the anterior choroidal artery has rich intracranial vascular anastomoses, the area supplied by the MCA lacks good communicating anastomoses and is prone to ischemia. The two anterior cerebral arteries on either side are connected by the anterior communicating artery.

The two vertebral arteries give rise to two posterior inferior cerebellar arteries on either side and then anastomose to form the basilar artery at the lower border of the pons. The major branches of the basilar artery are paramedian arteries and short and long circumferential arteries. The anterior inferior cerebellar artery and superior cerebellar artery, which originate from the basilar artery, along with posterior inferior cerebellar arteries, supply the cerebellum. The basilar artery then bifurcates to form the two posterior cerebral arteries on each side, which are connected to their ipsilateral ICA by the posterior communicating arteries.

Intracranial venous drainage

Most of the blood in the brain can be found in its venous system. Blood is drained into superficial and deep cerebral veins and veins of the posterior fossa. The superficial veins drain the surface of the brain cortex and lie within the cortical sulci. The deep cerebral veins drain the white matter, basal ganglia, diencephalon, cerebellum, and brainstem. The deep veins join to form the great vein of Galen. The veins of posterior fossa drain blood from the cerebellar tonsils and the posteroinferior cerebellar hemispheres. In addition, the diploic veins drain the blood between layers of bone in the skull. Emissary veins connect the veins near the surface of the skull to the diploic veins and venous sinuses. All the blood is drained into the meningeal sinuses, which mainly drain into the internal jugular vein. Usually, the right jugular vein is the dominant one receiving most of the blood from the brain. The veins and sinuses of the brain lack valves. Pressure of drainage vessels in the neck is directly transmitted to intracranial venous structures.

Physiologic and pharmacologic considerations

Continuous supply of oxygen and glucose by blood is essential for production of adenosine triphosphate, the source of energy in the brain. That is why the brain is a very vascular organ, receiving approximately 15% of cardiac output to supply its high demand for oxygen. On average, brain blood supply is about 50 mL/100 g/min, although this is higher in the cortical gray than white matter. Average weight of an adult brain is 1350 g. The blood content of the brain is about 50 mL, of which only 7 to 8 mL is arterial blood.

The average cerebral metabolic rate for oxygen ($CMRO_2$) is 3 to 3.5 mL/100 g/min, which varies from 2 mL/100 g/min in white matter to 6 mL/100 g/min in gray matter. About 60% of O_2 use in the brain is for maintenance of brain cell function including its electrophysiologic activity to generate action potentials and synthesis of neurotransmitters. Brain cell function can be clinically monitored by electroencephalography, evoked potentials, and neurologic examination. The remaining 40% of the brain's O_2 use is directed toward maintenance of the cellular integrity. Any intervention that can decrease cellular activity also decreases $CMRO_2$ and may protect the brain against ischemia. Certain anesthetics, such as barbiturates, can decrease O_2 requirements for the functional component by depressing electroencephalography activity. Hypothermia may protect brain cells by decreasing O_2 use for both the functional component and cellular integrity [1]. Managing $CMRO_2$ is an integral part of anesthetic management for temporary ischemia during neurovascular surgical procedures, even though clinical efficacy remains controversial.

Most IV anesthetics, except ketamine, decrease cerebral metabolic rate and cerebral blood flow (CBF). In humans, volatile anesthetics in doses less than 1 minimum alveolar concentration decrease CBF, coupled with a decrease in CMR. In doses above 1 minimum alveolar concentration, the vasodilatory effect of volatile agents on the cerebral vessels predominates and CBF increases despite further reduction in CMR [2]. An assessment of the adequacy of oxygen delivery to the brain can be achieved by measuring cerebral oxygen extraction. The oxygen saturation of blood in the jugular bulb in an adult with normal hematocrit is 65% to 70%. Monitoring the oxygen saturation in the jugular bulb can provide information about the ratio of global O_2 supply to demand in the brain and be useful in the detection of hypoperfusion states [3].

The main constituents of the cranium are brain and meninges, blood, and cerebrospinal fluid, which are located in a tight, bony skull. Intracranial elastance $[\Delta P/\Delta V]$ is high because a small change in intracranial volume, ΔV, can cause a large change in intracranial pressure (ICP), ΔP (Fig. 1). This concept is also known as "low intracranial compliance" $[\Delta V/\Delta P]$. According to the equation $CPP = MAP - ICP$, with an acute increase in ICP (eg, in SAH), cerebral perfusion pressure (CPP) decrease unless there is a concomitant increase in mean arterial pressure (MAP). Increasing the MAP, however, can in turn increase the amount of intracranial bleeding. Management of this vicious circle is one of the most difficult tasks for the anesthesiologist or intensivist. The goal for managing patients with increased ICP is a controlled reduction of the volume of each cranial constituent (eg, positioning the head elevated to improve venous drainage, hyperventilation to decrease intracranial blood volume, drainage of cerebrospinal fluid, administration of mannitol to decrease cerebral edema, and so forth). Although the CO_2 responsiveness of intracranial vessels and autoregulation of CBF play an important role in normal ICP modulation, these mechanisms are often disrupted after SAH [4,5]. Successful management of patients with intracranial pathology depends on knowledge of the pathophysiology of cerebral hypoperfusion, reliable and timely information

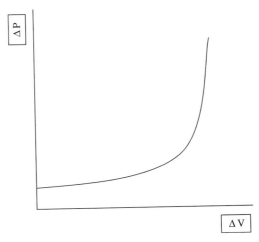

Fig. 1. Diagram showing relationship between changes in intracranial pressure (ΔP) with change in volume (ΔP).

from monitoring devices, and appropriate choice of therapeutic intervention.

Intracranial aneurysms

IAs are not uncommon, with autopsy studies showing an incidence of 0.2% to 9.9% in the general population [6]. Fortunately, not all aneurysms rupture. Bleeding from an IA can present as SAH; 85% of all SAH results from ruptured IAs [7]. The incidence of SAH is 5 to 10 per 100,000 person years [8]. SAH is a devastating disease with high mortality and morbidity accounting for 25% of cerebrovascular deaths [9]. About 25% to 50% of patients die as a result of initial bleeding. Many who survive become debilitated.

IAs typically occur at branch points throughout the cerebral vasculature (Fig. 2). Most IAs are at the anterior communicating artery and MCA, followed by ICA between posterior communicating artery and anterior choroidal artery. About 10% of the aneurysms are at the ICA bifurcation or the basilar artery bifurcation. About 30% of patients who present with SAH have multiple aneurysms [10]. Risk factors for multiple aneurysms in patients aged 15 to 60 years include cigarette smoking, female gender, and hypertension [11]. New IAs can grow in patients who have undergone aneurysm clipping at the site of clipping or at a new site [10].

Most cases of IA are sporadic, although some might present a familial pattern [12]. Recent genetic linkage studies have shown positive linkages for various regions and putative candidate genes, although causative mutations have not yet been proved [13]. A population-based study in Scotland showed a 4.7% lifetime risk of SAH in first-degree relatives and an even higher risk if there are two first-degree relatives with SAH [14]. Some hereditary disorders

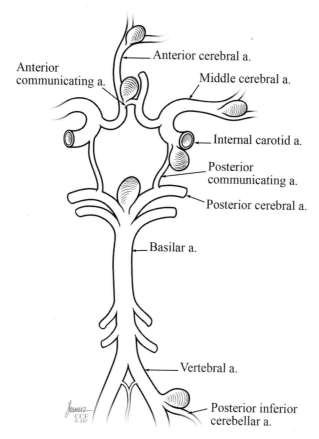

Fig. 2. Aneurysms around circle of Willis. (*Reprinted* with permission of the Cleveland Clinic Foundation.)

are associated with IA development. Ehlers-Danlos syndrome type IV, adult polycystic kidney disease, fibrous dysplasia, neurofibromatosis type 1, Marfan syndrome [15], and AVM are associated with IA [16]. With the development of noninvasive diagnostic methods, screening for IA has become easier [17]. Screening is indicated for patients with adult polycystic kidney disease [18] and those who have two immediate relatives with IA [19].

Certain factors increase risk of SAH in patients with IA. About 75% of patients with SAH are women [20]. Men with IA tend to have a higher risk of SAH before the fifth decade of life, after which women have a higher risk of rupture [21]. The mean age of patients with SAH from IA is 52 years, and incidence of hemorrhage increases with age until at least the eighth decade of life [21,22]. Rupture can also occur during pregnancy, most frequently during the thirtieth to fortieth week or in the postpartum period. Cigarette smoking [23], hypertension [24], and moderate to heavy alcohol consumption (especially binge drinking) [25] increase the risk of SAH.

Certain characteristics of IAs increase their likelihood of rupture. Aneurysm size and location are independent predictors of rupture. In patients with no history of SAH from other IAs, aneurysms less than 10 mm in diameter are less likely to rupture than those 10 to 24 mm in diameter [20]. Aneurysms located in the basilar tip, vertebrobasilar, or posterior cerebral distribution have a higher chance of bleeding [20]. Recently, it was shown that rebleeding is also more frequent in larger (> 10 mm) aneurysms [26]. The strength of the aneurysm wall, which is related to collagen type and reticular fibers in the medial layer of arteries [27], a history of previous rupture of another IA [20], and transmural pressure are also important in determining the risk of IA rupture [28]. Transmural pressure is the difference in pressure inside (blood pressure) and pressure applied from outside the aneurysmal wall (ICP or cerebrospinal fluid pressure). An increase in blood pressure resulting from exertion, activities involving Valsalva maneuver, and emotional strain can increase the blood pressure and cause rupture. Changes in cerebrospinal fluid pressure are mainly caused by Valsalva maneuver or postural changes [28].

Most IAs do not rupture and are asymptomatic; some of these are discovered incidentally with CT or MRI. Incidentally discovered IAs have an annual rate of rupture around 0.5% to 2% [29]. In larger IAs, mass effect can cause focal neurologic symptoms, such as third nerve palsy. Aneurysms in the ICA and posterior circulation are more likely to cause focal symptoms from mass effect than those in the anterior circulation or MCA aneurysms [30]. An IA can act as a nidus for thrombus formation and cause subsequent ischemic symptoms from emboli [31]. The most dramatic presentation of IA, however, is bleeding. Although intraparenchymal and intraventricular bleeding occurs, the most common presentation for bleeding is SAH. Severe headache ("worst headache of my life") is a common presentation. Some patients have had similar but less severe headaches days or weeks before SAH. This may be because of minor leaks in the aneurysm wall or leaks into the subarachnoid space [21]. These prodromal headaches are usually misdiagnosed for migraine or sinus problems. In addition to headache, patients may have meningeal irritation resulting in nuchal rigidity and vomiting. Focal neurologic deficits and change in mental status are the basis of the Hunt Hess grading scale, which has been used as a predictor for outcome (Table 1). A frequently overlooked part in this classification is that if patients have other medical comorbidities, such as hypertension, severe atherosclerotic disease, chronic pulmonary disease, diabetes, and severe vasospasm, the grade should be the next less favorable one. The World Federation of Neurosurgical Societies has introduced a new grading system [32] that has better prognostic value and is partially based on the Glasgow Comas Scale of patients on arrival (Table 2).

A detailed discussion of the relative merits of surgical treatment versus endovascular intervention [33] and its timing [20,34] is outside the scope of this article. There has been a substantial increase in the popularity of

Table 1
Hunt Hess classification of patients with intracranial aneurysm according to surgical risk

Grade[a]	Description
I	Asymptomatic or minimal headache and slight nuchal rigidity
II	Moderate to severe headache, nuchal rigidity but no focal deficit other than cranial nerve involvement
III	Drowsiness, confusion, or mild focal deficit
IV	Stupor, moderate to severe hemiparesis, possible early decerebrate rigidity, and vegetative disturbance
V	Deep coma, decerebrate rigidity, moribund appearance

[a] Serious systemic diseases, such as hypertension, severe arteriosclerosis, diabetes, chronic pulmonary diseases, and severe vasospasm, result in placement to the next grade with less favorable outcome.

endovascular treatment of IA [35]. Anesthetic considerations for interventional neuroradiology are discussed in the article by William Young of this volume.

Preoperative considerations

Similar to all other surgical procedures involving anesthesia, careful evaluation of a patient's medical history and physical examination are key to successful anesthetic planning and preoperative optimization. In patients who present with a ruptured IA there is less time for evaluation and medical optimization before surgery. A detailed history and physical examination can provide valuable information when deciding on an anesthetic plan. The World Federation of Neurosurgical Societies grade at presentation and before surgery should be used as a guide to understand clinical progress and outcome after surgery. Understanding patients' baseline functional class by their activity level is a good measure of their cardiac status. A history of asthma or chronic pulmonary disease can alert the anesthesiologist when planning for intubation and subsequent emergence. A family history of chronic renal failure or hypertension can alert to the possibility of adult polycystic kidney disease. Some SAH events occur after a surge in blood pressure (eg, following cocaine or methamphetamine use). Cocaine use can adversely affect both presentation and outcome after SAH [36], and

Table 2
World Federation of Neurological Surgeons grading for clinical features of intracranial aneurysm

Grade	Glasgow Coma Scale Score	Clinical Appearance
1	15	No motor deficit
2	13–14	No motor deficit
3	13–14	Motor deficit
4	7–12	With or without motor deficit
5	3–6	With or without motor deficit

should alert the practitioner to the possibility of coexistent drug or alcohol dependencies.

Laboratory and radiologic evaluation is essential before submitting the patient to an operation. A current blood type and screen should be available in all patients who consent to blood transfusion. If a patient is known to have positive antibodies for blood products, timely availability of cross-matched blood should be guaranteed. A recent study showed that advances in surgical technique have made routine cross-matching of blood in IA surgery unnecessary [37]. In patients who are absolutely opposed to autologous blood transfusion, cell salvage techniques may be appropriate. Information about platelet count and coagulation profile in patients on anticoagulants or those with chronic liver problems is important. A metabolic panel can reveal electrolyte abnormalities including hyponatremia in patients with SAH [38]. EKG changes are common with SAH [39]. These changes should not be misinterpreted and prevent the surgical procedure; however, further cardiac evaluation should be considered in patients with ongoing cardiac symptoms. Prophylactic antiepileptic treatment is not advocated by all experts [40] and craniotomy per se is not a reason for prophylactic antiepileptic therapy [41]. At the onset of SAH, 6.3% to 7.8% of patients have seizures [42,43].

In patients undergoing elective aneurysm clipping who are of conceiving age, a pregnancy test should be offered to the patient because this might change the surgical and anesthetic plan. There is a higher risk of IA rupture during pregnancy [44]. In the pregnant patient with a ruptured IA, the principles of surgical management are similar to nonpregnant patients [45]. The reader is referred to reviews of anesthetic considerations in pregnant patients undergoing nonobstetric surgeries [46,47].

Review of the CT scan determines the extent of bleeding in patients with SAH. Multiple grading scales have been introduced for determining the risk of vasospasm according to the CT scan evaluation of intracranial bleeding, the most famous [48] of which is the Fisher grading system (Table 3) [49]. Radiologic studies with CT angiogram, MR angiography, or angiography can also help in determining the size and location of an aneurysm and

Table 3
Fisher grading system for subarachnoid hemorrhage

Grade	Description
1	No blood
2	Diffuse deposition or thin layer, no clots >3 mm thick, or vertical layers >1 mm thick
3	Dense collection of blood >1 mm thick in the vertical plane (interhemispheric fissure, insular cistern, or ambient cistern), or >5 × 3 mm in longitudinal and transverse dimension in the horizontal plane (system of sylvian fissure, sylvian cistern, and interpeduncular cistern)
4	Intracerebral or intraventricular clots, but with only diffuse or no blood in basal cisterns

patient positioning on the operating table. No test, however, can replace communication with the surgeon regarding patient position, likelihood of temporary clip application, anticipated blood loss, and need for hemodynamic manipulations during the procedure.

Intracranial bleeding can decrease intracranial compliance and increase ICP. An adequate blood pressure is required to maintain adequate CPP, especially if vasospasm develops. High systolic blood pressure imposes shear forces on the aneurysm wall, however, and is thought to increase the risk of rebleeding after SAH [50], but this issue is controversial [51,52]. In some centers, hypertension is not treated unless MAP is above 130 mm Hg, whereas in others, tight blood pressure control is practiced with an upper systolic blood pressure target of 140 to 160 mm Hg, to prevent the high mortality rate from hypertension-induced rebleeding in SAH [53]. The American Heart Association notes that although antihypertensive therapy alone is not recommended to prevent rebleeding, it is frequently used in combination with monitored bed rest. The β-blockers labetalol and esmolol and the calcium channel blocker nicardipine can be used with minimal adverse cardiovascular and ICP effects [52]. Use of nitroprusside can increase ICP by causing intracranial vasodilation. Direct arterial blood pressure monitoring is required. Control of headache can assist with blood pressure control.

Most patients who present with SAH have already been admitted to the neurosurgical intensive care unit. Some may be intubated because they are obtunded and unable to protect their airway; others require mechanical ventilation to control elevated ICP either from diffuse brain swelling or hydrocephalus. It is useful to check electrolytes and serum osmolality in patients who have received mannitol. Patients with ventriculostomy should have their cerebrospinal fluid drains closed during transport to avoid unintended intracranial hypotension. Acute intracranial hypotension (acute reduction in ICP) can increase the transmural pressure in the aneurysm, causing its expansion and possible rebleeding.

Despite the trend toward early surgical intervention after SAH, some patients may have signs of clinical vasospasm when they are referred for surgery. In these patients, therapy includes specific calcium channel blockers and "triple H therapy" (induced hypertension, hypervolemia, and hemodilution). Hypervolemia, especially in patients with a poor cardiac reserve, can cause pulmonary edema. Careful preoperative assessment of cardiac function is particularly important in these patients.

Induction and intraoperative management

Transport of intensive care unit patients to the operating room may be dangerous and has been associated with a high rate of potentially detrimental complications [54]. The best practice is for the anesthesia team to meet the critically ill patient in the neurosurgical intensive care unit and plan for continued hemodynamic monitoring during transport. Transport help should be available because the anesthesia provider should focus on management of hemodynamic changes and ventilatory support and sedation in intubated patients. Extra care should be taken during transport to decrease the risk of extubation, monitoring disruption or IV displacement.

Standard American Society of Anesthesiologists monitoring and invasive arterial monitoring is necessary during surgery. Whether central venous pressure or pulmonary artery pressure should be monitored depends on several factors including patient medical history, size and location of the IA, use of inotropic agents, and the anesthesiologist's discretion. In patients receiving triple H therapy, a pulmonary artery or central venous pressure catheter should be considered to monitor the preload and cardiac performance. When adequate peripheral IV access is available, however, central venous cannulation cannot be justified only on the grounds that the patient is undergoing cranial surgery. Jugular bulb oxygen monitoring can also be helpful in patients at risk for global cerebral ischemia [55,56]. Rozet and colleagues [57] have used this method extensively as an indicator for global CBF; they also reported this monitoring tool useful to diagnose perioperative aneurysmal rupture before dural opening.

When surgical technique calls for placement of a spinal drain, it is essential to refrain from opening the drain before dural opening because sudden decrease in ICP can increase the aneurysm transmural pressure resulting in acute SAH. Before dural opening IV mannitol can be used to reduce ICP because this does not cause an acute change in transmural pressure.

Induction of general anesthesia and intubation should be accomplished in a smooth and controlled manner. Small doses of anxiolytics like midazolam can help to decrease patient anxiety preoperatively, although one should be aware that this can change neurologic evaluation and create suspicion of deteriorating mental status postoperatively, especially in elderly patients. Placement of an arterial line before induction can assist in the prompt diagnosis and treatment of sudden blood pressure changes during induction. Patients who are on antihypertensive medications may respond to standard induction doses with excessive hypotension. Severe hypertension can cause intracranial rebleeding with further increases in ICP, whereas hypotension may compromise CPP in patients with already increased ICP.

IV lidocaine can suppress sympathetic activation during intubation and positioning, and decrease $CMRO_2$. A variety of IV anesthetic agents may be used for induction; however, one should keep in mind the hemodynamic effect of these agents. Although etomidate does not affect MAP while decreasing CBF and $CMRO_2$ [58], it can produce some myoclonal activity that could be misinterpreted as a seizure. Also, etomidate is painful on injection and there have been accounts of an adrenocortical suppressive effect even with a single bolus dose [59]. Unless clinically indicated (eg, in patients with low cardiac output), the authors tend to avoid etomidate for induction. Ketamine increases $CMRO_2$, CBF, and ICP and is not recommended for these cases. Thiopental decreases $CMRO_2$ and ICP; although CBF also decreases with thiopental, the ratio of CBF to $CMRO_2$ remains stable. Even though MAP decreases with thiopental, CPP is improved because the ICP decreases to a greater extent than MAP [60]. Propofol also decreases $CMRO_2$, ICP, and CBF. A significant reduction in CPP occurs when propofol is administered to patients with high ICP [61]. When temporary clipping is anticipated and the need to administer barbiturate for brain protection is planned, one might consider using an agent other than thiopental for induction so that the total barbiturate dose is lessened and emergence facilitated.

In patients receiving antiepileptic medications, the half-life of muscle relaxants is shortened significantly because of a more rapid metabolism and increased volume of distribution. Atracurium or cisatracurium, with their alternate routes of metabolism, can be helpful in these patients [62] because their duration of action is more predictable in the presence of anticonvulsants. Atracurium administration is known to release histamine, however, with a potentially unfavorable effect on hemodynamic control. Laudanosine, a metabolite of atracurium, is a central nervous system stimulant and enhances stimulation-evoked release of norepinephrine [63], but the clinical importance of these effects is not clear.

Pinning the head in a Mayfield surgical frame is associated with a high sympathetic discharge, systemic hypertension, and potential aneurysm rupture. A bolus of opioids, such as sufentanil, 0.8 µg/kg, or fentanyl, 4.5 µg/kg [64], and scalp infiltration with a local anesthetic attenuates the hemodynamic changes during head pinning [65]. A bolus dose of IV anesthetics, such as propofol, immediately before skull pinning can also be used for this purpose. Scalp infiltration with local anesthetics may also decrease early postoperative pain [66].

Opioids limit the need for higher-dose volatile anesthetics [67] and may be useful in avoiding cerebral vasodilation and increased CBF. With their minimum alveolar concentration-sparing effect opioids are useful adjuncts for blood pressure control during aneurysm surgery. During maintenance of anesthesia opioids can be administered as intermittent boluses or by continuous infusion. If rapid emergence is desired to perform an early neurologic examination, a short-acting agent like remifentanil should be considered [68]. The short half-life of this agent and the induction of acute opioid tolerance may be associated, however, with severe early postoperative incision pain [69]. When using longer-acting opioids, clinicians are advised to decrease infusion dose early to achieve faster emergence and timely neurologic evaluation. Nitrous oxide is avoided by many neuroanesthesiologists because it can be associated with increased $CMRO_2$, CBF, and ICP, especially if used alone. In patients who have had a recent craniotomy, nitrous oxide can cause expansion of air pockets left from previous craniotomy within the cranium and is better avoided.

Total IV anesthesia affords rapid and predictable titration, swift recovery, and fewer respiratory complications [70]. Usually, total IV anesthesia consists of propofol infusion with an opioid. Propofol also decreases the risk of postoperative nausea [71]. The anesthetic method should be individualized for each patient, however, according to their condition. In patients who are not suffering from increased ICP, a volatile anesthetic that does not increase ICP, such as sevoflurane, is a good alternative to propofol; in a patient with increased ICP, use of propofol that decreases ICP may be a better choice [72], provided CPP can be monitored.

Brain protection

Temporary clips are used in situations where surgical exploration and exposure of the aneurysm carry a high risk of aneurysm rupture. With temporary clip application the risk of intraoperative bleeding from the aneurysm is lower. Temporary clips facilitate aneurysm dissection, excision, and arterial reconstruction [73]. The surgical decision to use temporary clipping should prompt the anesthesia team to consider measures for brain protection, because temporary clipping can cause a period of reversible focal cerebral ischemia.

Multiple methods have been suggested for preserving brain viability during hypoxic periods, although none have proved effective in the setting of temporary ischemia during aneurysm surgery. They include ischemic preconditioning, mild hypothermia, barbiturates, use of preoperative hyperbaric oxygen [74], diazoxide [75], statins, antihypertensives, and even antibiotics. Special attention has been directed toward the ischemic preconditioning action of recombinant human erythropoietin [76]. Although most studies of erythropoietin have investigated its potential for neuronal apoptosis after stroke, preoperative administration of erythropoietin in elective cases might reduce injury from reversible ischemia during temporary clipping for cerebral aneurysm surgery. The Intraoperative Hypothermia For Aneurysm Surgery Trial showed that short-duration intraoperative hypothermia did not improve 3-month neurologic outcome after craniotomy for good-grade patients with aneurysmal SAH [77]. Most agree that fever worsens outcome after SAH [78], however, and avoid and treat hyperthermia aggressively. Some avoid active heating unless the temperature decreases to less than 34°C, but actively normalize body temperature toward the end of the surgical procedure. Hypothermia can slow emergence by decreasing metabolism of medications used for anesthesia. It may also result in shivering with increased oxygen demand. Hypothermia is also associated with arrhythmias and cardiac ischemia, decreased platelet activity, prolonged coagulation, and increased infection rate. Hyperglycemia also has a deleterious effect on recovery from ischemic brain injury [79]. The prophylactic use of calcium antagonists like nimodipine in patients with SAH reduces the risk of brain damage [80]. The efficacy of magnesium in preventing delayed ischemic neurologic deficits in patients with SAH seems to be comparable with nimodipine [81]. There is no clear-cut standard of practice, however, for magnesium loading in IA surgery. Some in vitro and in vivo studies show lidocaine to be neuroprotective [82,83], possibly as a result of its ability to block Na^+ channels, which is important in the ischemic cascade of cell death.

Communication between the surgeon and anesthesiologist about timing of application and release of the temporary clip (ie, a clip on a cerebral artery as opposed to the aneurysm itself) is one of the most important factors in achieving optimal oxygenation and perfusion of the brain during this critical period. If temporary clips are used before placement of the permanent aneurysm clip, the anesthesiologist can decrease the $CMRO_2$ by giving a bolus of IV anesthetic (eg, thiopental) while blood pressure is maintained. If electroencephalography is monitored, barbiturate dosing can be titrated to achieve burst-suppression, although this end point is controversial. A moderate decrease in blood pressure can help the surgeon manipulate the artery for placement of the temporary clip. After temporary clip placement, however, a higher blood pressure is needed to promote collateral perfusion to the ischemic area. Duration of temporary clipping may vary. In prolonged cases, brain protective measures should be repeated, although there are no universally accepted guidelines about dosing and timing.

Postclip placement and emergence

After placement of the permanent clip and removal of the temporary clip a normal blood pressure is desired; however, occasionally the clip may require repositioning. Further, some surgeons may wish to "test" clip placement and request a brief period of hypertension to mimic levels expected to occur during emergence. Confirmation of correct clip placement may be done by applying Doppler ultrasound directly to the feeding vessels and the aneurysm itself. An adequate flow should be seen proximal and distal to the aneurysm, but not inside the aneurysm. In some institutions intraoperative angiography is used to assess for correct clip placement.

After surgical closure, decisions on emergence and final destination should be based on preoperative status, operative course, hemodynamic stability, and whether the patient can meet extubation criteria. The surgical team is always appreciative of a timely and smooth (ie, good blood pressure control and minimum of coughing) emergence so that an immediate postoperative neurologic examination can be performed. IV lidocaine (1 mg/kg) can help decrease the cough reflex temporarily, so that increases in ICP are minimized.

Many factors can delay emergence. A systematic method to explore the differential diagnosis of delayed emergence promotes timely diagnosis and treatment. First, adequate oxygenation and ventilation should be confirmed. The patient should have stable hemodynamics and normothermic body temperature. The anesthetic record should be reviewed for the medications used and adequate reversal from muscle relaxants confirmed. Anticonvulsive medication can cause depression in mental status and a slower emergence. Pharmacologic methods of brain protection, such as the administration of barbiturates, can also delay emergence. If depressed mental status or unexpected and new focal neurologic changes are seen, the surgical team may require a brain CT or MRI scan to investigate the possibility of a new stroke or intracranial bleed. Transportation to the radiology suite should be accomplished with close hemodynamic and ventilatory monitoring [84]. During transportation the anesthesia team should have adequate medications and equipment for emergency intubation. In patients who are being transported intubated, adequate sedation should be provided to decrease the stimulant effect of the endotracheal tube, which can result in inadvertent hypertension or straining. If there is a clinical suspicion of cerebral hypoperfusion, however, blood pressure may need to be elevated until definitive diagnosis is achieved. Once the patient is extubated, opioids should be titrated carefully to avoid hypoventilation from overdosing. Postoperative nausea and vomiting is common after craniotomy, especially after infratentorial surgery [85]. Although prophylactic administration of 5HT3 receptor antagonists, such as ondansetron, reduces the risk of vomiting, it does not have a significant effect on nausea [86]. It is essential to initiate timely communication with the physician and nursing team at the final destination (postanesthesia care or intensive care unit) about the patient's condition, ongoing therapy, and postoperative needs.

Arteriovenous malformations

Many of the anesthetic issues involved in the surgical clipping of IA are also applicable to surgery for AVM. The principle is to provide the brain with adequate perfusion and oxygenation. In AVMs, however, the normal physiology of artery-capillary-vein flow is altered causing an abnormal blood supply to brain. Knowledge of AVM pathophysiology is important in designing the anesthetic plan for these patients.

Cerebral AVMs are a tangle of thin-walled vessels called "nidus" that connect the high-pressure arterial circulation to the low-pressure venous system bypassing the normal capillary network (Fig. 3). Some patients have one or more aneurysms inside the AVM (Fig. 4). The etiology of AVM is thought to be congenital. Only about 12% are symptomatic, with bleeding as the most common form of presentation. Bleeding from AVM is intraparenchymal or intraventricular, unlike IA, which presents as SAH. Seizures, headache, and focal neurologic signs are alternate presentations. These symptoms result from brain ischemia (caused by AVM-induced steal phenomenon) or raised ICP (caused by venous engorgement or bleeding). An increase in pressure on the arterial side or any blockage of venous drainage can increase the risk of bleeding [87].

Treatment is directed toward prevention of hemorrhage and treatment of neurologic deficits or intractable seizures. Treatment methods include

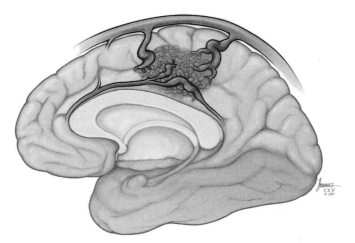

Fig. 3. Schematic view of an AVM showing a tangle of thin-walled vessels connecting the arteries to the venous system. (*Reprinted* with permission of the Cleveland Clinic Foundation.)

endovascular embolization, radiosurgery, and surgical excision. The choice of treatment modality depends on size, location, and pattern of venous drainage and age and medical condition of the patient. Spetzler and Martin [88] have introduced a grading system to help in decision making for the treatment of intracranial AVMs. In most instances embolization is

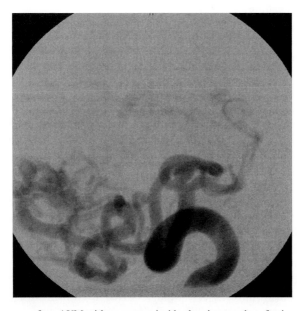

Fig. 4. Angiogram of an AVM with aneurysm inside showing tangles of veins connecting the arterial supply to the venous drainage (*Courtesy of* Raymond Turner, MD, Cleveland, OH).

performed before surgical excision to prevent excessive surgical bleeding, but sometimes embolization can be curative [89].

There are two major physiologic effects of an AVM. The low-pressure venous side provides a rapid outflow tract for the high-pressure arterial system. Instead of perfusing the adjacent brain tissue, arterial blood is shunted through the AVM resulting in a typical steal phenomenon. This in turn results in arterial hypotension in nearby regions. The degree of hypotension is below the range of normal autoregulation [90]. Because there is a preserved response to CO_2, it is believed that autoregulation still remains and its curve shifted to the left [91], consistent with adaptive changes observed in the presence of chronic hypoxic conditions [92]. Seizures in AVM patients who have not bled can be explained by epileptogenic foci caused by steal-induced hypoxia [91,93]. Focal neurologic deficits have also been attributed to local hypoperfusion, although local mass effect also may play a role [87].

The next important pathophysiologic characteristic of AVM is the occasional development of diffuse bleeding and brain swelling during the surgical procedure or postoperatively. The most accepted mechanism for this complication is referred to as "normal perfusion pressure breakthrough." Supporters of this mechanism agree that elimination of the arteriovenous shunt causes a redistribution of parenchymal blood flow to vasculature not accustomed to high pressure [94]. Another theory, the occlusive hyperemia theory by Al-Rodhan and colleagues [95], attributes brain swelling to the occlusion of the draining veins during surgery, which is thought to compromise normal venous drainage adjacent to the AVM, in turn resulting in vascular congestion and swelling.

Whatever the reason, excessive bleeding and edema after surgical excision or embolization of an AVM, although rare, can cause serious morbidity or even mortality. To decrease the risk of these complications, preoperative intravascular embolization is usually performed in multiple stages [96], so that a portion of the draining veins is obliterated each time. Recently, a new embolization material named Onyx (a mixture of ethylene-vinyl alcohol copolymer, dimethyl sulfoxide, and micronized tantalum) has been successfully used [97]. The anesthesiologist should know that use of this agent can cause a characteristic odor in a patient's breath. Patients may experience nausea and distress from this smell after emergence.

The most important anesthetic consideration in surgical AVM resection is attentiveness to treating excessive blood loss and cerebral edema. Adequate vascular access and timely availability of blood are essential, as is monitoring direct arterial pressure. The authors use a central line for large AVMs when substantial blood loss and aggressive fluid replacement are expected. Central access is also useful if vasoactive or vasodilator infusions are needed during the surgery or postoperatively. Jugular bulb venous oxygen saturation monitoring has been reported useful in both embolization [98] and surgical excision [99] of AVMs. Katayama and colleagues [98] reported the effectiveness of this monitoring method as a measure of shunt flow and real-time information about the progress of embolization. Because presence of the AVM causes higher venous oxygenation, elimination of abnormal arteriovenous fistulas during embolization is associated with progressive decreases in jugular venous oxygen saturation.

Brain relaxation is crucial for safe surgical dissection to proceed. This is accomplished by implementing moderate hypocapnia ($Paco_2$ 25–30 mm Hg); elevating the head position; adding diuretics and mannitol; draining spinal fluid; and avoiding cerebral vasodilators.

Unlike elsewhere in the body where oncotic pressure is the determinant of fluid shift between interstitial and intravascular space, in the brain osmotic pressure determines fluid movement across the blood-brain barrier, which is impermeable to electrolytes. Isosmolar or slightly hyperosmolar (normal saline) fluid is preferred in brain surgery to avoid movement of free water across the blood-brain barrier into brain cells. Because hyperglycemia can exacerbate cerebral injury, glucose-containing fluids should be restricted to patients with hypoglycemia. Perioperative steroids can increase the blood glucose level and make glycemic control more difficult. Hypoglycemia should be avoided through frequent monitoring of blood glucose concentration if insulin is administered. It is common practice to keep serum glucose level below 180 to 200 mg/dL.

During AVM resection the surgeon might need to place temporary clips on feeder arteries to visualize bleeding. Tight control of blood pressure can help the operator identify and control arterial bleeding. To accomplish this, short-acting agents, such as nitroprusside or esmolol, should be considered. The theoretic risk of vasodilator-induced steal is outweighed by benefits of blood pressure control on vasogenic edema and risk of bleeding. There may be a need to continue induced hypotension in the postoperative period to decrease the risk of brain edema from normal perfusion pressure breakthrough. There is no literature, however, to support a specific formula for determining ideal blood pressure values during the postoperative period. If prolonged blood pressure control is needed, the dose of nitroprusside needs to be limited to prevent cyanide toxicity.

Toward the end of the procedure and during surgical hemostasis the surgeon might request that blood pressure be raised to confirm adequacy of hemostasis. Intraoperative or immediate postoperative angiography may be performed to assess completeness of AVM resection. Similar to IA surgery, a smooth emergence is desirable to decrease risk of bleeding or cerebral edema. Furthermore, the decision to extubate should be individualized. If normal perfusion pressure breakthrough is suspected or continued mechanical ventilation is needed, close hemodynamic monitoring is required in the immediate postoperative period including patient transport. Any suspected intracranial pathology should trigger an immediate CT of the head. If continuous mechanical ventilation is required (eg, ongoing cerebral edema from normal perfusion pressure breakthrough), efforts should be directed toward improving patient tolerance of the endotracheal tube. Sedation with dexmedetomidine has been used effectively to attenuate tachycardia and plasma norepinephrine concentrations [100].

Extracranial-to-intracranial arterial bypass

During the 1970s and 1980s, extracranial-to-intracranial bypass surgery was common for treatment of intracranial carotid disease. It was abandoned, however, when a large trial showed no benefit from the procedure [101,102]. Recently, however, it has been suggested that this surgery can be beneficial in certain patients. Indications for extracranial-to-intracranial bypass presently include sacrifice of a large vessel planned as part of another surgical procedure (eg, excision of a large intracranial tumor) and flow augmentation for ongoing cerebral ischemia (eg, in moyamoya disease) [103]. This surgery is currently being re-evaluated in the ongoing Carotid Occlusion Surgery Study [104] and the Japanese Extracranial to Intracranial Bypass Trial [105].

In moyamoya disease (Fig. 5), where there is a progressive stenosis and occlusion of the supraclinoid ICA and its branches, several surgical techniques have been suggested for creating an extracranial-to-intracranial bypass. In the pediatric population, the procedure involves placing the superior temporal artery (STA), the dura, and the temporalis muscles on the brain surface to initiate collateralization of vessels from these structures to the brain. This procedure is referred to as "encephaloduroarteriomyosynangiosis." In adults

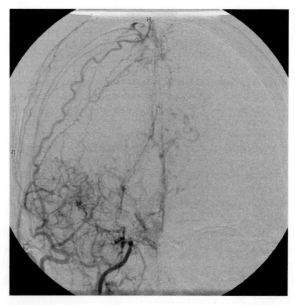

Fig. 5. Angiogram of moyamoya disease showing sparse vascular supply (*Courtesy of* Peter Rasmussen, MD, Cleveland, OH).

the STA is mobilized, rerouted intracranially, and connected end-to-side to the MCA.

Anesthetic management centers on the need to maintain adequate collateral perfusion of the brain at risk. A sudden decrease in blood pressure during induction can compromise perfusion to pressure-dependant regions in the brain. A preinduction arterial line is extremely helpful to identify hypotension quickly and initiate treatment. Hyperventilation should be avoided to decrease intracranial arterial constriction and subsequent ischemia. Although a large amount of blood loss is not expected in this procedure, good venous access is needed for volume therapy and transfusion in cases of incidentally excessive blood loss to ensure adequate cerebral perfusion. As with other intracranial vascular surgeries, inotropic agents should be available to manipulate blood pressure when temporary clips are placed during the STA-MCA anastomosis. Brain-protective measures mentioned should be considered because a period of potential local cerebral ischemia exists during the time when STA-MCA anastomosis is being established.

References

[1] Klementavicius R, Nemoto EM, Yonas H. The Q10 ratio for basal cerebral metabolic rate for oxygen in rats. J Neurosurg 1996;85:482–7.

[2] Kuroda Y, Murakami M, Tsuruta J, et al. Preservation of the ration of cerebral blood flow/metabolic rate for oxygen during prolonged anesthesia with isoflurane, sevoflurane, and halothane in humans. Anesthesiology 1996;84:555–61.

[3] Chan KH, Dearden NM, Miller JD, et al. Multimodality monitoring as a guide to treatment of intracranial hypertension after severe brain injury. Neurosurgery 1993;32:547–52.

[4] Tenjin H, Hirakawa K, Mizukawa N, et al. Dysautoregulation in patients with ruptured aneurysms: cerebral blood flow measurements obtained during surgery by a temperature-controlled thermoelectrical method. Neurosurgery 1988;23:705–9.

[5] Voldby B, Enevoldsen EM, Jensen FT. Cerebrovascular reactivity in patients with ruptured intracranial aneurysms. J Neurosurg 1985;62:59–67.

[6] Rinkel GJ, Djibuti M, Algra A, et al. Prevalence and risk of rupture of intracranial aneurysms: a systematic review. Stroke 1998;29:251–6.

[7] van Gijn J, Rinkel GJ. Subarachnoid haemorrhage: diagnosis, causes and management. Brain 2001;124:249–78.

[8] Linn FH, Rinkel GJ, Algra A, et al. Headache characteristics in subarachnoid haemorrhage and benign thunderclap headache. J Neurol Neurosurg Psychiatr 1998;65:791–3.

[9] Wardlaw JM, White PM. The detection and management of unruptured intracranial aneurysms. Brain 2000;123(Pt 2):205–21.

[10] Wermer MJ, Greebe P, Algra A, et al. Incidence of recurrent subarachnoid hemorrhage after clipping for ruptured intracranial aneurysms. Stroke 2005;36:2394–9.

[11] Juvela S. Risk factors for multiple intracranial aneurysms. Stroke 2000;31:392–7.

[12] Schievink WI, Parisi JE, Piepgras DG. Familial intracranial aneurysms: an autopsy study. Neurosurgery 1997;41:1247–51.

[13] Markus HS, Alberts MJ. Update on genetics of stroke and cerebrovascular disease 2005. Stroke 2006;37:288–90.

[14] Teasdale GM, Wardlaw JM, White PM, et al. The familial risk of subarachnoid haemorrhage. Brain 2005;128:1677–85.

[15] Schievink WI, Parisi JE, Piepgras DG, et al. Intracranial aneurysms in Marfan's syndrome: an autopsy study. Neurosurgery 1997;41:866–70.

[16] Brisman JL, Song JK, Newell DW. Cerebral aneurysms. N Engl J Med 2006;355:928–39.

[17] Rinkel GJ. Intracranial aneurysm screening: indications and advice for practice. Lancet Neurol 2005;4:122–8.

[18] Butler WE, Barker FG, Crowell RM. Patients with polycystic kidney disease would benefit from routine magnetic resonance angiographic screening for intracerebral aneurysms: a decision analysis. Neurosurgery 1996;38:506–15.

[19] Schievink WI. Genetics of intracranial aneurysms. Neurosurgery 1997;40:651–62.

[20] Unruptured intracranial aneurysms: risk of rupture and risks of surgical intervention. International study of unruptured intracranial aneurysms investigators. N Engl J Med 1998;339:1725–33.

[21] Schievink WI. Intracranial aneurysms. N Engl J Med 1997;336:28–40.

[22] Phillips LH, Whisnant JP, O'Fallon WM, et al. The unchanging pattern of subarachnoid hemorrhage in a community. Neurology 1980;30:1034–40.

[23] Juvela S, Hillbom M, Numminen H, et al. Cigarette smoking and alcohol consumption as risk factors for aneurysmal subarachnoid hemorrhage. Stroke 1993;24:639–46.

[24] Toftdahl DB, Torp-Pedersen C, Engel UH, et al. Hypertension and left ventricular hypertrophy in patients with spontaneous subarachnoid hemorrhage. Neurosurgery 1995;37: 235–9.

[25] Donahue RP, Abbott RD, Reed DM, et al. Alcohol and hemorrhagic stroke. The Honolulu Heart Program. JAMA 1986;255:2311–4.

[26] Machiel PC, Algra A, Velthuis BK, et al. Relation between size of aneurysms and risk of rebleeding in patients with subarachnoid haemorrhage. Acta Neurochir (Wien.) 2006; 148:1277–80.

[27] Ruigrok YM, Rinkel GJ, Wijmenga C. Genetics of intracranial aneurysms. Lancet Neurol 2005;4:179–89.

[28] Schievink WI, Karemaker JM, Hageman LM, et al. Circumstances surrounding aneurysmal subarachnoid hemorrhage. Surg Neurol 1989;32:266–72.

[29] Juvela S, Porras M, Poussa K. Natural history of unruptured intracranial aneurysms: probability and risk factors for aneurysm rupture. Neurosurg Focus 2000;8(5):preview1.

[30] Raps EC, Rogers JD, Galetta SL, et al. The clinical spectrum of unruptured intracranial aneurysms. Arch Neurol 1993;50:265–8.

[31] Przelomski MM, Fisher M, Davidson RI, et al. Unruptured intracranial aneurysm and transient focal cerebral ischemia: a follow-up study. Neurology 1986;36:584–7.

[32] Teasdale GM, Drake CG, Hunt W, et al. A universal subarachnoid hemorrhage scale: report of a committee of the World Federation of Neurosurgical Societies. J Neurol Neurosurg Psychiatr 1988;51:1457.

[33] Britz GW. Clipping or coiling of cerebral aneurysms. Neurosurg Clin N Am 2005;16: 475–85, v.

[34] Mitchell P, Gholkar A, Vindlacheruvu RR, et al. Unruptured intracranial aneurysms: benign curiosity or ticking bomb? Lancet Neurol 2004;3:85–92.

[35] Koebbe CJ, Veznedaroglu E, Jabbour P, et al. Endovascular management of intracranial aneurysms: current experience and future advances. Neurosurgery 2006;59: S93–102.

[36] Howington JU, Kutz SC, Wilding GE, et al. Cocaine use as a predictor of outcome in aneurysmal subarachnoid hemorrhage. J Neurosurg 2003;99:271–5.

[37] de Gray LC, Matta BF. The health economics of blood use in cerebrovascular aneurysm surgery: the experience of a UK centre. Eur J Anaesthesiol 2005;22:925–8.

[38] Sherlock M, O'Sullivan E, Agha A, et al. The incidence and pathophysiology of hyponatraemia after subarachnoid haemorrhage. Clin Endocrinol (Oxf) 2006;64:250–4.

[39] Sommargren CE. Electrocardiographic abnormalities in patients with subarachnoid hemorrhage. Am J Crit Care 2002;11:48–56.

[40] Varelas PN, Spanaki M. Management of seizures in the critically ill. Neurologist 2006;12: 127–39.

[41] Foy PM, Chadwick DW, Rajgopalan N, et al. Do prophylactic anticonvulsant drugs alter the pattern of seizures after craniotomy? J Neurol Neurosurg Psychiatr 1992;55: 753–7.

[42] Butzkueven H, Evans AH, Pitman A, et al. Onset seizures independently predict poor outcome after subarachnoid hemorrhage. Neurology 2000;55:1315–20.

[43] Pinto AN, Canhao P, Ferro JM. Seizures at the onset of subarachnoid haemorrhage. J Neurol 1996;243:161–4.

[44] Kittner SJ, Stern BJ, Feeser BR, et al. Pregnancy and the risk of stroke. N Engl J Med 1996; 335:768–74.

[45] Selo-Ojeme DO, Marshman LA, Ikomi A, et al. Aneurysmal subarachnoid haemorrhage in pregnancy. Eur J Obstet Gynecol Reprod Biol 2004;116:131–43.

[46] Kuczkowski KM. The safety of anaesthetics in pregnant women. Expert Opin Drug Saf 2006;5:251–64.

[47] Ni MR, O'Gorman DA. Anesthesia in pregnant patients for nonobstetric surgery. J Clin Anesth 2006;18:60–6.

[48] Klimo P Jr, Schmidt RH. Computed tomography grading schemes used to predict cerebral vasospasm after aneurysmal subarachnoid hemorrhage: a historical review. Neurosurg Focus 2006;21:e5.

[49] Fisher CM, Kistler JP, Davis JM. Relation of cerebral vasospasm to subarachnoid hemorrhage visualized by computerized tomographic scanning. Neurosurgery 1980;6: 1–9.

[50] Wijdicks E. Aneurysmal subarachnoid hemorrhage. The clinical practice of critical care neurology. 2nd edition. Oxford (NY): Oxford University Press; 2003. p. 185–220.

[51] Ohkuma H, Tsurutani H, Suzuki S. Incidence and significance of early aneurysmal rebleeding before neurosurgical or neurological management. Stroke 2001;32:1176–80.

[52] Rose JC, Mayer SA. Optimizing blood pressure in neurological emergencies. Neurocrit Care 2004;1:287–99.

[53] Naidech AM, Janjua N, Kreiter KT, et al. Predictors and impact of aneurysm rebleeding after subarachnoid hemorrhage. Arch Neurol 2005;62:410–6.

[54] Szem JW, Hydo LJ, Fischer E, et al. High-risk intrahospital transport of critically ill patients: safety and outcome of the necessary road trip. Crit Care Med 1995;23: 1660–6.

[55] Gunn HC, Matta BF, Lam AM, et al. Accuracy of continuous jugular bulb venous oximetry during intracranial surgery. J Neurosurg Anesthesiol 1995;7:174–7.

[56] Mayberg TS, Lam AM. Jugular bulb oximetry for the monitoring of cerebral blood flow and metabolism. Neurosurg Clin N Am 1996;7:755–65.

[57] Rozet I, Newell DW, Lam AM. Intraoperative jugular bulb desaturation during acute aneurysmal rupture. Can J Anaesth 2006;53:97–100.

[58] Cold GE, Eskesen V, Eriksen H, et al. CBF and CMRO2 during continuous etomidate infusion supplemented with N2O and fentanyl in patients with supratentorial cerebral tumour: a dose-response study. Acta Anaesthesiol Scand 1985;29:490–4.

[59] Allolio B, Dorr H, Stuttmann R, et al. Effect of a single bolus of etomidate upon eight major corticosteroid hormones and plasma ACTH. Clin Endocrinol (Oxf) 1985;22:281–6.

[60] Reves JG, Glass PSA, Lubarsky DA, et al. Intravenous nonopioid anesthetics. In: Miller RD, editor. Miller's anesthesia. 6th edition. Philadelphia: Elsevier Churchill Livingston; 2005. p. 317–61.

[61] Herregods L, Verbeke J, Rolly G, et al. Effect of propofol on elevated intracranial pressure: preliminary results. Anaesthesia 1988;43(Suppl):107–9.

[62] Ornstein E, Matteo RS, Schwartz AE, et al. The effect of phenytoin on the magnitude and duration of neuromuscular block following atracurium or vecuronium. Anesthesiology 1987;67:191–6.

[63] Kinjo M, Nagashima H, Vizi ES. Effect of atracurium and laudanosine on the release of 3H-noradrenaline. Br J Anaesth 1989;62:683–90.

[64] Jamali S, Archer D, Ravussin P, et al. The effect of skull-pin insertion on cerebrospinal fluid pressure and cerebral perfusion pressure: influence of sufentanil and fentanyl. Anesth Analg 1997;84:1292–6.

[65] Doblar DD, Lim YC, Baykan N, et al. A comparison of alfentanil, esmolol, lidocaine, and thiopental sodium on the hemodynamic response to insertion of headrest skull pins. J Clin Anesth 1996;8:31–5.

[66] Bloomfield EL, Schubert A, Secic M, et al. The influence of scalp infiltration with bupivacaine on hemodynamics and postoperative pain in adult patients undergoing craniotomy. Anesth Analg 1998;87:579–82.

[67] Glass PS, Gan TJ, Howell S, et al. Drug interactions: volatile anesthetics and opioids. J Clin Anesth 1997;9:18S–22S.

[68] Coles JP, Leary TS, Monteiro JN, et al. Propofol anesthesia for craniotomy: a double-blind comparison of remifentanil, alfentanil, and fentanyl. J Neurosurg Anesthesiol 2000;12: 15–20.

[69] Bilotta F, Caramia R, Paoloni FP, et al. Early postoperative cognitive recovery after remifentanil-propofol or sufentanil-propofol anaesthesia for supratentorial craniotomy: a randomized trial. Eur J Anaesthesiol 2007;24:122–7.

[70] Wong AY, O'Regan AM, Irwin MG. Total intravenous anaesthesia with propofol and remifentanil for elective neurosurgical procedures: an audit of early postoperative complications. Eur J Anaesthesiol 2006;23:586–90.

[71] Apfel CC, Stoecklein K, Lipfert P. PONV: a problem of inhalational anaesthesia? Best Pract Res Clin Anaesthesiol 2005;19:485–500.

[72] Engelhard K, Werner C. Inhalational or intravenous anesthetics for craniotomies? Pro inhalational. Curr Opin Anaesthesiol 2006;19:504–8.

[73] Taylor CL, Selman WR. Temporary vascular occlusion during cerebral aneurysm surgery. Neurosurg Clin N Am 1998;9:673–9.

[74] Dong H, Xiong L, Zhu Z, et al. Preconditioning with hyperbaric oxygen and hyperoxia induces tolerance against spinal cord ischemia in rabbits. Anesthesiology 2002;96: 907–12.

[75] Liu RG, Wang WJ, Song N, et al. Diazoxide preconditioning alleviates apoptosis of hippocampal neurons induced by anoxia-reoxygenation in vitro through up-regulation of Bcl-2/Bax protein ratio. Sheng Li Xue Bao 2006;58:345–50.

[76] Sharples EJ, Thiemermann C, Yaqoob MM. Novel applications of recombinant erythropoietin. Curr Opin Pharmacol 2006;6:184–9.

[77] Todd MM, Hindman BJ, Clarke WR, et al. Mild intraoperative hypothermia during surgery for intracranial aneurysm. N Engl J Med 2005;352:135–45.

[78] Wartenberg KE, Schmidt JM, Claassen J, et al. Impact of medical complications on outcome after subarachnoid hemorrhage. Crit Care Med 2006;34:617–23.

[79] Kagansky N, Levy S, Knobler H. The role of hyperglycemia in acute stroke. Arch Neurol 2001;58:1209–12.

[80] Barker FG, Ogilvy CS. Efficacy of prophylactic nimodipine for delayed ischemic deficit after subarachnoid hemorrhage: a metaanalysis. J Neurosurg 1996;84:405–14.

[81] Schmid-Elsaesser R, Kunz M, Zausinger S, et al. Intravenous magnesium versus nimodipine in the treatment of patients with aneurysmal subarachnoid hemorrhage: a randomized study. Neurosurgery 2006;58:1054–65.

[82] Lei B, Popp S, Capuano-Waters C, et al. Effects of delayed administration of low-dose lidocaine on transient focal cerebral ischemia in rats. Anesthesiology 2002;97:1534–40.

[83] Niiyama S, Tanaka E, Tsuji S, et al. Neuroprotective mechanisms of lidocaine against in vitro ischemic insult of the rat hippocampal CA1 pyramidal neurons. Neurosci Res 2005; 53:271–8.

[84] Waydhas C. Intrahospital transport of critically ill patients. Crit Care 1999;3:R83–9.

[85] Leslie K, Williams DL. Postoperative pain, nausea and vomiting in neurosurgical patients. Curr Opin Anaesthesiol 2005;18:461–5.

[86] Neufeld SM, Newburn-Cook CV. The efficacy of 5-HT3 receptor antagonists for the prevention of postoperative nausea and vomiting after craniotomy: a meta-analysis. J Neurosurg Anesthesiol 2007;19:10–7.

[87] Hashimoto T, Young WL. Anesthesia-related considerations for cerebral arteriovenous malformations. Neurosurg Focus 2001;11:e5.

[88] Spetzler RF, Martin NA. A proposed grading system for arteriovenous malformations. J Neurosurg 1986;65:476–83.

[89] Clatterbuck RE, Hsu FP, Spetzler RF. Supratentorial arteriovenous malformations. Neurosurgery 2005;57:164–7.

[90] Fogarty-Mack P, Pile-Spellman J, Hacein-Bey L, et al. The effect of arteriovenous malformations on the distribution of intracerebral arterial pressures. AJNR Am J Neuroradiol 1996;17:1443–9.

[91] Young WL, Prohovnik I, Ornstein E, et al. The effect of arteriovenous malformation resection on cerebrovascular reactivity to carbon dioxide. Neurosurgery 1990;27:257–66.

[92] Kader A, Young WL. The effects of intracranial arteriovenous malformations on cerebral hemodynamics. Neurosurg Clin N Am 1996;7:767–81.

[93] Turjman F, Massoud TF, Sayre JW, et al. Epilepsy associated with cerebral arteriovenous malformations: a multivariate analysis of angioarchitectural characteristics. AJNR Am J Neuroradiol 1995;16:345–50.

[94] Spetzler RF, Wilson CB, Weinstein P, et al. Normal perfusion pressure breakthrough theory. Clin Neurosurg 1978;25:651–72.

[95] al Rodhan NR, Sundt TM Jr, Piepgras DG, et al. Occlusive hyperemia: a theory for the hemodynamic complications following resection of intracerebral arteriovenous malformations. J Neurosurg 1993;78:167–75.

[96] Taylor CL, Dutton K, Rappard G, et al. Complications of preoperative embolization of cerebral arteriovenous malformations. J Neurosurg 2004;100:810–2.

[97] Song DL, Leng B, Zhou LF, et al. Onyx in treatment of large and giant cerebral aneurysms and arteriovenous malformations. Chin Med J (Engl) 2004;117:1869–72.

[98] Katayama Y, Tsubokawa T, Hirayama T, et al. Continuous monitoring of jugular bulb oxygen saturation as a measure of the shunt flow of cerebral arteriovenous malformations. J Neurosurg 1994;80:826–33.

[99] Wilder-Smith OH, Fransen P, de Tribolet N, et al. Jugular venous bulb oxygen saturation monitoring in arteriovenous malformation surgery. J Neurosurg Anesthesiol 1997;9:162–5.

[100] Talke P, Chen R, Thomas B, et al. The hemodynamic and adrenergic effects of perioperative dexmedetomidine infusion after vascular surgery. Anesth Analg 2000;90:834–9.

[101] Failure of extracranial-intracranial arterial bypass to reduce the risk of ischemic stroke: results of an international randomized trial. The EC/IC bypass study group. N Engl J Med 1985;313:1191–200.

[102] Grubb RL Jr. Extracranial-intracranial arterial bypass for treatment of occlusion of the internal carotid artery. Curr Neurol Neurosci Rep 2004;4:23–30.

[103] Amin-Hanjani S, Charbel FT. Is extracranial-intracranial bypass surgery effective in certain patients? Neurol Clin 2006;24:729–43.

[104] Grubb RL Jr, Powers WJ, Derdeyn CP, et al. The Carotid Occlusion Surgery Study. Neurosurg Focus 2003;14(3):article 9.

[105] Mizumura S, Nakagawara J, Takahashi M, et al. Three-dimensional display in staging hemodynamic brain ischemia for JET study: objective evaluation using SEE analysis and 3D-SSP display. Ann Nucl Med 2004;18:13–21.

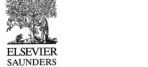

ANESTHESIOLOGY
CLINICS

Anesthesiology Clin
25 (2007) 465–481

Perioperative Management of Pediatric Patients with Craniosynostosis

Jeffrey L. Koh, MD, MBA[a,b,*], Heike Gries, MD, PhD[a]

[a]*Department of Anesthesiology and Perioperative Medicine, Oregon Health and Sciences University, 3181 SW Sam Jackson Park Road, Portland, OR 97201, USA*
[b]*Division of Pediatric Anesthesia and Pain Management, Doernbecher Children's Hospital, Portland, OR, USA*

The growth of an infant's skull is intimately intertwined with the growth of the infant's brain. At birth, a term newborn will have nearly 40% of his adult brain size and the nine-year-old brain and skull will be approximately 90% of its adult size [1]. A normal newborn skull accommodates this rapid growth via the presence of unfused sutures and open fontanelles. The skull has two sets of paired sutures, the coronal sutures and the lamboid sutures. There are also two single sutures, the metopic suture and the sagittal suture (Fig. 1). Premature closure of these sutures results in craniosynostosis and can result in a dysmorphic appearance if left untreated. Impaired brain growth and cognitive development may be another untoward effect of uncorrected craniosynostosis.

Although reported frequency varies, the incidence of craniosynostosis is believed to be approximately 0.6 per 1000 births [2] and the exact sutures involved differ somewhat between patients. There are a variety of ways that these different presentations can be categorized. One of the most common is nonsyndromic versus syndromic. Nonsyndromic craniosynostosis typically affects only one suture and is not associated with any other syndrome. The most common form of craniosynostosis (approximately 50% of cases) affects only the sagittal suture [1,3]. This form is also called scaphocephaly. The next most common is fusion of the coronal suture or plagiocephaly. This form accounts for approximately 20% of craniosynostosis. Finally, fusion of the metopic suture accounts for 10% of cases and is also called trigonocephaly (Fig. 2). Fusion of the lamboid suture has been

* Corresponding author. Department of Anesthesiology and Perioperative Medicine, Oregon Health and Sciences University, 3181 Sam Jackson Park Road, Portland, OR 97239.
E-mail address: kohj@ohsu.ed (J.L. Koh).

1932-2275/07/$ - see front matter © 2007 Elsevier Inc. All rights reserved.
doi:10.1016/j.anclin.2007.05.008 *anesthesiology.theclinics.com*

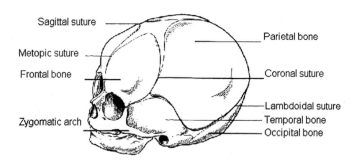

Fig. 1. Cranial Sutures. (*Reprinted from* Deshpande, Kelly, Baker. Anesthesia for Pediatric Plastic Surgery. In: Motoyama EK, Davis PJ, editors. Smith's Anesthesia for Infants and Children. 7th edition. Philadelphia, PA: Mosby; 2006. p. 724; with permission.)

reported but is extremely rare. A familial pattern of nonsyndromic craniosynostosis has been identified and has been shown to be an autosomal dominant disorder. Two to six percent of infants with sagittal synostosis and 8% to 14% of infants with coronal synostosis are familial in nature [1].

Syndromic craniosynostosis accounts for approximately 20% of cases and usually affects two or more sutures. Over 150 syndromes have been identified that can include craniosynostosis as part of their presentation, but the most common are Apert's syndrome and Crouzon's syndrome. Both coronal sutures are usually affected (brachycephaly) in patients with these syndromes. In addition, patients with Apert's or Crouzon's syndrome may have midface hypoplasia and obstructive apnea because of their abnormal airway anatomy, which requires consideration when making plans for airway management.

Although not truly craniosynostosis, deformational plagiocephaly is another form of cranial deformity that is often discussed along with craniosynostosis. In this case, there is no suture fusion that has occurred. Rather, frequent positioning of an infant on their back results in the distinctively misshaped skull. The distinguishing feature of deformational plagiocephaly is the lack of suture fusion and a different pattern of cranial deformation as compared with true lamboid synostosis. Although initially felt to require surgical intervention, surgery is no longer felt to be indicated for this problem.

Other causes of craniosynostosis are much less common and are often termed "secondary" forms. These include metabolic disorders (hypothyroidism), fetal teratogen exposure (phenytoin, valproic acid) and certain forms of mucopolysaccharidosis (Hurler's syndrome). Finally, congenital malformations involving the brain or skull can have associated craniosynostosis.

Researchers examining children with both syndromic and nonsyndromic craniosynostosis have recently identified a possible underlying genetic

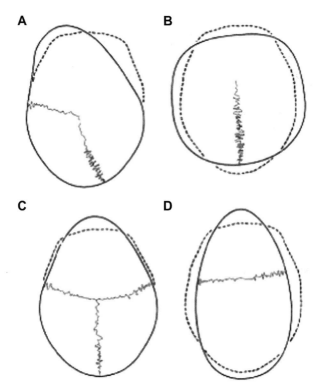

Fig. 2. Deformity patterns due to cransiosynostosis: (*A*) bilateral coronal synostosis, (*B*) unilateral fusion of coronal suture, (*C*) saggital synostosis, (*D*) metopic synostosis. (*Reprinted from* Deshpande, Kelly, Baker. Anesthesia for Pediatric Plastic Surgery. In Motoyama EK, Davis PJ, editors. Smith's Anesthesia for Infants and Children. 7th edition. Philadelphia, PA: Mosby; 2006. p. 724; with permission.)

alteration in some patients. Mutations have been found in genes involved in the osteogenic process of the skull [4]. Although a full discussion is beyond the scope of this article, it is clear that the development of craniosynostosis is part of a complex process that is likely multifactorial in nature.

Craniosynostosis and cognitive function

Early intervention has traditionally been recommended in an effort to maximize the opportunity for normal brain growth and cognitive development. Traditionally, it has been believed that infants with nonsyndromic craniosynostosis had otherwise normal brains and cognitive function that would be negatively affected by the restriction caused with craniosynostosis. There has been a growing amount of research over the past few years that has sought to clarify the influence of craniosynostosis, brain development, and cognitive development.

The largest body of research has attempted to explore the neurodevelopmental status of children with nonsyndromic craniosynostosis, with somewhat varied results. Kapp-Simon [5] reported a longitudinal study, evaluating mental development and learning disorders of infants and young children with single suture craniosynostosis (nonsyndromic). This study found that most of the children had mental development within the normal range for infancy; however, a high rate of learning disorders was identified. Becker and colleagues [6] found that nonsyndromic craniosynostosis was associated with cognitive, speech, and behavioral abnormalities, regardless of which sutures were fused. This study included both patients who had surgical repair and those who did not. Magge and colleagues [7] found that 50% of children with nonsyndromic sagittal craniosynostosis had learning disabilities that affected their reading or spelling. However, similar to the findings of Kapp-Simon, the children in the study group were found to fall in the normal range of intelligence. Panchal and colleagues [8] evaluated the neurodevelopment of infants with single suture craniosynostosis and children with deformational plagiocephaly. Neither group had undergone surgical intervention at the time of the study. Results indicated that both groups demonstrated delay in cognitive and psychomotor development. The investigators suggest that postintervention assessment is required to determine if these delays can be reversed with treatment.

In contrast to the studies described above, Warchausky and colleagues [9] found no difference in cognitive and motor development between children with untreated metopic craniosynostosis and normative data. The severity of synostosis did not seem to influence development negatively. In another study, Da Costa and colleagues [10] used global intellectual evaluations to test intellectual outcomes of children and adolescents with both syndromic and nonsyndromic craniosynostosis. This study found that the children with nonsyndromic craniosynostosis had no intellectual impairment, as compared with normative data. This study also observed that the majority of children with syndromic craniosynostosis were of normal intelligence.

There has been much less work evaluating the potential benefit of surgical intervention on cognitive development in patients with craniosynostosis. Virtanen and colleagues [11] examined the cognitive outcome of children who had undergone surgical repair of scaphocephaly. This study found that the neurocognitive performance of these children did not reach the same level as matched controls on follow up at school age. The investigators also found that a small subgroup of children who were repaired before 1 month of age tended to have better neurocognitive outcome, suggesting early repair may be important to long-term cognitive performance. Cohen and colleagues [12] performed a prospective study seeking to evaluate the effect of surgical intervention on cognitive development for children with nonsyndromic craniosynostosis. This study showed that the study group had mild baseline (preoperative) deficits in both motor and mental development. Improvement in motor function was found on follow up one year after surgery, however mental function remained delayed. There was no correlation between patient age at the time of surgical intervention and outcome. Finally, Gewalli and colleagues [13] evaluated the effect of dynamic cranioplasty repair of sagittal synostosis on cognitive development. They found no difference in pre- and postoutcome measurements.

In summary, it appears that children with nonsyndromic craniosynostosis may suffer from underlying neurodevelopmental deficits that can lead to learning disabilities once school age is reached. Overall intelligence seems to be in the normal range. It is unclear whether the underlying etiology of this cognitive dysfunction is a result of abnormal brain development unrelated to the presence of craniosynostosis, a comorbid condition caused by some of the same factors that cause craniosynostosis, or the impairment of growth of an otherwise normal brain due to the premature fusion of sutures. The impact of surgery is unclear at this point; however, performing a true randomized controlled trial to evaluate the effect of surgery on outcome is difficult to do because of ethical considerations. Therefore, most clinicians recommend repair of craniosynostosis as early as feasible after the diagnosis is made.

Anesthetic management

Preoperative assessment

As with any surgery, preoperative assessment is an extremely important part of the anesthetic care for cranial vault surgery. The basics are the same as any preoperative assessment: evaluating preexisting medical conditions, medication history, allergies, problems with previous anesthetics, family history of problems with anesthetics, and a physical exam. These patients should have had a complete multidisciplinary evaluation by a craniofacial team before surgery and the anesthesiologist should take advantage of this process by reviewing the records and recommendations from this evaluation. In addition, special attention should be directed to signs of increased intracranial pressure, such as visual difficulties, nausea and vomiting, somnolence, or headaches. These findings are unusual in infants presenting with craniosynostosis, but may be seen in older children or in cases with fusion of multiple sutures [3].

Patients with nonsyndromic craniosynostosis are usually otherwise healthy infants. However, patients with syndromic craniosynostosis can have associated anomalies that will need to be considered when planning a safe anesthetic. For instance, patients with Crouzon's syndrome or Apert's syndrome can have very abnormal airway anatomy and may require fiberoptic intubation. In addition, identifying a history of obstructive apnea will be important in planning the postoperative care. A history of congenital heart disease should also be sought, as many syndromes, including Apert's syndrome, can have associated congenital cardiac defects.

Laboratory evaluation usually includes a preoperative hematocrit (Hct), platelet count, and coagulation studies. Appropriate additional laboratory evaluations should be obtained based on the patient's medical history. Probably the most important laboratory evaluation is a type and cross for packed red blood cells. The availability of an appropriate volume of packed red blood cells must be confirmed before surgery is started.

As with any preoperative evaluation, adequate time should be dedicated to addressing parental concerns and questions. The surgical repair of craniosynostosis is a major procedure and the parents deserve whatever reassurances the anesthesia team can provide. The parents should also be fully informed about the likelihood of transfusion, as well as the possibility of postoperative mechanical ventilation. Assistance from a child life specialist is often very helpful in helping parents to understand the process and ensure appropriate communication.

Intraoperative management

Many patients undergoing craniosynostosis repair will be young infants and will not require any premedication. For patients old enough to display separation or situational anxiety, a discussion with the parents about the best way to ease the transition from parents to the operating room may be helpful to both the anesthesiologist and the parents. These children may benefit from premedication, such as oral midazolam, before separation from parents, or a parent present during induction of anesthesia may be preferable. The use of nonpharmacologic interventions, such as video games, has also proven useful. A history of obstructive apnea may limit the option for pharmacologic premedication; however, nonpharmacologic means can still be used. Patients with a potentially difficult airway may also need an intravenous tube (IV) placed before induction. In this case, topical anesthetic creams can be used to decrease pain associated with IV placement.

Monitoring should include standard monitoring (American Society of Anesthesiologists guidelines), as well as blood pressure measurement with an arterial line. Central venous pressure monitoring is not routine, but can be considered should especially large blood loss be anticipated. Venous air embolism has been a reported complication of craniosynostosis repair. Fabrowski and colleagues [14] reported an 83% incidence of venous air embolism in a prospective study of 23 patients undergoing craniosynostosis repair, although most were without hemodynamic symptoms. The investigators recommended routine use of a precordial Doppler to increase the chance of early diagnosis. Careful patient positioning should also be considered to minimize the occurrence of venous air entrainment, as surgical indications allow [15].

Finally, adequate venous access is critical, with two large bore IVs being most common. For an infant less than 6 months old, 22- to 20-gauge catheters are adequate. Central access is not routine, but is used if adequate peripheral access cannot be obtained. Central venous access can also be considered if concern of venous air embolus is high.

There are few studies in the literature evaluating different anesthetic techniques for craniosynostosis repair. One study has reported the safe use of remifentanil during repair [16]. Another compared the use of sevoflurane and remifentanil to isoflurane and remifentanil [17]. Outcome variables in both study groups, including intraoperative physiologic parameters and time to wake up, did not differ significantly. A balanced neurosurgical technique using opioid and inhalation agents is often chosen as the anesthetic of choice. In most circumstances, the real focus of anesthetic clinical care is on management of intraoperative blood loss.

Intraoperative blood loss management

The most challenging part of the anesthetic management for craniosynostosis repair is managing the inevitable blood loss that occurs with these procedures. Management can be especially tricky, given that most of these surgeries are performed on small infants. Even though the majority of patients will be infants who weigh more than 5 kg, the blood volume in these infants is still very limited: only 80 mL/kg. In a retrospective study, Meyer and colleagues [18] found a red cell volume loss of 91 in plus or minus 66% of patient's estimated red blood cell volume during the perioperative period in surgical repair of craniosynostosis. Kearney and colleagues [19] reported a mean blood loss of 24% of the estimated blood volume for sagittal suture repair, 21% for unicoronal, 65% for bicoronal suture repair and 42% for metopic suture repair. Another study reported that 96.3% of their patients received a blood transfusion and concluded that transfusion for craniosynostosis repair is almost unavoidable [20]. Finally, in a retrospective review, Eaton and colleagues [21] found that transfusion rates differed among types of suture repair, but also varied between neurosurgeons and anesthesiologists caring for the patients. Mean intraoperative transfusion in Eaton and colleagues' investigation was 72.1 in plus or minus 55.6% estimated red cell mass.

Blood loss not only varies depending on type of craniosynostosis, but also differs with surgical technique. In general, techniques associated with more bony dissection (and therefore more blood loss) are associated with better cosmetic outcome [22]. The spring-mediated cranioplasty, a newer technique for sagittal craniosynostosis repair, might be an exception. Several investigators have found that spring-mediated cranioplasty required less blood product replacement than cranial vault remodeling and might provide the same cosmetic outcome as cranial vault remodeling [23–25]. However, other studies have shown that complex calvarial vault remodeling provides the better outcome, in comparison to less invasive procedures like synostectomy or strip craniectomy, for sagittal craniosynostosis repair [22,26].

Moreover, accurate assessment and replacement of blood loss in cranial vault repair is difficult. Most blood loss occurs during elevation of the vascular periosteum and a significant percentage is lost on the surgical gowns and drapes. Once the osteotomy is performed, blood loss is usually slow and continuous. Yet another source of bleeding can be from dural sinuses. Bleeding from the sinuses can be dramatic and require an immediate response.

Transfusion guidelines

There are no randomized trials of transfusion algorithms available for pediatric surgical patients, but it has been shown that institutional protocols might decrease the number of transfusions [27]. The American Society of Anesthesiologists Task Force on Blood Component Therapy excluded infants and children from the published practice guidelines in 1996 [28]. Other authorities consider adults and children older than 4 months of age equivalent, despite missing reliable data on perioperative transfusion in this population [29–31]. The British Committee for Standards in Hematology Transfusion [31] stated that for neonates and older children:

- All components other than granulocytes should be leukocyte depleted.
- Blood transfused in the first year of life should be cytomegalovirus seronegative.
- A screen filter (170μ–200μ) or alternative filtration system should be used during transfusion, for all components.
- Red blood cells stored less than 2 or 3 weeks should be used in young children.

Red blood cell transfusion

Red blood cell (RBC) transfusion is rarely indicated when the hemoglobin (Hb) concentration is greater than 10 g/dL and is almost always indicated when it is less than 6 g/dL. For patients more than 4 months of age, transfusion is indicated if the intraoperative blood loss is greater or equal to 15% of the total blood volume, and if the hematocrit is less than 24% in the perioperative period, with signs and symptoms of anemia [29]. Using the formula of desired Hb (g/dL) − actual Hb × weight (kg) × 3, will result in an appropriate volume (usually 10–20 mL RBC/kg).

In the intraoperative setting, it is useful to estimate the maximal allowable blood loss (MABL) by using the formula MABL = EBV (Ho − Hl): Ho, where EBV is estimated total blood volume, Ho is initial Hct and Hl is the lowest acceptable Hct (in percentage). Sometimes red blood cells need to be given before the maximal allowable blood loss is reached: for example, if hemodynamic instability occurs despite adequate volume replacement, or if rapid blood loss occurs [30]. In many institutions, red cell transfusion is begun on incision (before the patient meeting guidelines for transfusion) for cases with a high likelihood for significant blood loss, especially in young infants. This is done by experienced care teams to prevent hemodynamic instability at times when the rate of blood loss is greater than the rate at which blood can be returned to the patient (because of the relative small size of the intravenous catheters). In addition, one might decide to transfuse the whole unit of RBC once the patient is exposed to the unit, thereby minimizing the need to transfuse a second unit postoperatively.

Platelet transfusion

Surgical patients with microvascular bleeding usually require platelet transfusion if the platelet count is less than $50 \times 10^9/L$, and rarely require therapy if it is greater than $100 \times 10^9/L$. The usual therapeutic dose is one platelet concentrate per 10 kg body weight [29,30]. In children under 10 kg bodyweight, 5 mL/kg to 10 mL/kg of a random donor or apheresis unit should result in a rise of platelets of 50 to $100 \times 10^9/L$.

It is useful to use ABO matched platelets, especially in small children, where the plasma volume is relatively large compared with the patient's total blood volume [30].

Fresh frozen plasma

Fresh frozen plasma (FFP) is indicated for correction of microvascular bleeding when prothrombin and partial thromboplastin times are greater than 1.5 times normal, or for correction of microvascular bleeding in the setting of massive transfusion when coagulation tests cannot be obtained in a timely manner. It should be given in doses calculated to achieve a minimum of 30% of plasma factor concentration, which is usually achieved with administration of 10 mL/kg to 15 mL/kg FFP. Reference values for coagulation tests are essentially identical for children older than 6 months and adults. Nevertheless, the activated partial thromboplastin time is often prolonged in the first 6 months of life because of the lower concentrations of coagulation factors IX, X and XI in newborns and young infants.

Cryoprecipitate

Cryoprecipitate should be considered when microvascular bleeding is present and fibrinogen levels are below 80 mg/dL to 100 mg/dL. One unit of cryoprecipitate per 10 kg body weight raises plasma fibrinogen concentration by approximately 50 mg/dL, in the absence of massive bleeding or consumption.

Regardless of the kind of craniosynostosis repair, the transfusion of red blood cells is very common, whereas the need for platelets, fresh frozen plasma and cryoprecipitate is rare. The risks of transfusion are well known. Besides transfusion related morbidity from posttransfusion hepatitis, acquired immunodeficiency syndrome, hemolytic transfusion reactions, and allergic reactions, transfusion-related acute lung injury and leukocyte-platelet allogenic immunization are complications associated with massive and rapid transfusions. Rapid blood transfusion in an infant can result in hyperkalemia and cardiac arrest, primarily because of the high concentration of potassium in stored blood [31]. Furthermore, coagulopathy is associated with blood loss approaching 1.5 times of estimated blood volume [32].

Strategies for decreasing homologous transfusion

Preoperative autologous donation

Preoperative autologous donation is usually not feasible in children younger than 3 years and is, therefore, very uncommon. Beside concerns related to smaller blood volumes, younger children usually do not tolerate repeated vascular access and donation procedures without deep or general sedation.

Directed donations and limited-exposure blood donor programs

When parents wish to be a directed donor for their children, it is presumably because they believe that blood from themselves is less likely to be a source of transfusion-transmitted diseases than blood from an anonymous volunteer blood donor pool. Whether this is true or not has been a source of controversy in the literature. Several studies have shown no statistically significant differences in the results of infectious disease markers (human immunodeficiency virus, hepatitis C, hepatitis B, syphilis) in directed donors versus anonymous volunteer donors. Other studies have shown an increased frequency of positive infectious disease markers among directed donors, which could be attributed to the relatively larger number of first time donors [30,33,34].

Potential risks of parental blood transfusion are chimerism and graft-versus-host diseases (GVHD). Therefore, all cellular blood components obtained from biologic relatives must be gamma-irradiated before transfusion. In addition, it is also possible that the added complexity of providing directed donations could lead to an increased frequency of human error [35].

Acute normovolemic hemodilution

Acute normovolemic hemodilution (ANH) is a difficult strategy to use in small children because they have a lower hemoglobin level than adults, which translates to a smaller red cell volume available to dilute on a per kilogram basis. In addition, infants less than 4 to 6 months may not be good candidates because the compensatory increased cardiac output, seen in adults during hemodilution, can be absent or decreased in infants of this age. Moreover, only small volumes of whole blood can be harvested before a postdilutional target Hct (usually 25% Hct) is reached. Hans and colleagues [36] investigated the potential benefit of ANH in the surgical repair of craniosynostosis. The investigators randomly assigned 34 infants undergoing craniosynostosis repair over a 4-year period to receive ANH or standard fluid management, and found that ANH reduces neither the incidence of homologous transfusion nor the amount of homologous blood transfused.

Perioperative blood salvage

There are several studies that have evaluated perioperative blood salvage for children undergoing craniosynostosis surgery. For instance, Deva and colleagues [37] did not find significant benefit in using autologous blood recovery and transfusion during primary cranial vault remodeling. For this study, the investigators used the Cobe-Bret 2 autologous blood recovery system for 11 subjects (mean age 8.8 months) and an equal number of consecutive comparable subjects who did not receive intraoperative autotransfusion. In addition to the autologous blood, the autotransfusion group received 34.1 mL/kg of homologous blood, and the control group 32.1 mL/kg. Four subjects did not receive recovered autologous blood because of inadequate recovery [37].

However, outcomes from other studies have shown some benefit for using perioperative blood salvage techniques. For instance, a retrospective, nonrandomized study by Dahmani and coworkers [38] found that the use of continuous autotransfusion system (CATS) was associated with a reduction in homologous transfusion during the surgical correction of craniosynostosis in infants. The use of CATS did not prevent the need for transfusion completely and all 20 infants studied received intraoperative transfusions. Using a prospective nonrandomized study design, Fearon [39] evaluated 60 consecutive children undergoing major cranial vault remodeling. The average age was 4 years old; the mean estimated blood loss was 28% of the estimated total blood volume. Only 30% of their study group required homologous blood transfusion. Likewise, in a nonrandomized prospective trial, Jimenez and Barone [40] demonstrated a cell-salvage reduced need for blood transfusion in children undergoing craniosynostosis repair.

Intraoperative blood salvage presents inherent risks, including coagulopathy, hemolysis, bacterial contamination, and damage to platelets. Studies demonstrated that cultures of blood harvested for recycling yielded positive results for up to 30% of patients. The most common microorganism isolated was coagulase-negative staphylococci. However, none of the patients who received the culture-positive autotransfusion blood showed clinical signs or laboratory findings of bacteremia [41]. Innenhofer and colleagues [42] found, in their pilot study with adolescent and adult patients, that polymorphonuclear leukocytes, which may induce endothelial damage and increase vascular permeability or coagulopathy, are neither impaired nor activated to the priming threshold, and concluded that the use of intraoperative blood salvage is safe. There is no similar data currently available for younger children.

Autotransfusion, by using a postoperative blood salvaging system like the CBCII ConstaVac system, has the potential to be useful because of the common occurrence of postoperative oozing. Although the feasibility of this technique is not clearly established, Orliaguet and colleagues compared CATS intraoperative blood salvaging with the postoperative use of the CBCII Consta Vac system in a retrospective nonrandomized study [43]. They found the postoperative blood salvaging system was equally effective as the perioperative use of the CATS system for reducing homologous blood transfusion during craniosynostosis repair in infants weighing less than 10 kg.

Other blood saving techniques

Induced hypotension

Induced hypotension has not gained acceptance for craniosynostosis repair. Reasons include increased risk of venous air embolism and potential added hemodynamic instability associated with blood loss [3].

Preoperative administration of recombinant human erythropoietin

A few investigators have studied recombinant human erythropoietin (RHEPO) in craniosynostosis surgery in an attempt to decrease the need for homologous transfusion. Helfaer and colleagues [44] administered 300 U/kg erythropoietin every other day for 3 weeks to 31 children scheduled for craniosynostosis repair. The children also received additional elemental iron (6 mg/kg per day divided into three portions a day) during this period. They found that children who received RHEPO had significantly higher Hct values (43%) before surgery, compared with the control group (Hct 35%). The estimated blood loss in the erythropoietin group was about one third less than in the control group, and there was a 36% reduction in homologous transfusion for the study group. The investigators speculated that the reduction in blood loss might be caused by the higher hematocrit level and therefore associated with higher viscosity. In another prospective randomized, single blinded controlled trial by Fearon and Weinthal [45], the study group received 3 weeks of preoperative erythropoietin at a dose of 600 U/kg per week. Both the study group and the control group received supplemental iron (4 mg/kg per day). Fifty-seven percent of the patients given erythropoietin and 93% of the control group needed blood transfusion. These studies suggest that erythropoietin may reduce the transfusion requirements, but cannot eliminate the need for transfusion.

Combination of blood sparing modalities

Meneghini and colleagues [46] performed a retrospective study to evaluate whether pretreatment with erythropoietin and iron combined with ANH could decrease homologous blood transfusion in craniosynostosis surgery. The study group consisted of 16 infants who were given erythropoietin at a dosage of 300 U/kg two times a week, and 10 mg/kg per day of iron for 3 weeks before surgery. Acute normovolemic hemodilution (Hct target 25%) was performed in all 16 subjects at the time of surgery. Five out of the 16 infants in the study group required homologous transfusion, while 7 out of 9 infants in the control group (no treatment) received homologous transfusion. In a similar retrospective study, Meara and colleagues [47] found that transfusion requirements were lower in the study group that received recombinant human erythropoietin and iron in conjunction with other blood conserving modalities (ANH, hypervolemic hemodilution, controlled hypotension) versus the control group, that was not pretreated with erythropoietin but was managed with blood conserving techniques. The investigators concluded that erythropoietin pretreatment combined with blood-conservation modalities was associated with a decreased need for blood transfusion. They also found that when ANH was used in combination with preoperative erythropoietin, the allowable blood loss was doubled, which might present a major advantage of preoperative erythropoietin. Finally, Rohling and colleagues [48] found that a multimodal strategy using erythropoietin, preoperative autologous donation, ANH, intraoperative blood salvage and deliberate hypotension for craniofacial procedures in a large cohort of children and adults (between 8 and 71 years) resulted in a significant reduction in homologous transfusions. Interestingly, they also reported that no transfusion was required in any of the subjects who received erythropoietin in combination with other blood conserving modalities. This finding is similar to the results of Helfaer and colleagues [44] noted above.

Colloid versus crystalloid fluid replacement

In addition to blood replacement, children undergoing craniofacial surgery require additional fluid administration to provide maintenance fluid, replace third space losses, and potentially to replace a portion of the blood loss. The decision about using colloid versus crystalloid is always present, but unfortunately there are few studies comparing colloids versus crystalloids in the pediatric population undergoing surgery. Oca and colleagues [49] did perform a randomized trial in newborns with acute hypotension. They found that administration of normal saline was as effective as 5% albumin for the treatment of neonatal hypotension.

Studies in the adult population have failed to clearly support the benefit of colloid replacement as compared with crystalloid [49–51]. In their consensus statement, the American Thoracic Society stated that the influence of albumin and synthetic colloids on microvascular integrity is still uncertain [52]. Jones and colleagues [53] investigated the influence of crystalloid and colloid replacement solutions in ANH and found changes in factor VIII, activated partial thromboplastin time, and thromboelastography in the group receiving hetastarch and dextran 70. The investigators hypothesized that these changes may attenuate hypercoagulability related to surgery.

In light of the lack of empirical evidence, it seems most prudent in the circumstance of craniofacial reconstructive surgery to replace blood loss with packed red blood cells if necessary, and to use crystalloid for other fluid replacement. Colloid can be used for acute volume resuscitation when packed red blood cells are not indicated or not available.

Postoperative course

Postoperative management varies by surgeon and institution. In most circumstances, the patient can be extubated at the end of surgery and transported to the perioperative anaesthetic care unit. If the patient has been particularly unstable, has undergone an unusually lengthy surgery, or has a history of a difficult airway, it may be prudent to leave the endotracheal tube in place for a period postoperatively to allow more time for stabilization. The patient's hematocrit should be followed postoperatively, as continued oozing is common. Coagulation studies may be indicated should postoperative bleeding be excessive. Often, the patient will undergo a postoperative computed tomography at some point after leaving the operating room.

As with any postoperative patient, pain management is crucial. Appropriate dosing of an opioid is usually required, with follow-up to ensure adequate analgesia is achieved. A careful balance may be required for patients with a difficult airway or obstructive apnea. Patients are routinely watched in the pediatric intensive care unit for at least 24 hours, to insure close nursing care. The use of nonsteroidal anti-inflammatory drugs is usually deferred because of the fear of platelet inhibition and increased postoperative bleeding. Acetaminophen can be a useful adjunct to intravenous opioids.

Summary

Craniosynostosis is a complex condition that is most likely caused by multiple influencing factors. There is now some evidence that even patients with nonsyndromic craniosynostosis may have some underlying abnormality in brain development that can lead to learning disorders or more severe cognitive disabilities. The impact of early repair of craniosynostosis on the incidence of cognitive delay remains to be clearly determined. Nonetheless, it is the current standard of care to consider early surgical intervention for most forms of craniosynostosis. The young age of most patients, combined with the high likelihood of significant blood loss, make these some of the most challenging cases for a pediatric anesthesiologist. With proper preoperative planning, and careful attention to intravascular volume status during the case, patient outcome is usually excellent.

References

[1] Kabbani H, Raghuveer TS. Craniosynostosis. Am Fam Physician 2004;69(12):2863–70.

[2] Shuper A, Merlob P, Grunebaum M, et al. The incidence of craniosynostosis in the newborn infant. Am J Dis Child 1985;139(1):85–6.

[3] Faberowski LW, Black S, Mickle JP. Craniosynostosis: an overview. Am J Anesthesiol 2000; 27(2):76–82.

[4] Morris-Kay GM, Wilkie AOM. Growth of the normal skull vault and its alteration in craniosynostosis: insights from human genetics and experimental studies. J Anat 2005;207: 637–53.

[5] Kapp-Simon KA. Mental development and learning disorders in children with single suture craniosynostosis. Cleft Palate Craniofac J 1998;35(3):197–203.

[6] Becker DB, Petersen JD, Kane AA, et al. Speech, cognitive, and behavioral outcomes in nonsyndromic craniosynostosis. Plast Reconstr Surg 2005;116(2):400–7.

[7] Magge NS, Westerveld M, Pruzinsky T, et al. Long-term neuropsychological effects of sagittal craniosynostosis on child development. J Craniofac Surg 2002;13(1):99–104.

[8] Panchal J, Amirsheybani H, Gurwitch R, et al. Neurodevelopment in children with single-suture craniosynostosis and plagiocephaly without synostosis. Plast Reconstr Surg 2001; 108:1492–8.

[9] Warschausky S, Angobaldo J, Kewman D, et al. Early development of infants with untreated metopic craniosynostosis. Plast Reconstr Surg 2005;115:1518–23.

[10] Da Costa AC, Walters I, Savarirayan R, et al. Intellectual outcomes in children and adolescents with syndromic and nonsyndromic craniosynostosis. Plast Reconstr Surg 2006;118: 175–81.

[11] Virtanen R, Korhonen T, Fagerholm J, et al. Neurocognitive sequelae of scaphocephaly. Pediatrics 1999;103(4):791–5.

[12] Cohen SR, Cho DC, Nichols SL, et al. American Society of Maxillofacial Surgeons Outcome Study: preoperative and postoperative neurodevelopmental findings in single-suture craniosynostosis. Plast Reconstr Surg 2004;114:841–7.

[13] Gewalli F, da Silva Guimaraes-Ferreira JP, Sahlin P, et al. Mental development after modified pi procedure: dynamic cranioplasty for sagittal synostosis. Ann Plast Surg 2001;46: 415–20.

[14] Faberowksi LW, Black S, Mickle JP. Incidence of venous air embolism during craniectomy for craniosynostosis repair. Anesthesiology 2000;92:20–3.

[15] Rancel P, Bell A, Jane JA. Operative postioning for patients undergoing repair of craniosynostosis. Neurosurgery 1994;35(2):304–6.

[16] Chiaretti A, Pietrini D, Piastra M, et al. Safety and efficacy of remifentanil in craniosynostosis repair in children less than 1 year old. Pediatr Neurosurg 2000;33(2):83–8.

[17] Pietrini D, Ciano F, Forte E, et al. Sevoflurane-remifentanil vs. isoflurane-remifentanil for the surgical correction of craniosynostosis in infants. Pediatr Anaesth 2005;15:653–62.

[18] Meyer P, Renier D, Arnaud E, et al. Blood loss during repair of craniosynostosis. Br J Anaesth 1993;71(6):854–7.

[19] Kearney RA, Rosales JK, Howes WJ. Craniosynostosis: an assessment of blood loss and transfusion practices. Can J Anaesth 1989;36(4):473–7.

[20] Faberowski LW, Black S, Mickle JP. Blood loss and transfusion practice in the perioperative management of craniosynostosis repair. J Neurosurg Anesthesiol 1999;11(3):167–72.

[21] Eaton AC, Marsh JL, Pilgram TK. Transfusion requirements for craniosynostosis surgery in infants. Plast Reconstr Surg 1995;95(2):277–83.

[22] Boop FA, Shewmake K, Chadduck WM. Synostectomy versus complex cranioplasty for the treatment of sagittal synostosis. Childs Nerv Syst 1996;12(7):371–5.

[23] Ririe DG, David LR, Glazier SS, et al. Surgical advancement influences perioperative care: a comparison of two surgical techniques for sagittal craniosynostosis repair. Anesth Analg 2003;97:699–703.

[24] Guimaraes-Ferreira J, Gewalli F, David L, et al. Spring-mediated cranioplasty compared with the modified pi-plasty for sagittal synostosis. Scand J Plast Reconstr Surg Hand Surg 2003;37(4):208–15.

[25] David LR, Proffer P, Hurst WJ, et al. Spring-mediated cranial reshaping for craniosynostosis. J Craniofac Surg 2004;15(5):810–6.

[26] Maugans TA, McComb JG, Levy ML. Surgical management of sagittal synostosis: a comparative analysis of strip craniectomy and calvarial vault remodeling. Pediatr Neurosurg 1997;27(3):137–48.

[27] Mallett SV, Peachey TD, Sanehi O, et al. Reducing red blood cell transfusion in elective surgical patients: the role of audit and practice guidelines. Anesthesia 2000;55(10): 1013–9.

[28] Practice guidelines for blood component therapy: a report by the American Society of Anesthesiologists Task Force on Blood Component Therapy. Anesthesiology 1996;84(3): 732–47.

[29] Roseff SD, Luban NLC, Manno CS. Guidelines for assessing appropriateness of pediatric transfusion. Transfusion 2002;42:1398–413.

[30] Hume HA, Limoges P. Perioperative blood transfusion therapy in pediatric patients. Am J Ther 2002;9(5):396–405.

[31] British Committee for Standards in Hematology Transfusion (bjh). Transfusion guidelines for neonates and older children. Br J Haematol 2004;124:433–53.

[32] Williams GD, Ellenbogen RG, Gruss JS. Abnormal coagulation during pediatric craniofacial surgery. Pediatr Neurosurg 2001;35:5–12.

[33] Pink J, Thomson A, Wylie B. Infectious disease markers in autologous and directed donations. Transfus Med 1994;4(2):35–8.

[34] Myhre BA, Figueroa PI. Infectious disease markers in various groups of donors. Ann Clin Lab Sci 1995;25(1):39–43.

[35] Goldman M, Remy-Prince S, Trepanier A, et al. Autologous donation error rates in Canada. Transfusion 1997;37(5):523–7.

[36] Hans P, Collin V, Bonhomme V, et al. Evaluation of acute normovolemic hemodilution for surgical repair of craniosynostosis. J Neurosurg Anesthesiol 2000;12(1):33–6.

[37] Deva AK, Hopper RA, Landecker A, et al. The use of intraoperative autotransfusion during cranial vault remodeling for craniosynostosis. Plast Reconstr Surg 2001;109:58–63.

[38] Dahmani S, Orliaguet GA, Meyer PG, et al. Perioperative blood salvage during surgical correction of craniosynostosis in infants. Br J Anaesth 2000;85(4):550–5.

[39] Fearon JA. Reducing allogenic blood transfusions during pediatric cranial vault surgical procedures: a prospective analysis of blood recycling. Plast Reconstr Surg 2004;113: 1126–30.

[40] Jimenez DF, Barone CM. Intraoperative autologous blood transfusion in the surgical correction of craniosynostosis. Neurosurgery 1995;37(6):1075–9.

[41] Sugai Y, Sugai K, Fuse KA. Current status of bacterial contamination of autologous blood for transfusion. Transfus Apher Sci 2001;24(3):255–9.

[42] Innenhofer P, Wiedermann FJ, Tiefenthaler W, et al. Are leucocytes in salvaged washed autologous blood harmful for the recipient? The results of a pilot study. Anesth Analg 2001;93:566–72.

[43] Orliaguet GA, Bruyere M, Meyer PG, et al. Comparison of perioperative blood salvage and postoperative reinfusion of drained blood during surgical correction of craniosynostosis in infants. Paediatr Anaesth 2003;13:797–804.

[44] Helfaer MA, Carson BS, James CS, et al. Increased hematocrit and decreased transfusion requirements in children given erythropoietin before undergoing surgery. J Neurosurg 1998; 88:704–8.

[45] Fearon JA, Weinthal J. The use of recombinant erythropoietin in the reduction of blood transfusion rates in craniosynostosis repair in infants and children. Plast Reconstr Surg 2002;109:2190–6.

[46] Meneghini L, Zadra N, Aneloni V, et al. Erythropoietin therapy and acute preoperative normovolaemic haemodilution in infants undergoing craniosynostosis surgery. Paediatr Anaesth 2003;13:392–6.

[47] Meara JG, Smith EM, Harshbarger RJ, et al. Blood-conservation techniques in craniofacial surgery. Ann Plast Surg 2005;54:525–9.

[48] Rohling RG, Haers PE, Zimmerman AP, et al. Multimodal strategy for reduction of homologous transfusions in cranio-maxillofacial surgery. Int J Oral Maxillofac Surg 1999;28(2): 137–42.

[49] Oca MJ, Nelson M, Donn SM. Randomized trial of normal Saline versus 5% albumin for the treatment of neonatal hypotension. J Perinatol 2003;23:473–6.

[50] Verheij J, Van Lingen A, Raijmakers GHM, et al. Effect of fluid loading with saline or colloids on pulmonary permeability, oedema and lung injury score after cardiac and major vascular surgery. Br J Anaesth 2006;96:21–30.

[51] Roberts I, Alderson P, Bunn F, et al. Colloids versus crystalloids for fluid resuscitation in critically ill patients. Cochrane Rev 2006;4:1–59.

[52] American Thoracic Society. Evidence-based colloid use in the critically ill: American Thoracic Society consensus statement. Am J Respir Crit Care Med 2004;170:1247–59.

[53] Jones SB, Whitten CW, Despotis GJ, et al. The influence of crystalloid and colloid replacement solutions in acute normovolemic hemodilution: a preliminary survey of hemostatic markers. Anesth Analg 2003;96:363–8.

ELSEVIER
SAUNDERS

Anesthesiology Clin
25 (2007) 483–509

ANESTHESIOLOGY
CLINICS

Perioperative Care of Patients with Neuromuscular Disease and Dysfunction

Ansgar M. Brambrink, MD, PhD*,
Jeffrey R. Kirsch, MD

Department of Anesthesiology and Perioperative Medicine, Oregon Health and Sciences University, 3181 Sam Jackson Park Road, Portland, OR 97239–3098, USA

Although neuromuscular disease and neuromuscular dysfunction (NMD) may present with clinical similarities, the underlying pathophysiologic processes can be located in different anatomic compartments of the neuromuscular unit (ie, the central nervous system, the peripheral nerves, the neuromuscular junction, or the muscle fibers). The underlying mechanisms, affected muscle groups, time of onset, progression, and prognosis all are used ultimately to distinguish different disease entities.

Several of the classical NMDs (eg, amyotrophic lateral sclerosis [ALS]; hereditary polyneuropathies, such as Charcot-Marie-Tooth disease or Friedreich's ataxia; myasthenia gravis [MG]; or Lambert-Eaton syndrome [LES]) are rare and the individual anesthesiologist may encounter affected patients only a few times in his or her entire career. Other entities that regularly are associated with neuromuscular dysfunction, such as multiple sclerosis (MS), spinal cord injury, or critical illness polyneuropathy (CIP), are more frequent and respective patients are more commonly treated by a variety of different interventions, especially in large health care centers.

Patients affected with NMDs often present a challenge, even to the very experienced practitioner. Some classical diseases are associated with myocardial irregularities, such as malignant arrhythmias (myotonic dystrophy, Friedreich's ataxia), or cardiomyopathy (Duchenne's muscular dystrophy [DMD]), or they result in respiratory dysfunction. Several NMDs affect the functionality of cranial nerves (MG, ALS) or the autonomic nervous system (Guillain-Barré syndrome [GBS]), resulting in chronic aspiration

---

* Corresponding author.
E-mail address: brambrin@ohsu.edu (A.M. Brambrink).

1932-2275/07/$ - see front matter © 2007 Elsevier Inc. All rights reserved.
doi:10.1016/j.anclin.2007.05.005   *anesthesiology.theclinics.com*

or cardiovascular dysfunction. Moreover, some types are also associated with developmental delay and cognitive dysfunction (eg, DMD) [1].

Perioperative management of patients with NMD may become complex. Agents with known effect on muscular function (eg, muscle relaxants, volatile anesthetics, barbiturates, or benzodiazepines) may be used only with great caution or need to be omitted altogether. Potential life-threatening complications include malignant arrhythmia, congestive heart failure, and severe hyperkalemia leading to cardiac arrest, and in other cases rhabdomyolysis, malignant hyperthermia, or postoperative respiratory insufficiency [2–5]. In addition, it is not uncommon that affected patients receive their first general anesthesia before the NMD is diagnosed [6–9]. This is particularly relevant for the pediatric anesthesiologist.

A detailed history is probably the best tool to identify individuals who may suffer from an undiagnosed NMD. Additional tests (eg, ECG, echocardiography, chest radiography, pulmonary function tests, or blood tests [electrolytes]), may complete the preoperative work-up [10,11]. It is of utmost importance that the individual NMD be identified, because the anesthetic management varies significantly between diseases (ie, the choice of muscle relaxants). As an example, although succinylcholine is strictly contraindicated in patients presenting with DMD or myotonic dystrophy, it may be administered to patients with MG or LES.

This article summarizes the characteristic pathophysiologic aberrations and the anesthetic implications of some of the more common NMDs. It is beyond the scope of this article to comment on the specifics of all known NMDs. Instead, each affected anatomic compartment of the neuromuscular unit (ie, central nervous system, motor neuron, and peripheral nerve [prejunctional]; neuromuscular junction [junctional]; muscle fiber [postjunctional]) is represented with one or more typical examples.

Prejunctional neuromuscular disease

Several pathologies affect the motor neurons either in the central nervous system or the periphery and result in phenotypes summarized as NMDs. Examples for disease processes that destroy the functionality of the primary or secondary motor neuron are ALS, spinal muscular atrophy (SMA), MS, and spinal cord injury. Examples for peripheral neuropathies that result in NMD phenotype are the Charcot-Marie-Tooth syndrome, Friedreich's ataxia, GBS, toxic polyneuropathy, and CIP.

The denervation of the respective muscle groups results in reduced levels of acetylcholine at the neuromuscular junction and more acetylcholine receptor (AChR) of fetal phenotype expressed on extrajunctional membrane aspects of the muscle fibers. The overall increased number and their diffuse expression pattern of the AChR and their fetal phenotype of a higher conductivity for potassium ions allow a profound potassium release secondary to the application of succinylcholine, which can result in cardiac arrhythmias or even cardiac arrest. It is important to know that the described morphologic changes are initiated immediately after the denervation, and become clinically relevant as early as 48 hours after the insult (eg, a spinal injury or a complete immobilization secondary to an acute illness). The degree of the succinylcholine-triggered hyperkalemia is determined by the muscle mass affected. The risk for hyperkalemia may persist for up to 1 year.

Degeneration or injury of central neurons

Distinct pathologies of the central nervous system disrupt the functionality of the neuromuscular unit, which are characterized by weakness and degeneration of skeletal muscle secondary to the absence of neuronal stimulation based on central denervation. Sensory nerves may be involved or not depending on the disease process. Suggested modifications to the anesthetic plan may involve meticulous discussion about the risk and benefits of muscular paralysis and regional anesthesia.

Amyotrophic lateral sclerosis and spinal muscular atrophy

Both ALS and SMA are characterized by progressive muscular atrophy secondary to degeneration of cortical, brainstem, and spinal motor neurons [12]. ALS (Lou Gehrig's disease) usually is diagnosed in men during the fourth to fifth decade of life, and is considered to result from a combination of genetic and environmental risk factors (incidence about 1:100.000). ALS is a diagnosis of exclusion, because no specific test is available. Most recently, however, a set of cerebral spinal fluid biomarkers was suggested to allow an early and definitive diagnosis [13]. ALS initially may only affect single muscles of the extremities, but it later generalizes and eventually also affects the bulbar muscles resulting in speech and swallowing problems, with secondary pulmonary aspiration. There is no specific cure for ALS, but one drug (riluzole) was recently introduced, which may reduce the neuronal deterioration by decreasing the release of glutamate. Extensive physical therapy may extend the independence of the patient and prevent early complications; later, the use of ventilator support (eg, intermittent positive airway pressure, bi-level positive airway pressure) may help patients to overcome the progressive loss of intercostal muscle strength and vital capacity for some time. ALS is a progressive disease, however, and patients finally are limited by severe pulmonary complications.

SMA summarizes a number of genetic disorders (in most cases chromosome 5 is affected, duplication and malfunction of the "survival motor neuron gene; autosomal recessive; combined incidence of all forms 1:6000) that affect the motor neurons in the spinal cord and the brainstem [14]. The phenotype allows separating four general forms of the disease: (1) infantile (first year of life, Werdnig-Hoffmann disease, never able to sit independently); (2) intermediate (1–2 year old, able to sit but never able to walk); (3) juvenile (<2 years, Kugelberg-Welander syndrome, able to walk at some period of their life); and (4) adult SMA (type IV, often affects control of the tongue and extremities first). The earlier the onset, the shorter is the life span of the patient. Affected infants may not survive the first 2 years, whereas the adult form progresses much slower and frequently does not impact life expectancy. Intellectual functions remain unaffected, and in the adult, sexual function and sphincter control remain intact. There is no specific therapy available, although some drugs are under investigation for SMA. The focus of medical intervention is generally on prevention and treatment of respiratory complications, such as pneumonia, which is the leading cause of death in these patients. Physical therapy and nutritional care play a dominant role.

Anesthetic challenges in amyotrophic lateral sclerosis and spinal muscular atrophy patients. The specific concerns influencing the anesthetic plan are similar for both diseases, and relate to regional anesthesia and muscular paralysis. The perioperative risks result from the individual limitation of pulmonary function, and the extent of the bulbar muscle paralysis. Profoundly limited patients may require prolonged postoperative ventilation in an ICU to address both ventilatory and bulbar weakness. Case reports describing the safe use of either general or regional anesthesia exist in the literature [15–17]. Patients are not at an increased risk for malignant hyperthermia or rhabdomyolysis. Regional anesthesia seems not to result in clinical deterioration, but it is suggested carefully to limit the neuroaxial block levels to limit the impact on the patient's respiration. In contrast, the use of muscle relaxants is of concern. Succinylcholine is strictly contraindicated in patients with ALS and SMA because of the risk for a profound potassium release. Nondepolarizing muscle relaxants may be used, although depending on the individual case, prolonged activity has been described for both ALS and SMA patients [18]. Reduced dosing, continuous neuromuscular monitoring, and the use of antagonists (cholinesterase inhibitors [eg, neostigmine]) is suggested [19]. Anesthesia in an outpatient setting cannot be recommended for these patients.

Spinal cord injury
    There are about 285,000 people in the United States who have survived a spinal cord injury (prevalence 700–900:1,000,000, about 1:1100). According to the National Spinal Cord Injury Statistical Center at the University of Birmingham, Alabama (http://www.spinalcord.uab.edu/), about 11,000 patients are added to this group each year, almost exclusively secondary to traumatic events (incidence 40:1,000,000 [20]; for further detail see the article by Crosby elsewhere in this issue). Spinal cord injury can be considered a prejunctional disease process, which accounts for many of the perioperative management challenges. In contrast to other prejunctional NMDs, however, the challenges are different in the acute and the chronic phase.

Anesthetic concerns after spinal cord injury. The acute phase is dominated by associated injuries (eg, traumatic injuries to the head or other organs). In many cases there is an early need for ventilatory support and airway management, which may be complicated by a full stomach, blood in the airway, and the need for cervical spine immobilization (see the article by Crosby elsewhere in this issue) [21,22]. Frequently, patients require hemodynamic stabilization in the early phase because of blood loss or "spinal shock" with vasodilatation and bradycardia, secondary to interrupted sympathetic outflow, which is frequently seen with lesions above T4. These patients require invasive hemodynamic monitoring and rapid therapeutic intervention to prevent, among other problems, a worsening of their spinal cord injury secondary to hypoxemia and low perfusion (ischemia). The interrupted sympathetic outflow also may result in an unbalanced and overwhelming parasympathetic influence to the heart when initiated, for example, with laryngoscopy during endotracheal intubation. Cardiac arrest may result requiring myocardial pacing. Although pretreatment with anticholinergic agents may prevent the profound bradycardia with laryngoscopy, efficacy is limited after cardiac arrest because of the inability to get the drug to the heart. Head-injured patients may experience profound autonomic discharge with hypertension and bradycardia, (Cushing's response), which may lead to pulmonary edema [21]; others may suffer pulmonary edema from extensive fluid resuscitation in response to low blood pressure. The administration of adequate amounts of synthetic catecholamines after adequate fluid replacement is suggested as an alternative in these situations. High-dose methylprednisolone has been advocated for spinal cord–injured patients during the first 48 hours after the insult to limit secondary damage, [23]. There has been continuous controversy, however, around this practice [20,24–28]. Spinal cord injury also results in a loss of temperature control below the lesion, and measures need to be taken to prevent the patient from becoming hypothermic or hyperthermic. Communication between peripheral temperature sensors and the hypothalamus may be interrupted and vasoconstriction, shivering, and perspiration are not initiated. The postoperative management may vary significantly between individual patients and is determined by the additional injury and hemodynamic stability.

In the chronic phase the anesthesiologist is faced with different problems, the most important being the changes in the patient's sensitivity to muscle relaxants, and the management of autonomic dysreflexia. As with ALS and SMA, denervation of the neuromuscular unit after spinal cord injury results in expression changes of nicotinic receptors [29], with the risk of a profound release of potassium from the respective musculature after the application of succinylcholine, which immediately may lead to cardiac arrest [30–32]. Although succinylcholine is safe during the first 24 hours after the insult, it should be avoided 48 hours after the onset of symptoms [33]. This hypersensitivity has been reported up to 6 months after injury, and its duration may even be longer. In contrast, nondepolarizing muscle relaxants are safe to use; however, some patients may be relatively resistant and require higher doses.

With the reappearance of sympathetic tone some weeks after injury and following the phase of spinal shock, most patients (84%) with lesions above T6 (above the splanchnic outflow) develop autonomic dysreflexia, which is characterized by sympathetic overshoot (ie, massive sympathetic discharge in response to visceral stimulation, such as bladder or rectal distention, uterus contraction, or surgical stimulation). Autonomic dysreflexia is unlikely to occur in patients with lesions below T10. Afferent impulses by intact peripheral fibers ascend into the spinal cord (spinothalamic and posterior columns) below the lesion and stimulate sympathetic neurons (intermediolateral gray). The inhibitory outflow of cerebral vasomotor centers is generally increased but cannot pass below the block caused by the spinal cord injury. The resulting disproportional sympathetic outflow causes sudden elevation in blood pressure and compensatory vasodilation above the level of injury. There is also increased parasympathetic outflow with subsequent bradycardia; sweating; and vasodilatation (skin flushing).

The practitioner should consider all patients at risk who are a few days to several weeks after the acute spinal cord injury and who undergo surgical procedures below the level of the lesion, including vaginal deliveries and extracorporeal shockwave lithotripsy [34–38], although these may be painless for the individual. The classical symptoms, such as hypertension and headaches, are frequently mistaken for preeclampsia in the parturient. To prevent potentially life-threatening complications, affected patients need either regional or general anesthesia. The spread of a regional block using local anesthetics may be difficult to evaluate, and the sympathetic block of large vessels of the lower extremity may result in unwanted hemodynamic effects. Spinal and epidural opioids alone, however, may be very effective. Acute treatment involves use of antihypertensive drugs with rapid onset and short duration (eg, nifedipine or nitroglycerine) and treatment of the underlying cause.

Multiple sclerosis

Demyelization of neuronal fibers is the hallmark of MS, which is a chronic disease of the central nervous system and spares the peripheral nerves. It is the most frequent cause of neurologic disability of early to middle adulthood. MS affects about 1 in every 1000 citizens in northern Europe, North America, and Australia and New Zealand (highest on Orkney and Shetland Islands) [39–41], but the prevalence is very low near the equator [42,43]. The exact cause of MS is still unknown, but climate, diet, sunlight exposure, toxins, genetic background, and infections have all been implicated [39–44]. According to the most prevalent theory, myelin sheets are attacked by T-cells, which identify healthy nervous system structures as foreign material. This triggers an inflammatory process involving other immunocompetent cells (eg, macrophages), cytokines, antibodies, and other destructive proteins (eg, matrix metalloproteinases), ultimately resulting in the complete destruction of the myelin sheet of attacked neurons. Remyelination also occurs in MS, especially early in the disease, and is most likely responsible for remissions, when symptoms decrease or disappear. The brain can compensate for some of the damage by functional reorganization and by cellular plasticity. Remyelination is often only partially successful and after several such remissions scar-like plaques result with functional loss and subsequent degeneration for the respective axons and neurons [45–48]. The clinical symptoms of MS develop as the cumulative result of multiple lesions in the spinal cord and the brain. They may include changes in sensation of arms, leg, or face (33%); visual problems (optic neuritis 16%, double vision 7%); muscle weakness (13%); difficulty with coordination and balance (unsteady gait 5%); speech problems; severe fatigue; cognitive impairment (eg, inability to multitask, short-term memory loss); or depression [49–57]. The incidence of epileptic seizures is increased with MS [58]. Many patients present with a wide range of findings. Symptoms may develop over the course of some days, and last for a week followed by a remission. In most patients MS occurs in such a relapsing-remitting course (80%–90%). Most patients eventually experience a worsening of the course (secondary progressive) without any remission between their acute attacks, whereas a small number of individuals (10%) experience a primary progressive course from the initial manifestation of their symptoms. There is no known cure for MS, but some therapies have been shown to be helpful to support the return of function and prevent new attacks and disability [59–61]. Suggested drug therapies include high-dose corticosteroids, interferons, and other immunotherapies, and supportive drugs, such as specific amino acids and vitamins. Patients with further progressed clinical presentation may receive benzodiazepines or dantrolene for muscle spasticity [59,61].

Anesthetic challenges in multiple sclerosis patients. Preoperative evaluation should focus on the neurologic deficit and on potential secondary diseases or complications related to pharmacologic treatment [62–64]. The cardiovascular system may be impaired because of autonomic dysfunction secondary to disease in the high thoracic spinal cord (abnormal Valsalva's response, marked hypotension with reduced response to fluid or vasopressors). History of syncope, bladder and bowel dysfunction, and orthostasis should alert the clinician. Cardiotoxicity may also result from anti-inflammatory drugs (eg, cyclophosphamide) and should trigger appropriate evaluation (EKG, echocardiography) if functional impairment is suspected. The respiratory function may be limited secondary to overall neuromuscular dysfunction; kyphoscoliosis; or lung fibrosis (secondary to anti-inflammatory drugs) [65]. The results of a thorough neurologic examination should be documented preoperatively. Specific laboratory tests should evaluate hepatic and adrenal function if patients are treated with particular drugs (eg, dantrolene, steroids).

The choice between general and neuraxial anesthesia is a matter of debate among specialists. The main concern is the potential for neurologic deterioration. Lumbar puncture per se was shown to be not harmful in MS patients, whereas postoperative decline of neurologic function has been demonstrated after spinal anesthesia [62,64,66,67] potentially secondary to toxic effects of the local anesthetics to unmyelinated nerve roots (relative higher concentrations). In contrast, epidural anesthesia (lower intrathecal doses) and regional nerve block are considered to be safe by most authors [62,64,67–71]. In a scenario where regional anesthesia is desired (eg, during an obstetric procedure), epidural anesthesia is suggested. Efforts should be made to reduce the dose of the local anesthetic, which may be possible by considering opioids as part of the solution. In addition, the exposure time of the local anesthetic should be limited to a minimum (long-term epidural infusions should be avoided).

For premedication purposes there are no primary restrictions on any drug. Benzodiazepines may be helpful because they may reduce muscular spasticity in affected patients. Drugs with unwanted anticholinergic effects may further aggravate the autonomic dysfunction and impair temperature regulation.

Induction of general anesthesia can safely be achieved using propofol or thiopental [62–64]. Volatile anesthetics can be used for maintenance of anesthesia without any restrictions. The use of muscle relaxants, however, requires specific considerations. Succinylcholine should be avoided because it has been associated with hyperkalemia in patients with MS [72]. Only patients with motor nuclei affection (flaccidity, spasticity, hyperreflexia), however, are at risk [72,73]. The response to nondepolarizing agents may also vary; some patients may present with an increased requirement, which could be explained by (1) the additional acetylcholine receptors (this also explains the increased risk for hyperkalemia after succinylcholine); (2) faster metabolism of the paralytic drugs secondary to induction of liver enzymes; or (3) differences in the binding kinetics of the muscle relaxants to plasma proteins (reduced free fraction) [74].

Routine American Society of Anesthesiologists (ASA) monitoring should be applied and more invasive hemodynamic monitoring should be considered in patients with evidence of abnormal autonomic regulation. Body temperature should be controlled continuously, and hyperpyrexia avoided. Twitch monitoring should be applied in all MS patients who received muscle relaxants. The use of anticholinergic drugs in conjunction with reversal agents should be limited to a minimum.

Postoperative observation should be tailored to the individual requirements of the patient and is organized around the preoperative presentation (blood pressure variability, hypoventilation, residual neuromuscular block). There is a risk for postoperative decline of the patient's neurologic function, which cannot be attributed to any particular anesthetic technique. The risk is elevated threefold in the parturient. Frequent neurologic examinations should be conducted to assess for the need for specific interventions (neurologic consult, steroids). Elevated body temperature should be anticipated and should be prevented (perioperative antibiotics, active temperature control) or aggressively treated (antipyretics, cold air), because postoperative fever has been associated with MS exacerbation. MS patients frequently have evidence for increased platelet aggregation and require effective thromboembolic prophylaxis [75,76]. Cranial nerve involvement exposes the patient at risk for aspiration.

Peripheral neuropathies

Damage to nerves of the peripheral nervous system may be secondary to diseases of the nerve or systemic illness. Peripheral neuropathies are characterized by motor, sensory, and autonomic dysfunction. Myelin cells or the axons may be damaged by infections; autoimmune processes (eg, GBS); hereditary gene defects (eg, Charcot-Marie-Tooth disease, Friedreich's ataxia [77–85]); intoxications (eg, alcohol [86,87]); or other disease states (eg, prolonged critical illness [critical care neuropathy] or diabetes mellitus). Beside the loss of motor and sensory control in affected regions, cardiovascular and gastrointestinal symptoms may be apparent indicating involvement of the autonomous nervous system. Critical issues for the anesthesia provider are whether to provide muscle relaxants to these patients, and if neuraxial or regional anesthesia can safely be performed. In this article the focus is on GBS and critical care neuropathy as examples of peripheral nerve diseases and their impact on perioperative management.

Guillain-Barré syndrome

GBS is an acute, autoimmune neuropathy (several subtypes are known, incidence about 1:50,000) that is usually triggered by an acute infectious process [88,89]. GBS usually exhibits as an ascending paralysis noted by weakness in the legs that spreads to the upper limbs and the face along with complete loss of deep tendon reflexes. The morphologic correlate of GBS is an inflammatory demyelinating process of peripheral nerves resulting from an autoimmune attack on gangliosides (glycosphingolipids), which are present in large quantities in the myelin cells, especially in the nodes of Ranvier. The destruction of these structures quickly results in a conduction block, leading to a rapidly evolving flaccid paralysis with or without accompanying sensory or autonomic disturbances. Organisms frequently associated with GBS include *Campylobacter jejuni, Mycoplasma*, Epstein-Barr virus, and cytomegalovirus. Patients often report a preceding mild upper respiratory or gastrointestinal tract infection. GBS has also been described after epidural anesthesia [90–93]. GBS is often associated with autonomic dysfunction and significant muscle pain. Diagnosis is by exclusion of other causes of muscle weakness, such as MG or primary spinal cord diseases. Nerve conduction studies determine demyelination and axonal degeneration in the affected regions.

Plasmapheresis and intravenous immunoglobulins have been shown to be effective treatment [89,94–96]. Steroid treatment has not been shown to be effective. Symptomatic treatment includes analgesics (especially nonsteroidal anti-inflammatory drugs, but also opioids if necessary or local anesthetics [eg, by epidural or peripheral catheters]) and respiratory support (ventilatory and bulbar weakness). Tracheostomy should be considered early. Efficient thromboembolic prophylaxis and enteral nutrition are of paramount importance as part of the temporary intensive care treatment plan, which is basically targeted to support and protect vital functions during the plateau phase of the disease [88,89,97,98].

Anesthetic challenges in patients with Guillain-Barré syndrome. The characteristic changes relevant to anesthesia practice secondary to GBS are the risk for abnormal response to muscle relaxants and the potential for hemodynamic instability. The latter is a consequence of abnormal autonomic function and results in similar problems as described for MS patients. The degree of the former is determined by the proliferation of extrajunctional acetylcholine receptors in response to the denervation, and a potential for a life-threatening hyperkalemic response to succinylcholine. This has been reported even after resolution of the clinical symptoms of GBS [99–101], and poses a significant risk for affected patients. The response to nondepolarizing neuromuscular blockers may also be affected in that patients with GBS can be more resistant or more sensitive to conventional doses [102,103].

Critical illness neuropathy

In the course of prolonged intensive care treatment, patients independent of their initial disease may develop a specific form of neuromuscular dysfunction. It is characterized by muscle weakness, failure to wean or problems during weaning from the ventilator, or a protracted recovery [104–109]. The incidence of CIP is considered to be rather high: critical care neuropathy affects about 1.7% of pediatric intensive care patients, and is estimated to be present to some degree in 50% of adult ICU patients after 1 week, and in about 70% of patients with sepsis and multiorgan failure [109–111]. Patients present with muscle atrophy, flaccid tetraparesis, and most of them have reduced reflexes [112,113] because predominately motor neurons seem to be involved [114]. If CIP is suspected electrophysiologic evaluation is necessary to determine the diagnosis. Positive recordings show fibrillation potentials and sharp waves, both indicating axonal damage [104–107]. The final diagnosis, however, requires the exclusion of other neurologic causes of muscle weakness. Among the factors that are discussed to trigger CIP are long-term administration of muscle relaxants, steroids, malnutrition, and hyperglycemia, although the true etiology of CIP is still unclear. CIP is frequently seen in patients who recover from multiorgan failure secondary to sepsis, and the axonal degeneration in CIP may share similar pathomechanisms. A likely scenario is one of disrupted microcirculation induced by circulating levels of cytokines, histamine, or toxic metabolites (eg, arachidonic acid) altogether leading to endoneural ischemia and subsequent damage of peripheral nerves [104–107,109–112]. So far, no specific treatment or prophylaxis has been described for CIP other than symptomatic treatment; the strict avoidance of potentially worsening factors (eg, hypoxemia and hypotension); and aggressive treatment of sepsis.

Anesthetic challenges in patients with critical illness neuropathy. It is frequently observed that neuromuscular blockade is prolonged in critically ill patients, and in many cases this can be explained by coexisting factors, such as electrolyte abnormalities; antibiotic treatment (aminoglycosides); or liver and renal failure (resulting in accumulation of muscle relaxants and active metabolites). As with other demyelinating diseases, CIP patients may experience hyperkalemia following administration of succinylcholine [115,116]. Likewise, patients may be resistant to nondepolarizing neuromuscular blockers [117–119].

Junctional neuromuscular diseases

These diseases are characterized by a dysfunction of the neuromuscular conduction. The best known entities are MG and LES. There are other very rare congenital syndromes with similarities to MG where neuromuscular transmission is compromised by one or more mechanisms, and some medications that benefit one type can be detrimental in another type [120]. Common among all diseases affecting the neuromuscular transmission is the pronounced muscular weakness and a high sensitivity to the effects of neuromuscular blocking agents. Several other drugs, however, may cause worsening of the clinical presentation. Among those are various antibiotics (eg, aminoglycoside, macrolides, β-lactams) and calcium antagonists; β-blockers; local anesthetics (eg, lidocaine); phenytoin; or iodine-based contrast mediums [121–124].

Myasthenia gravis

This NMD is characterized by muscle weakness and an overall fatigability that increases with exertion and over the course of the day. MG currently affects about 14:100,000 patients in the United States, with an onset commonly between age 10 and 40. Females are more frequently diagnosed with MG [125–129]. The clinical manifestation in most cases is marked by diplopia and ptosis resulting from weakness of the ocular muscles. The disease may then slowly spread to bulbar muscles, which may lead to aspiration and respiratory failure, and later affect the proximal extremities. The Myasthenia Gravis Foundation of America (www.myasthenia.org) classifies the clinical presentation according to a modified scale initially presented by Osserman and Genkins [131]: class I (ocular muscles only); class II (eye symptoms plus mild generalize weakness); class III (eye plus moderate weakness); class IV (eye plus severe weakness); and class V (intubation, ventilation) [125,127].

MG is an autoimmune disorder caused by circulating antibodies to nicotinic acetylcholine receptors at the neuromuscular junction [129–132]. The antibodies reduce the numbers of receptors available for muscular stimulation by acetylcholine, apparently by blockade and increased degradation of the receptor (different antibody subtypes). There is no competition between the antibodies and acetylcholine, however, because the binding sites at the receptor molecule are different. In patients with long-term MG the number of receptors is decreased to approximately 30%, and many of the residual receptors are bound by an antibody [133]. There is no correlation between the antibody titer and the severity of the disease. Up to 25% of patients have a concurrent thymoma, and about 10% have evidence for other autoimmune diseases [126,129]. More recently, antibodies against the MuSK receptor, which is involved in the formation of the neuromuscular junction, have been identified in MG patients [131,132]. The specific diagnosis involves blood tests for antibodies; electromyographic recordings; cholinesterase inhibitor test (edrophonium test); and imaging (to identify thymoma). Long-term therapeutic interventions aim to improve muscular weakness and to suppress the autoimmune mechanism. Cholinesterase inhibitors (neostigmine, pyridostigmine) are applied for the former and corticosteroids and immunosuppressive drugs (cyclosporine, azathioprine) are used for the latter [134]. In some patients, plasmapheresis is indicated to decrease circulating antibodies (four to eight treatments over 2 weeks) [128,131,134]. In addition, thymectomy is performed in most patients leading to improvement in clinical symptoms in most patients, and in some patients to a complete remission, which sometimes requires several months to determine [135,136]. In general, MG is not a progressive disease, and the symptoms may fluctuate or even spontaneously disappear within several years. With appropriate therapy the life expectancy is normal.

Anesthetic challenges in patients with myasthenia gravis. Respiratory and bulbar functions should be carefully evaluated during the preoperative evaluation. Although the respiratory drive and the CO_2 response are usually intact, patients may have a profoundly diminished vital capacity [137]. Efforts should be made to determine the absence of a larger thymoma, which may cause tracheal compression or even airway collapse during induction of general anesthesia. Cardiac arrhythmias and myocarditis have been described in MG patients, suggesting that preoperative ECG recordings should be part of the preoperative work-up [138–141]. While assessing the airway, the degree of bulbar involvement requires special attention. Medical management before surgery aims to optimize the patient's muscular function. The decision to continue or hold immediate preoperative anticholinergic medication is based on an individual basis. Patients with severe MG should receive preoperative anticholinergic medication (to prevent myasthenic crisis) despite the increased risk of potentiation of vagal responses and decreasing metabolism of local anesthetics and succinylcholine in the intraoperative period [137,142]. Preoperative plasmapheresis has been shown to be very effective preoperatively in severe MG for improving pulmonary function. The reduction in plasma esterases by plasmapheresis, however, prolongs the duration of action of drugs like succinylcholine, esmolol, mivacurium, and remifentanil [142]. Sedative drugs may be dosed very carefully or even avoided completely in MG patients because of the risk for respiratory compromise [121–123,143].

Patients can safely undergo regional anesthesia, and it seems to be the preferential regimen in MG patients whenever possible. The doses of local anesthetics (ester types and amides) should be reduced in patients receiving cholinesterase inhibitors to avoid prolonged blocks and the potential for a myasthenic crisis [140,141,144,145]. If general anesthesia is planned, induction and maintenance may involve intravenous agents, such as propofol, thiopental, and etomidate, and volatile anesthetics. Volatile anesthetics exert muscular relaxation by impairing the neuromuscular transmission, with isoflurane being twice as potent as halothane in MG patients, and independent of the severity of the disease [136,137,142].

Neuromuscular blockers may be used cautiously in MG patients, but their differential effects need to be considered. Compared with patients without MG, succinylcholine has decreased efficacy at low doses and a higher incidence of phase-two block at high doses. At a dose of 1 to 1.5 mg/kg, succinylcholine can be expected to achieve clinical efficacy and duration as expected in a normal patient (1.5–2.0 mg/kg is safe for rapid sequence induction in MG patients) [146]. In contrast, MG patients show high sensitivity to nondepolarizing muscular blocking agents. The reduced number of acetylcholine receptors may require only 10% of the normal dose to elicit a reasonable neuromuscular block. Even then the duration of the block may be prolonged, especially if long-acting drugs, such as pancuronium or rocuronium [147–150], and medium-acting drugs, such as vecuronium (ED95 = 56%) or atracurium, are preferred, although producing a longer than normal block [151–153]. The effects of reversal drugs are unpredictable, especially in patients on chronic anticholinergic treatment, and the excessive administration may precipitate a cholinergic crisis (generalized muscle weakness, bradycardia, increased secretion, and gut motility). The variability in sensitivity to muscular blocking agents does not correlate with the clinical severity of MG, but some report predictability by perioperative monitoring of the train-of-four, which may guide the dosing regime [153]. In addition, drug interactions need to be considered, because substances that are known to exacerbate the clinical symptoms of muscular weakness (aminoglycosides, vancomycin, quinidine, ester-type local anesthetics, furosemide, calcium antagonists, β-blockers) may also amplify the clinical effects of neuromuscular blocking agents [121–123,143].

The two most important concerns during the postoperative period are mechanical ventilation and sufficient pain management. Predictors of the need for postoperative ventilations have been suggested for patients undergoing thymectomy [147]. Postoperative pain control may be a challenge because of the sensitivity of MG patients to any drug with respiratory depressant effects, such as opioids and benzodiazepines. Regional anesthesia may be beneficial for the management of postoperative pain. Neuraxial techniques using epidural opioids were shown to be safe and effective, reduced the overall requirements for systemic narcotics, provided excellent pain relief, and resulted in improved postoperative respiratory function in patients with MS after thymectomy [154]. It is recommended to resume the anticholinergic therapy as soon as possible after surgery. The postoperative requirements may be different from the routine preoperative dose and careful titration is suggested because the IV dose is only about 1/30 to 1/120 of the oral dose because of differences in bioavailability of the two preparations [121–123,143].

Lambert-Eaton syndrome

This is a rare neuromuscular disorder that shares some similarities with MG, but substantial differences in clinical presentations and pathogenetic features characterize the two distinct disorders. It is estimated that LES affects about 1:100,000 individuals in the United States, but it may frequently remain undiagnosed as such. For example, prolonged neuromuscular blockade or general weakness must invoke the thought of LES for all cancer patients who have surgery. About 50% of LES patients have a tumor, and 3% of all patients with small cell lung carcinoma (prevalence in the United States of 1:200,000) are affected by LES [155]. Similar to MG, LES is considered an autoimmune disease. LES, however, is associated with a reduced release of acetylcholine at the presynaptic terminal [129,155–157] secondary to circulating antibodies against voltage-gated calcium channels at the presynaptic neuron. It is currently unknown whether the number, the function, or the location of postsynaptic acetylcholine receptors is also affected. Some patients have no circulating antibodies and the pathomechanism in these cases is currently unknown. Approximately 50% of patients with LES have evidence of malignant tumors, such as lung cancer (frequently small cell type), lymphoma, leukemia, prostate, or bladder cancer [155,158]. Patients present with muscle weakness and hyporeflexia predominantly affecting the proximal extremities (legs more than arms) [127]. In contrast to MG, it rarely affects ocular or bulbar muscles, and muscular strength frequently improves with activity. Autonomic dysfunction is common with dry mouth, dry skin, orthostatic hypotension, and bladder and bowel dysfunction. The diagnostics include clinical evaluation, tests for antibodies to calcium channels, electromyograms, and imaging for possible malignancies. Treatment options are limited: application of anticholinesterases has no effect, but 3,4-diaminopyridine, which blocks potassium channels resulting in a prolonged calcium channel opening and a subsequent increase in acetylcholine release from the presynaptic membrane to stimulate the muscle fiber, has been successfully used [159,160]. Other strategies include treatment with immunosuppressive drugs, such as corticosteroids and azathioprine; plasma exchange; or intravenous immunoglobulin infusions.

Anesthetic challenges in patients with Lambert-Eaton syndrome. The main concern for the anesthesia provider is that patients affected by LES are highly sensitive to depolarizing and nondepolarizing neuromuscular blockers. If muscle relaxants are given, muscle weakness and paralysis may last for days and cannot be antagonized with anticholinesterase, even with doses that are 5% of typical [158,161,162]. If possible, neuromuscular blockers should be avoided, and if needed twitch monitoring may guide dosing. If regional anesthesia is an option it should be preferred. General anesthesia can safely be performed using intravenous or volatile anesthetics. Volatile anesthetics may be of advantage during surgery because the muscular relaxing effects may be sufficient to produce adequate paralysis if desired. As with MG, drugs that may precipitate worsening of neuromuscular transmission should be avoided.

Postjunctional neuromuscular diseases

Disruption of the neuromuscular unit may also result from primary muscular diseases. These comprise a heterogeneous group of at least 30 different diseases that share the common pathophysiologic motive of disruption of the cellular integrity of muscular tissue. Currently, the different disease entities are distinguished basically according to their pathomechanisms in primary muscular dystrophies (eg, DMD, myotonic [163–165], Becker's [166,167], Emery-Dreifuss [168–172]); inflammatory myopathies (eg, dermatomyositis [173–176], polymyositis [177,178]); metabolic muscular dystrophies (eg, mitochondrial myopathy [179–182], lactate dehydrogenase deficiency, phosphofructokinase deficiency [183–186], lipid myopathy [187–189]); and other rare muscular myopathies (eg, nemaline myopathy [190–195], central core disease [196–199]). Most of these are congenital diseases and for several muscular dystrophies the genetic disruption and the affected genetic product have been identified. The disease affects the muscle itself, whereas the neuronal circuitry is intact. Frequently, the myocardium is also affected by the cellular dysfunction. Anesthetic concerns are focused on the use of neuromuscular blockers (succinylcholine must be omitted, nondepolarizing drugs require careful dosing and meticulous monitoring); volatile anesthetics (association with malignant hyperthermia, rhabdomyolysis); and the perioperative respiratory function. The anesthetic implications associated with DMD are described to illustrate the general issues that need to be considered in patients with disease of postjunctional muscle diseases.

Duchenne's muscular dystrophy

This X chromosome–linked recessive disorder is characterized by progressive weakness and atrophy of the skeletal muscles, which initially affects the legs and pelvic area and later spreads to the muscles of shoulder and neck and finally affects the upper extremities and the respiratory muscles. The onset of symptoms is usually around age 5 years and delays motor development. Cardiomyopathy becomes apparent ultimately in about 70% of the patients and cardiac complications and respiratory compromise frequently are responsible for early death in the third decade [200–202].

DMD is the most frequent muscular dystrophy, and it affects about 1:3300 males [203]. DMD is caused by a defective Xp21 gene, which encodes the protein dystrophin that is part of a large protein complex connecting muscle fibers to the extracellular matrix, thereby stabilizing the muscular cytoskeleton [203,204]. In DMD, dystrophin is absent resulting in continuous damage of the sarcolemma by shearing forces and ultimately muscular necrosis and replacement with adipose and connective tissue. In addition, dystrophin seems to play a role in clustering of acetylcholine receptors on the postsynaptic membrane, and DMD patients have large numbers of extrajunctional receptors of fetal phenotype. Finally, dystrophin may have a direct modulating effect on ion channels, and the absence of dystrophin is associated with a larger calcium influx into the muscle cell [205–208]. Dystrophin deficiency seems also to affect neuronal function because approximately 30% of the patients show signs of mental retardation [1].

The diagnosis is based on clinical signs; laboratory tests (serum creatine phosphokinase, myoglobin); electromyography; genetic testing; and muscle biopsy. There is no established causal therapy available for patients with DMD, although high-dose steroid therapy has been reported to reduce symptoms and maintain muscular strength for a time [209–212].

Anesthetic challenges in patients with Duchenne's muscular dystrophy. Patients with DMD frequently present for orthopedic surgery to correct scoliosis or contractures. Some patients with undiagnosed disease at the time of surgery may suffer significant complications from anesthesia including cardiac arrest, rhabdomyolysis, or malignant hyperthermia [213–223]. A thorough history including questions about anesthesia complications in the family, and a careful physical examination, are of paramount importance as an effective screening method. In patients with known DMD the preoperative evaluation should include appropriate tests for respiratory and cardiac performance (pulmonary function tests, echocardiography) [224–226]. Premedication may involve careful dosing of benzodiazepines to treat anxiety, with careful monitoring of respiratory function. Regional anesthesia is the preferred technique when appropriate for the surgery being performed.

If general anesthesia is chosen, any potential trigger for malignant hyperthermia should be avoided [227,228]. Induction should be tailored toward the results of the preoperative cardiac evaluation, and total intravenous anesthesia is suggested for maintenance of general anesthesia [229,230]. Nondepolarizing neuromuscular blockers can safely be applied if necessary, but require neuromuscular monitoring to guide dosing. According to recent reports, the time for onset and the duration of rocuronium and mivacurium was prolonged after conventional doses. In contrast, dose reduction resulted in incomplete paralysis [231–233]. DMD patients are at risk for larger perioperative blood loss because of platelet function deficiency [234,235] and require active temperature control because reduced muscular mass allows more rapid heat loss during surgery.

Summary

A wide range of pathologic conditions can affect the functionality of the neuromuscular unit. Affected patients may require anesthesia management either for problems relevant to the disorders or for comorbid conditions. The different diseases often have specific problems that can usually be predicted from their pathophysiology. The key concerns of the anesthesia provider relate to the potential of an undiagnosed NMD, especially in children; the involvement of vital organ systems; the choice of anesthetic technique; anesthetics drugs; and particularly the effects of neuromuscular blocking agents. Thorough preoperative assessment is essential to develop an appropriate anesthetic plan, the degree of perioperative monitoring, and the extent of postoperative care. With these considerations the patient with NMD, although challenging, can be given anesthetic care in a safe fashion.

References

[1] D'Angelo MG, Bresolin N. Cognitive impairment in neuromuscular disorders. Muscle Nerve 2006;34(1):16–33.

[2] Girshin M, Mukherjee J, Clowney R, et al. The postoperative cardiovascular arrest of a 5-year-old male: an initial presentation of Duchenne's muscular dystrophy. Paediatr Anaesth 2006;16(2):170–3.

[3] Gronert GA. Cardiac arrest after succinylcholine: mortality greater with rhabdomyolysis than receptor upregulation. Anesthesiology 2001;94(3):523–9.

[4] Larach MG, Rosenberg H, Gronert GA, et al. Did anesthetics trigger cardiac arrests in patients with occult myopathies? Anesthesiology 2001;94(5):933–5.

[5] Mathieu J, Allard P, Gobeil G, et al. Anesthetic and surgical complications in 219 cases of myotonic dystrophy. Neurology 1997;49(6):1646–50.

[6] Klinge L, Eagle M, Haggerty ID, et al. Severe phenotype in infantile facioscapulohumeral muscular dystrophy. Neuromuscul Disord 2006;16(9–10):553–8.

[7] Bushby KM, Hill A, Steele JG. Failure of early diagnosis in symptomatic Duchenne muscular dystrophy. Lancet 1999;353(9152):557–8.

[8] Zanette G, Robb N, Zadra N, et al. Undetected central core disease myopathy in an infant presenting for clubfoot surgery. Paediatr Anaesth 2007;17(4):380–2.

[9] Zanette G, Manani G, Pittoni G, et al. Prevalence of unsuspected myopathy in infants presenting for clubfoot surgery. Paediatr Anaesth 1995;5(3):165–70.

[10] Kernstine KH. Preoperative preparation of the patient with myasthenia gravis. Thorac Surg Clin 2005;15(2):287–95.

[11] Franklin JA, Lalikos JF, Wooden WA. A case of mitochondrial myopathy and cleft palate. Cleft Palate Craniofac J 2005;42(3):327–30.

[12] Rowland LP, Shneider NA. Amyotrophic lateral sclerosis. N Engl J Med 2001;344(22): 1688–700.

[13] Pasinetti GM, Ungar LH, Lange DJ, et al. Identification of potential CSF biomarkers in ALS. Neurology 2006;66(8):1218–22.

[14] Monani UR. Spinal muscular atrophy: a deficiency in a ubiquitous protein; a motor neuron-specific disease. Neuron 2005;48(6):885–96.

[15] Moser B, Lirk P, Lechner M, et al. General anaesthesia in a patient with motor neuron disease. Eur J Anaesthesiol 2004;21(11):921–3.

[16] Otsuka N, Igarashi M, Shimodate Y, et al. [Anesthetic management of two patients with amyotrophic lateral sclerosis (ALS)]. Masui 2004;53(11):1279–81, [in Japanese].

[17] Veen A, Molenbuur B, Richardson FJ. Epidural anaesthesia in a child with possible spinal muscular atrophy. Paediatr Anaesth 2002;12(6):556–8.

[18] Fiacchino F, Gemma M, Bricchi M, et al. Sensitivity to curare in patients with upper and lower motor neurone dysfunction. Anaesthesia 1991;46(11):980–2.

[19] Kuisma MJ, Saarinen KV, Teirmaa HT. Undiagnosed amyotrophic lateral sclerosis and respiratory failure. Acta Anaesthesiol Scand 1993;37(6):628–30.

[20] Leypold BG, Flanders AE, Schwartz ED, et al. The impact of methylprednisolone on lesion severity following spinal cord injury. Spine 2007;32(3):373–8.

[21] Dutton RP. Anesthetic management of spinal cord injury: clinical practice and future initiatives. Int Anesthesiol Clin 2002;40(3):103–20.

[22] Crosby ET. Airway management in adults after cervical spine trauma. Anesthesiology 2006;104(6):1293–318.

[23] Bracken MB, Shepard MJ, Collins WF, et al. A randomized, controlled trial of methylpred-nisolone or naloxone in the treatment of acute spinal-cord injury. Results of the Second National Acute Spinal Cord Injury Study. N Engl J Med 1990;322(20):1405–11.

[24] Bracken MB. Steroids for acute spinal cord injury. Cochrane Database Syst Rev 2002;3: CD001046.

[25] Qian T, Campagnolo D, Kirshblum S. High-dose methylprednisolone may do more harm for spinal cord injury. Med Hypotheses 2000;55(5):452–3.

[26] Tator CH. Review of treatment trials in human spinal cord injury: issues, difficulties, and recommendations. Neurosurgery 2006;59(5):957–82.

[27] Tsutsumi S, Ueta T, Shiba K, et al. Effects of the Second National Acute Spinal Cord Injury Study of high-dose methylprednisolone therapy on acute cervical spinal cord injury-results in spinal injuries center. Spine 2006;31(26):2992–6.

[28] Sipski ML, Pearse DD. Methylprednisolone and other confounders to spinal cord injury clinical trials. Nat Clin Pract Neurol 2006;2(8):402–3.

[29] Martyn JA, White DA, Gronert GA, et al. Up-and-down regulation of skeletal muscle acetylcholine receptors: effects on neuromuscular blockers. Anesthesiology 1992;76(5): 822–43.

[30] Stone WA, Beach TP, Hamelberg W. Succinylcholine–danger in the spinal-cord-injured patient. Anesthesiology 1970;32(2):168–9.

[31] Tobey RE. Paraplegia, succinylcholine and cardiac arrest. Anesthesiology 1970;32(4): 359–64.

[32] John DA, Tobey RE, Homer LD, et al. Onset of succinylcholine-induced hyperkalemia following denervation. Anesthesiology 1976;45(3):294–9.

[33] Gronert GA. Use of suxamethonium in cord patients: whether and when. Anaesthesia 1998;53(10):1035–6.

[34] Pope CS, Markenson GR, Bayer-Zwirello LA, et al. Pregnancy complicated by chronic spinal cord injury and history of autonomic hyperreflexia. Obstet Gynecol 2001;97(5 Pt 2): 802–3.

[35] Burns R, Clark VA. Epidural anaesthesia for caesarean section in a patient with quadriplegia and autonomic hyperreflexia. Int J Obstet Anesth 2004;13(2):120–3.

[36] Pereira L. Obstetric management of the patient with spinal cord injury. Obstet Gynecol Surv 2003;58(10):678–87.

[37] Khan A, Haque S, Hyder Z. Outcome from percutaneous nephrolithotomy in patients with spinal cord injury, using a single-stage dilator for access. BJU Int 2005;96(9): 1423.

[38] Cosman BC, Vu TT. Lidocaine anal block limits autonomic dysreflexia during anorectal procedures in spinal cord injury: a randomized, double-blind, placebo-controlled trial. Dis Colon Rectum 2005;48(8):1556–61.

[39] Kantarci O, Wingerchuk D. Epidemiology and natural history of multiple sclerosis: new insights. Curr Opin Neurol. 2006 Jun;19(3):248–54.

[40] Langer-Gould A, Popat RA, Huang SM, et al. Clinical and demographic predictors of long-term disability in patients with relapsing-remitting multiple sclerosis: a systematic review. Arch Neurol 2006;63(12):1686–91.

[41] Fog M, Hyllested K. Prevalence of disseminated sclerosis in the Faroes, the Orkneys and Shetland. Acta Neurol Scand 1966;42(Suppl 19):9–11.

[42] Wasay M, Khatri IA, Khealani B, et al. MS in Asian countries. Int MS J 2006;13(2):58–65.

[43] Marrie RA. Environmental risk factors in multiple sclerosis aetiology. Lancet Neurol 2004; 3(12):709–18.

[44] Sadovnick AD, Dyment D, Ebers GC. Genetic epidemiology of multiple sclerosis. Epidemiol Rev 1997;19(1):99–106.

[45] Imitola J, Chitnis T, Khoury SJ. Insights into the molecular pathogenesis of progression in multiple sclerosis: potential implications for future therapies. Arch Neurol 2006;63(1): 25–33.

[46] Fawcett JW, Asher RA. The glial scar and central nervous system repair. Brain Res Bull 1999;49(6):377–91.

[47] Correale J, de los Milagros Bassani Molinas M. Oligoclonal bands and antibody responses in multiple sclerosis. J Neurol 2002;249(4):375–89.

[48] Calza L, Fernandez M, Giuliani A, et al. Thyroid hormone and remyelination in adult central nervous system: a lesson from an inflammatory-demyelinating disease. Brain Res Brain Res Rev 2005;48(2):339–46, [Epub 2005 Jan 26].

[49] Vedula SS, Brodney-Folse S, Gal RL, et al. Corticosteroids for treating optic neuritis. Cochrane Database Syst Rev 2007;1:CD001430.

[50] Pirko I, Lucchinetti CF, Sriram S, et al. Gray matter involvement in multiple sclerosis. Neurology 2007;68(9):634–42.

[51] Pierson SH, Griffith N. Treatment of cognitive impairment in multiple sclerosis. Behav Neurol 2006;17(1):53–67.

[52] Ameis SH, Feinstein A. Treatment of neuropsychiatric conditions associated with multiple sclerosis. Expert Rev Neurother 2006 Oct;6(10):1555–67.

[53] Feinstein A. Mood disorders in multiple sclerosis and the effects on cognition. J Neurol Sci 2006;245(1–2):63–6, [Epub 2006 Apr 27].

[54] Rickards H. Depression in neurological disorders: an update. Curr Opin Psychiatry 2006; 19(3):294–8.

[55] Navarro S, Mondejar-Marin B, Pedrosa-Guerrero A, et al. Aphasia and parietal syndrome as the presenting symptoms of a demyelinating disease with pseudotumoral lesions. Rev Neurol 2005;41(10):601–3.

[56] Jongen PJ. Psychiatric onset of multiple sclerosis. J Neurol Sci 2006;245(1–2):59–62.

[57] Rees PM, Fowler CJ, Maas CP. Sexual function in men and women with neurological disorders. Lancet 2007;369(9560):512–25.

[58] Poser CM, Brinar VV. Epilepsy and multiple sclerosis. Epilepsy Behav 2003;4(1):6–12.

[59] Kleinschnitz C, Meuth SG, Kieseier BC, et al. Immunotherapeutic approaches in MS: update on pathophysiology and emerging agents or strategies 2006. Endocr Metab Immune Disord Drug Targets 2007;7(1):35–63.

[60] Taylor NF, Dodd KJ, Shields N, et al. Therapeutic exercise in physiotherapy practice is beneficial: a summary of systematic reviews 2002-2005. Aust J Physiother 2007;53(1): 7–16.

[61] De Jager PL, Hafler DA. New therapeutic approaches for multiple sclerosis. Annu Rev Med 2007;58:417–32.

[62] Dorotta IR, Schubert A. Multiple sclerosis and anesthetic implications. Curr Opin Anaesthesiol 2002;15(3):365–70.

[63] Schneider KM. AANA Journal course: update for nurse anesthetists–an overview of multiple sclerosis and implications for anesthesia [review]. AANA J 2005;73(3):217–24.

[64] Ferrero S, Pretta S, Ragni N. Multiple sclerosis: management issues during pregnancy. Eur J Obstet Gynecol Reprod Biol 2004;115(1):3–9.

[65] Smeltzer SC, Skurnick JH, Troiano R, et al. Respiratory function in multiple sclerosis: utility of clinical assessment of respiratory muscle function. Chest 1992;101(2):479–84.

[66] Rabadan Diaz JV, Lopez Moreno JA, Soria Quiles A, et al. Neurological deficit during recovery from cesarean section under spinal anesthesia after the appearance of undiagnosed multiple sclerosis. Rev Esp Anestesiol Reanim 2006;53(10):673–4.

[67] Perlas A, Chan VW. Neuraxial anesthesia and multiple sclerosis. Can J Anaesth 2005;52(5): 454–8.

[68] Finucane BT, Terblanche OC. Prolonged duration of anesthesia in a patient with multiple sclerosis following paravertebral block. Can J Anaesth 2005;52(5):493–7.

[69] Marshak DS, Neustein SM, Thomson J. The use of thoracic epidural analgesia in a patient with multiple sclerosis and severe kyphoscoliosis. J Cardiothorac Vasc Anesth 2006;20(5): 704–6, [Epub 2006 May 30].

[70] Drake E, Drake M, Bird J, et al. Obstetric regional blocks for women with multiple sclerosis: a survey of UK experience. Int J Obstet Anesth 2006;15(2):115–23, [Epub 2006 Feb 20].

[71] Ingrosso M, Cirillo V, Papasso A, et al. Femoral and sciatic nerves block (BiBlock) in orthopedic traumatologic lower limbs surgery in patients with multiple sclerosis. Minerva Anestesiol 2005;71(5):223–6.

[72] Cooperman LH. Succinylcholine-induced hyperkalemia in neuromuscular disease. JAMA 1970;213(11):1867–71.

[73] Brett RS, Schmidt JH, Gage JS, et al. Measurement of acetylcholine receptor concentration in skeletal muscle from a patient with multiple sclerosis and resistance to atracurium. Anesthesiology 1987;66(6):837–9.

[74] Kim CS, Arnold FJ, Itani MS, et al. Decreased sensitivity to metocurine during long-term phenytoin therapy may be attributable to protein binding and acetylcholine receptor changes. Anesthesiology 1992;77(3):500–6.

[75] Couch JR, Hassanein RS. Platelet hyperaggregability in multiple sclerosis. Trans Am Neurol Assoc 1977;102:62–4.

[76] Feuillet L, Guedj E, Laksiri N, et al. Deep vein thrombosis after intravenous immunoglobulins associated with methylprednisolone. Thromb Haemost 2004;92(3):662–5.

[77] Krajewski KM, Lewis RA, Fuerst DR, et al. Neurological dysfunction and axonal degeneration in Charcot-Marie-Tooth disease type 1A. Brain 2000;123(Pt 7):1516–27.

[78] Baloh RH, Schmidt RE, Pestronk A, et al. Altered axonal mitochondrial transport in the pathogenesis of Charcot-Marie-Tooth disease from mitofusin 2 mutations. J Neurosci 2007;27(2):422–30.

[79] Delatycki MB, Holian A, Corben L, et al. Surgery for equinovarus deformity in Friedreich's ataxia improves mobility and independence. Clin Orthop Relat Res 2005;430: 138–41.

[80] Schapira AH. Mitochondrial disease. Lancet 2006;368(9529):70–82.

[81] Rudnik-Schoneborn S, Rohrig D, Nicholson G, et al. Pregnancy and delivery in Charcot-Marie-Tooth disease type 1. Neurology 1993;43(10):2011–6.

[82] Antognini JF. Anaesthesia for Charcot-Marie-Tooth disease: a review of 86 cases. Can J Anaesth 1992;39(4):398–400.

[83] Kotani N, Hirota K, Anzawa N, et al. Motor and sensory disability has a strong relationship to induction dose of thiopental in patients with the hypertropic variety of Charcot-Marie-Tooth syndrome. Anesth Analg 1996;82(1):182–6.

[84] Schmitt HJ, Muenster T, Schmidt J. Central neural blockade in Charcot-Marie-Tooth disease. Can J Anaesth 2004;51(10):1049–50.

[85] Schmitt HJ, Wick S, Munster T. Onset and duration of mivacurium-induced neuromuscular blockade in children with Charcot-Marie-Tooth disease: a case series with five children. Paediatr Anaesth 2006;16(2):182–7.

[86] He X, Sullivan EV, Stankovic RK, et al. Interaction of thiamine deficiency and voluntary alcohol consumption disrupts rat corpus callosum ultrastructure. Neuropsychopharmacology 2007; [Epub ahead of print].

[87] Okamoto H, Miki T, Lee KY, et al. Oligodendrocyte myelin glycoprotein (OMgp) in rat hippocampus is depleted by chronic ethanol consumption. Neurosci Lett 2006;406(1–2): 76–80.

[88] Kuwabara S. Guillain-Barré syndrome. Curr Neurol Neurosci Rep 2007;7(1):57–62.

[89] Douglas MR, Winer JB. Guillain-Barre syndrome and its treatment. Expert Rev Neurother 2006;6(10):1569–74.

[90] Steiner I, Argov Z, Cahan C, et al. Guillain-Barre syndrome after epidural anesthesia: direct nerve root damage may trigger disease. Neurology 1985;35(10):1473–5.

[91] Wiertlewski S, Magot A, Drapier S, et al. Worsening of neurologic symptoms after epidural anesthesia for labor in a Guillain-Barre patient. Anesth Analg 2004;98(3):825–7.

[92] Otermin Maya I, Pereda Garcia A, Lopez Aldaz M, et al. Post-anesthesia recurrence of Guillain-Barre syndrome. Med Clin (Barc) 2006;127(3):118–9.

[93] Flores-Barragan JM, Martinez-Palomeque G, Ibanez R, et al. Guillain-Barre syndrome as a complication of epidural anaesthesia. Rev Neurol 2006;42(10):631–2.

[94] Lehmann HC, Hartung HP, Hetzel GR, et al. Plasma exchange in neuroimmunological disorders: Part 1: rationale and treatment of inflammatory central nervous system disorders. Arch Neurol 2006;63(7):930–5.

[95] Lehmann HC, Hartung HP, Hetzel GR, et al. Plasma exchange in neuroimmunological disorders: part 2. Treatment of neuromuscular disorders. Arch Neurol 2006;63(8):1066–71.

[96] Koski CL, Patterson JV. Intravenous immunoglobulin use for neurologic diseases. J Infus Nurs 2006;29(3 Suppl):S21–8.

[97] Chan LY, Tsui MH, Leung TN. Guillain-Barre syndrome in pregnancy. Acta Obstet Gynecol Scand 2004;83(4):319–25.

[98] Brooks H, Christian AS, May AE. Pregnancy, anaesthesia and Guillain Barre syndrome. Anaesthesia 2000;55(9):894–8.

[99] Dalman JE, Verhagen WI. Cardiac arrest in Guillain-Barre syndrome and the use of suxamethonium. Acta Neurol Belg 1994;94(4):259–61.

[100] Reilly M, Hutchinson M. Suxamethonium is contraindicated in the Guillain-Barre syndrome. J Neurol Neurosurg Psychiatry 1991;54(11):1018–9.

[101] Feldman JM. Cardiac arrest after succinylcholine administration in a pregnant patient recovered from Guillain-Barre syndrome. Anesthesiology 1990;72(5):942–4.

[102] Dhand UK. Clinical approach to the weak patient in the intensive care unit. Respir Care 2006;51(9):1024–40.

[103] Fiacchino F, Gemma M, Bricchi M, et al. Hypo- and hypersensitivity to vecuronium in a patient with Guillain-Barre syndrome. Anesth Analg 1994;78(1):187–9.

[104] Visser LH. Critical illness polyneuropathy and myopathy: clinical features, risk factors and prognosis. Eur J Neurol 2006;13(11):1203–12.

[105] Hund E. Critical illness polyneuropathy. Curr Opin Neurol 2001;14(5):649–53.

[106] Leijten FS, de Weerd AW. Critical illness polyneuropathy, facts and controversies. J Peripher Nerv Syst 1996;1(1):28–33.

[107] Leijten FS, de Weerd AW. Critical illness polyneuropathy: a review of the literature, definition and pathophysiology. Clin Neurol Neurosurg 1994;96(1):10–9.

[108] Williams S, Horrocks IA, Ouvrier RA, et al. Critical illness polyneuropathy and myopathy in pediatric intensive care: a review. Pediatr Crit Care Med 2007;8(1):18–22.

[109] Banwell BL, Mildner RJ, Hassall AC, et al. Muscle weakness in critically ill children. Neurology 2003;61(12):1779–82.

[110] Leijten FS, De Weerd AW, Poortvliet DC, et al. Critical illness polyneuropathy in multiple organ dysfunction syndrome and weaning from the ventilator. Intensive Care Med 1996; 22(9):856–61.

[111] Witt NJ, Zochodne DW, Bolton CF, et al. Peripheral nerve function in sepsis and multiple organ failure. Chest 1991;99(1):176–84.

[112] Hund E. Neurological complications of sepsis: critical illness polyneuropathy and myopathy. J Neurol 2001;248(11):929–34.

[113] Hough CL. Neuromuscular sequelae in survivors of acute lung injury. Clin Chest Med 2006;27(4):691–703.

[114] Hund E, Genzwurker H, Bohrer H, et al. Predominant involvement of motor fibres in patients with critical illness polyneuropathy. Br J Anaesth 1997;78(3):274–8.

[115] Nates JL, Cooper DJ, Day B, et al. Acute weakness syndromes in critically ill patients: a re-appraisal. Anaesth Intensive Care 1997;25(5):502–13.

[116] Biccard BM, Grant IS, Wright DJ, et al. Suxamethonium and critical illness polyneuropathy. Anaesth Intensive Care 1998;26(5):590–1.

[117] Geller TJ, Kaiboriboon K, Fenton GA, et al. Vecuronium-associated axonal motor neuropathy: a variant of critical illness polyneuropathy? Neuromuscul Disord 2001;11(6–7): 579–82.

[118] Hara K, Minami K, Takamoto K, et al. The prolonged effect of a muscle relaxant in a patient with chronic inflammatory demyelinating polyradiculoneuropathy. Anesth Analg 2000;90(1):224–6.

[119] Tuxen DV, Day BJ, Scheinkestel CD. Acute respiratory failure neuropathy: a variant of critical illness polyneuropathy. Crit Care Med 1993;21(12):1986–7.

[120] Engel AG. The therapy of congenital myasthenic syndromes. Neurotherapeutics 2007;4(2): 252–7.

[121] Wittbrodt ET. Drugs and myasthenia gravis: an update. Arch Intern Med 1997;157(4): 399–408.

[122] Rajasekaran D, Chandrasekar S, Rajendran M. Drug related crisis in myasthenia gravis. J Assoc Physicians India 2006;54:820–1, [erratum in: J Assoc Physicians India. 2006 Nov; 54:889].

[123] Feldman S, Karalliedde L. Drug interactions with neuromuscular blockers. Drug Saf 1996; 15(4):261–73.

[124] Ferrero S, Pretta S, Nicoletti A, et al. Myasthenia gravis: management issues during pregnancy. Eur J Obstet Gynecol Reprod Biol 2005;121(2):129–38.

[125] Scherer K, Bedlack RS, Simel DL. Does this patient have myasthenia gravis? JAMA 2005; 293:1906–14.

[126] Phillips LH. The epidemiology of myasthenia gravis. Semin Neurol 2004;24(1):17–20.

[127] Evoli A. Clinical aspects of neuromuscular transmission disorders. Acta Neurol Scand Suppl 2006;183:8–11.

[128] Conti-Fine BM, Milani M, Kaminski HJ. Myasthenia gravis: past, present, and future. J Clin Invest 2006;116(11):2843–54.

[129] Vincent A. Immunology of disorders of neuromuscular transmission. Acta Neurol Scand Suppl 2006;183:1–7.

[130] Vincent A, Leite MI. Neuromuscular junction autoimmune disease: muscle specific kinase antibodies and treatments for myasthenia gravis. Curr Opin Neurol 2005;18(5):519–25.

[131] Osserman KE, Genkins G. Studies in myasthenia gravis: review of a twenty-year experience in over 1200 patients. Mt Sinai J Med 1971;38:497–537.

[132] Vincent A, Rothwell P. Myasthenia gravis. Autoimmunity 2004;37(4):317–9.

[133] Lindstrom JM. Acetylcholine receptors and myasthenia. Muscle Nerve 2000;23(4):453–77.

[134] Sieb JP. Myasthenia gravis: emerging new therapy options. Curr Opin Pharmacol 2005; 5(3):303–7.

[135] Gronseth GS, Barohn RJ. Thymectomy for myasthenia gravis. Curr Treat Options Neurol 2002;4(3):203–9.

[136] White MC, Stoddart PA. Anesthesia for thymectomy in children with myasthenia gravis. Paediatr Anaesth 2004;14(8):625–35.

[137] Dillon FX. Anesthesia issues in the perioperative management of myasthenia gravis. Semin Neurol 2004;24(1):83–94.

[138] Mygland A, Aarli JA, Hofstad H, et al. Heart muscle antibodies in myasthenia gravis. Autoimmunity 1991;10(4):263–7.

[139] de Jongste MJ, Oosterhuis HJ, Lie KI. Intractable ventricular tachycardia in a patient with giant cell myocarditis, thymoma and myasthenia gravis. Int J Cardiol 1986;13(3):374–8.

[140] Lin TC, Hsu CH, Kong SS, et al. Ventricular asystole and complete heart block after thoracic epidural analgesia for thymectomy. Eur J Anaesthesiol 2002;19(6):460–2.

[141] Inoue S, Shiomi T, Furuya H. Severe bradycardia in a patient with myasthenia gravis during transurethral ureterolithotripsic procedure under spinal anaesthesia. Anaesth Intensive Care 2002;30(3):387.

[142] Abel M, Eisenkraft JB. Anesthetic implications of myasthenia gravis. Mt Sinai J Med 2002; 69(1–2):31–7.

[143] Barrons RW. Drug-induced neuromuscular blockade and myasthenia gravis. Pharmacotherapy 1997;17(6):1220–32.

[144] de Jose Maria B, Carrero E, Sala X. Myasthenia gravis and regional anaesthesia. Can J Anaesth 1995;42(2):178–9.

[145] Mekis D, Kamenik M. Remifentanil and high thoracic epidural anaesthesia: a successful combination for patients with myasthenia gravis undergoing transsternal thymectomy. Eur J Anaesthesiol 2005;22(5):397–9.

[146] Levitan R. Safety of succinylcholine in myasthenia gravis. Ann Emerg Med 2005;45(2): 225–6.

[147] Kadoi Y, Hinohara H, Kunimoto F, et al. Is the degree of sensitivity to nondepolarizing muscle relaxants related to requirements for postoperative ventilation in patients with myasthenia gravis? Anaesth Intensive Care 2004;32(3):346–50.

[148] De Haes A, Proost JH, De Baets MH, et al. Decreased number of acetylcholine receptors is the mechanism that alters the time course of muscle relaxants in myasthenia gravis: a study in a rat model. Eur J Anaesthesiol 2005;22(8):591–6.

[149] de Lemos JM, Carr RR, Shalansky KF, et al. Paralysis in the critically ill: intermittent bolus pancuronium compared with continuous infusion. Crit Care Med 1999;27(12):2648–55.

[150] De Haes A, Proost JH, Kuks JB, et al. Pharmacokinetic/pharmacodynamic modeling of rocuronium in myasthenic patients is improved by taking into account the number of unbound acetylcholine receptors. Anesth Analg 2002;95(3):588–96, table of contents.

[151] Tripathi M, Kaushik S, Dubey P. The effect of use of pyridostigmine and requirement of vecuronium in patients with myasthenia gravis. J Postgrad Med 2003;49(4):311–4, [discussion: 314–15].

[152] Itoh H, Shibata K, Nitta S. Sensitivity to vecuronium in seropositive and seronegative patients with myasthenia gravis. Anesth Analg 2002;95(1):109–13.

[153] Mann R, Blobner M, Jelen-Esselborn S, et al. Preanesthetic train-of-four fade predicts the atracurium requirement of myasthenia gravis patients. Anesthesiology 2000;93(2):346–50.

[154] Kirsch JR, Diringer MN, Borel CO, et al. Preoperative lumbar epidural morphine improves postoperative analgesia and ventilatory function after transsternal thymectomy in patients with myasthenia gravis. Crit Care Med 1991;19(12):1474–9.

[155] Mareska M, Gutmann L. Lambert-Eaton myasthenic syndrome. Semin Neurol 2004;24(2): 149–53.

[156] Wirtz PW, Bradshaw J, Wintzen AR, et al. Associated autoimmune diseases in patients with the Lambert-Eaton myasthenic syndrome and their families. J Neurol 2004;251(10):1255–9.

[157] Sidnev DV, Karganov MY, Shcherbakova NI, et al. Antibodies to acetylcholine receptors in patients with different clinical forms of myasthenia and Lambert-Eaton myasthenic syndrome. Neurosci Behav Physiol 2007;37(2):129–31.

[158] O'Neill GN. Acquired disorders of the neuromuscular junction. Int Anesthesiol Clin 2006; 44(2):107–21.

[159] Verschuuren JJ, Wirtz PW, Titulaer MJ, et al. Available treatment options for the management of Lambert-Eaton myasthenic syndrome. Expert Opin Pharmacother 2006;7(10): 1323–36.

[160] Maddison P, Newsom-Davis J. Treatment for Lambert-Eaton myasthenic syndrome. Cochrane Database Syst Rev 2005;2:CD003279.

[161] Small S, Ali HH, Lennon VA, et al. Anesthesia for an unsuspected Lambert-Eaton myasthenic syndrome with autoantibodies and occult small cell lung carcinoma. Anesthesiology 1992;76(1):142–5.

[162] Telford RJ, Hollway TE. The myasthenic syndrome: anaesthesia in a patient treated with 3.4 diaminopyridine. Br J Anaesth 1990;64(3):363–6.

[163] Trip J, Drost G, van Engelen BG, et al. Drug treatment for myotonia. Cochrane Database Syst Rev 2006;1:CD004762.

[164] Huang CC, Kuo HC. Myotonic dystrophies. Chang Gung Med J 2005;28(8):517–26.

[165] White RJ, Bass SP. Myotonic dystrophy and paediatric anaesthesia. Paediatr Anaesth 2003;13(2):94–102.

[166] Novakovic I, Bojic D, Todorovic S, et al. Proximal dystrophin gene deletions and protein alterations in Becker muscular dystrophy. Ann N Y Acad Sci 2005;1048:406–10.

[167] Drouet A, Leturcq F, Guilloton L, et al. Muscular exercise intolerance syndrome in Becker muscular dystrophy. Presse Med 2002;31(5):197–201.

[168] Muchir A, Worman HJ. Emery-Dreifuss muscular dystrophy. Curr Neurol Neurosci Rep 2007;7(1):78–83.

[169] Ifergane G, Al-Sayed I, Birk O, et al. Co-morbidity of Emery-Dreifuss muscular dystrophy and a congenital myasthenic syndrome possibly affecting the phenotype in a large Bedouin kindred. Eur J Neurol 2007;14(3):305–8.

[170] English KM, Gibbs JL. Cardiac monitoring and treatment for children and adolescents with neuromuscular disorders. Dev Med Child Neurol 2006;48(3):231–5.

[171] Choudhry DK, Mackenzie WG. Anesthetic issues with a hyperextended cervical spine in a child with Emery-Dreifuss syndrome. Anesth Analg 2006;103(6):1611–3.

[172] Shende D, Agarwal R. Anaesthetic management of a patient with Emery-Dreifuss muscular dystrophy. Anaesth Intensive Care 2002;30(3):372–5.

[173] Callen JP, Wortmann RL. Dermatomyositis. Clin Dermatol 2006;24(5):363–73.

[174] Rockelein S, Gebert M, Baar H, et al. Neuromuscular blockade with atracurium in dermatomyositis. Anaesthesist 1995;44(6):442–4.

[175] Ganta R, Campbell IT, Mostafa SM. Anaesthesia and acute dermatomyositis/polymyositis. Br J Anaesth 1988;60(7):854–8.

[176] Quain RD, Werth VP. Management of cutaneous dermatomyositis: current therapeutic options. Am J Clin Dermatol 2006;7(6):341–51.

[177] Briani C, Doria A, Sarzi-Puttini P, et al. Update on idiopathic inflammatory myopathies. Autoimmunity 2006;39(3):161–70.

[178] Saarnivaara LH. Anesthesia for a patient with polymyositis undergoing myectomy of the cricopharyngeal muscle. Anesth Analg 1988;67(7):701–2.

[179] Sasano N, Fujita Y, So M, et al. Anesthetic management of a patient with mitochondrial myopathy, encephalopathy, lactic acidosis, and stroke-like episodes (MELAS) during laparotomy. J Anesth 2007;21(1):72–5.

[180] Allison KR. Muscular dystrophy versus mitochondrial myopathy: the dilemma of the undiagnosed hypotonic child. Paediatr Anaesth 2007;17(1):1–6.

[181] Shipton EA, Prosser DO. Mitochondrial myopathies and anaesthesia. Eur J Anaesthesiol 2004;21(3):173–8.

[182] Driessen J, Willems S, Dercksen S, et al. Anesthesia-related morbidity and mortality after surgery for muscle biopsy in children with mitochondrial defects. Paediatr Anaesth 2007; 17(1):16–21.

[183] Mastaglia FL. Neuromuscular disorders: molecular and therapeutic insights. Lancet Neurol 2005;4(1):6–7.

[184] Nakajima H, Raben N, Hamaguchi T, et al. Phosphofructokinase deficiency; past, present and future. Curr Mol Med 2002;2(2):197–212.

[185] Servidei S, DiMauro S. Disorders of glycogen metabolism of muscle. Neurol Clin 1989;7(1): 159–78.

[186] Ing RJ, Cook DR, Bengur RA, et al. Anaesthetic management of infants with glycogen storage disease type II: a physiological approach. Paediatr Anaesth 2004;14(6):514–9.

[187] Klingler W, Lehmann-Horn F, Jurkat-Rott K. Complications of anaesthesia in neuromuscular disorders. Neuromuscul Disord 2005;15(3):195–206, [Epub 2005 Jan 28].

[188] Darras BT, Friedman NR. Metabolic myopathies: a clinical approach; part II. Pediatr Neurol 2000;22(3):171–81.

[189] Cwik VA. Disorders of lipid metabolism in skeletal muscle. Neurol Clin 2000;18(1): 167–84.

[190] Wallgren-Pettersson C, Laing NG. 109th ENMC International Workshop: 5th workshop on nemaline myopathy, 11th-13th October 2002, Naarden, The Netherlands. Neuromuscul Disord 2003;13(6):501–7.

[191] Udd B, Meola G, Krahe R, et al. 140th ENMC International Workshop: Myotonic Dystrophy DM2/PROMM and other myotonic dystrophies with guidelines on management. Neuromuscul Disord 2006;16(6):403–13.

[192] Wallgren-Pettersson C. Nemaline and myotubular myopathies. Semin Pediatr Neurol 2002;9(2):132–44.

[193] Ryan MM, Schnell C, Strickland CD, et al. Nemaline myopathy: a clinical study of 143 cases. Ann Neurol 2001;50(3):312–20.

[194] Stackhouse R, Chelmow D, Dattel BJ. Anesthetic complications in a pregnant patient with nemaline myopathy. Anesth Analg 1994;79(6):1195–7.

[195] Shenkman Z, Sheffer O, Erez I, et al. Spinal anesthesia for gastrostomy in an infant with nemaline myopathy. Anesth Analg 2000;91(4):858–9.

[196] Talwalkar SS, Parker JR, Heffner RR, et al. Adult central core disease. Clinical, histologic and genetic aspects: case report and review of the literature. Clin Neuropathol 2006;25(4): 180–4.

[197] Priori SG, Napolitano C. Cardiac and skeletal muscle disorders caused by mutations in the intracellular Ca2+ release channels. J Clin Invest 2005;115(8):2033–8.

[198] Avila G. Intracellular Ca2+ dynamics in malignant hyperthermia and central core disease: established concepts, new cellular mechanisms involved. Cell Calcium 2005;37(2):121–7.

[199] McCarthy TV, Quane KA, Lynch PJ. Ryanodine receptor mutations in malignant hyperthermia and central core disease. Hum Mutat 2000;15(5):410–7.

[200] Townsend D, Yasuda S, Metzger J. Cardiomyopathy of Duchenne muscular dystrophy: pathogenesis and prospect of membrane sealants as a new therapeutic approach. Expert Rev Cardiovasc Ther 2007;5(1):99–109.

[201] Simonds AK. Recent advances in respiratory care for neuromuscular disease. Chest 2006; 130(6):1879–86.

[202] Finsterer J. Cardiopulmonary support in Duchenne muscular dystrophy. Lung 2006; 184(4):205–15.

[203] Deconinck N, Dan B. Pathophysiology of Duchenne muscular dystrophy: current hypotheses. Pediatr Neurol 2007;36(1):1–7.

[204] Anderson JE, Hansen LL, Mooren FC, et al. Methods and biomarkers for the diagnosis and prognosis of cancer and other diseases: towards personalized medicine. Drug Resist Updat 2006;9(4–5):198–210.

[205] Allard B. Sarcolemmal ion channels in dystrophin-deficient skeletal muscle fibres. J Muscle Res Cell Motil 2006;27(5–7):367–73.

[206] Gissel H. The role of Ca2+ in muscle cell damage. Ann N Y Acad Sci 2005;1066:166–80.

[207] Naguib M, Flood P, McArdle JJ, et al. Advances in neurobiology of the neuromuscular junction: implications for the anesthesiologist. Anesthesiology 2002;96(1):202–31.

[208] Sekiguchi M. The role of dystrophin in the central nervous system: a mini review. Acta Myol 2005;24(2):93–7.

[209] Wagner KR, Lechtzin N, Judge DP. Current treatment of adult Duchenne muscular dystrophy. Biochim Biophys Acta 2007;1772(2):229–37.

[210] Patel K, Macharia R, Amthor H. Molecular mechanisms involving IGF-1 and myostatin to induce muscle hypertrophy as a therapeutic strategy for Duchenne muscular dystrophy. Acta Myol 2005;24(3):230–41.

[211] Ames WA, Hayes JA, Crawford MW. The role of corticosteroids in Duchenne muscular dystrophy: a review for the anesthetist. Paediatr Anaesth 2005;15(1):3–8.

[212] Blake DJ, Kroger S. The neurobiology of Duchenne muscular dystrophy: learning lessons from muscle? Trends Neurosci 2000;23(3):92–9.

[213] Allen GC. Malignant hyperthermia and associated disorders. Curr Opin Rheumatol 1993; 5(6):719–24.

[214] Ali SZ, Taguchi A, Rosenberg H. Malignant hyperthermia. Best Pract Res Clin Anaesthesiol 2003;17(4):519–33.

[215] Smelt WL. Cardiac arrest during desflurane anaesthesia in a patient with Duchenne's muscular dystrophy. Acta Anaesthesiol Scand 2005;49(2):267–9.

[216] Nathan A, Ganesh A, Godinez RI, et al. Hyperkalemic cardiac arrest after cardiopulmonary bypass in a child with unsuspected Duchenne muscular dystrophy. Anesth Analg 2005;100(3):672–4.

[217] Tokunaga C, Hiramatsu Y, Noma M, et al. Delayed onset malignant hyperthermia after a closure of ventricular septal defect. Kyobu Geka 2005;58(3):201–5.

[218] Hayes JA, Ames WA. Acute heart failure during spinal surgery in a boy with Duchenne muscular dystrophy. Br J Anaesth 2004;92(1):149.

[219] Takagi A. [Malignant hyperthermia of Duchenne muscular dystrophy: application of clinical grading scale and caffeine contracture of skinned muscle fibers]. Rinsho Shinkeigaku 2000;40(5):423–7, [in Japanese].

[220] Breucking E, Reimnitz P, Schara U, et al. Anesthetic complications: the incidence of severe anesthetic complications in patients and families with progressive muscular dystrophy of the Duchenne and Becker types. Anaesthesist 2000;49(3):187–95.

[221] Hu J, Higuchi I, Inose M, et al. Characteristic expression of thrombomodulin in the muscle sarcoplasm in patients with the acute phase of rhabdomyolysis. Eur Neurol 2000;43(3): 174–80.

[222] Takahashi H, Shimokawa M, Sha K, et al. Sevoflurane can induce rhabdomyolysis in Duchenne's muscular dystrophy. Masui 2002;51(2):190–2.

[223] Flick RP, Gleich SJ, Herr MM, et al. The risk of malignant hyperthermia in children undergoing muscle biopsy for suspected neuromuscular disorder. Paediatr Anaesth 2007; 17(1):22–7.

[224] Pruijs JE, van Tol MJ, van Kesteren RG, et al. Neuromuscular scoliosis: clinical evaluation pre- and postoperative. J Pediatr Orthop B 2000;9(4):217–20.

[225] Harper CM, Ambler G, Edge G. The prognostic value of pre-operative predicted forced vital capacity in corrective spinal surgery for Duchenne's muscular dystrophy. Anaesthesia 2004;59(12):1160–2.

[226] Almenrader N, Patel D. Spinal fusion surgery in children with non-idiopathic scoliosis: is there a need for routine postoperative ventilation? Br J Anaesth 2006;97(6):851–7.

[227] Yemen TA, McClain C. Muscular dystrophy, anesthesia and the safety of inhalational agents revisited, again. Paediatr Anaesth 2006;16(2):105–8.

[228] Schmitt HJ, Schmidt J, Muenster T. Dystrophin deficiency, inhalational anesthetics, and rhabdomyolysis. Paediatr Anaesth 2007;17(1):94–5.

[229] Kawaai H, Tanaka K, Yamazaki S. Continuous infusion propofol general anesthesia for dental treatment in patients with progressive muscular dystrophy. Anesth Prog 2005; 52(1):12–6.

[230] Molyneux MK. Anaesthetic management during labour of a manifesting carrier of Duchenne muscular dystrophy. Int J Obstet Anesth 2005;14(1):58–61.

[231] Schmidt J, Muenster T, Wick S, et al. Onset and duration of mivacurium-induced neuromuscular block in patients with Duchenne muscular dystrophy. Br J Anaesth 2005;95(6): 769–72.

[232] Wick S, Muenster T, Schmidt J, et al. Onset and duration of rocuronium-induced neuromuscular blockade in patients with Duchenne muscular dystrophy. Anesthesiology 2005; 102(5):915–9.

[233] Muenster T, Schmidt J, Wick S, et al. Rocuronium 0.3 mg × kg-1 (ED95) induces a normal peak effect but an altered time course of neuromuscular block in patients with Duchenne's muscular dystrophy. Paediatr Anaesth 2006;16(8):840–5.

[234] Turturro F, Rocca B, Gumina S, et al. Impaired primary hemostasis with normal platelet function in Duchenne muscular dystrophy during highly-invasive spinal surgery. Neuromuscul Disord 2005;15(8):532–40.

[235] Forst J, Forst R, Leithe H, et al. Platelet function deficiency in Duchenne muscular dystrophy. Neuromuscul Disord 1998;8(1):46–9.

ANESTHESIOLOGY
CLINICS

Anesthesiology Clin
25 (2007) 511–533

Considerations for Airway Management for Cervical Spine Surgery in Adults

Edward T. Crosby, MD, FRCPC

Department of Anesthesiology, University of Ottawa, The Ottawa Hospital–General Campus, Suite 1401, 501 Smyth Road, Ottawa, Ontario K1H 8L6, Canada

Surgery on the cervical spine runs the gamut from minor interventions done in a minimally invasive fashion on a short-stay or ambulatory basis, to major surgical undertakings of a high-risk, high-threat nature done to stabilize a degraded skeletal structure to preserve and protect neural elements. Planning for optimum airway management and anesthesia care is facilitated by an appreciation of the disease processes that affect the cervical spine and their biomechanical implications and an understanding of the imaging and operative techniques used to evaluate and treat these conditions. This article provides some of the background information and evidence to allow the anesthesia practitioner to develop a conceptual framework within which to develop strategies for care when a patient is presented for surgery on the cervical spine.

The adult cervical spine: anatomy and stability

Anatomy of the cervical spine

The first cervical vertebra, the atlas, is a ring-shaped structure with thick anterior and posterior arches that merge with large lateral masses (Fig. 1). Large kidney-shaped depressions on the upper aspects of the lateral masses articulate with the occipital condyles of the skull. The flatter interior surfaces of the lateral masses transmit the weight of the skull onto the superior facet joints of the axis, the second cervical vertebra. The body of the axis extends upward to form the odontoid process; the narrowed waist of the odontoid process is tethered posteriorly by the transverse ligament. Alar and apical ligaments fan upward from the odontoid process to insert on the anterior margins of the foramen magnum of the skull.

E-mail address: ecrosby@sympatico.ca

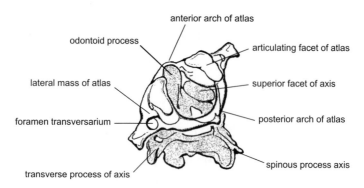

Fig. 1. Detail of atlantoaxial (C1-C2) articulation with skull removed.

The subaxial cervical vertebrae from C3 to C5 are anatomically more typical vertebra. There is an intervertebral disk between C2 and C3 and each subjacent pair of vertebra, and these disks account for about 25% of total spinal length at maturity. The disks are composed of peripheral fibrocartilage, the annulus fibrosis, surrounding a soft central core, the nucleus pulposus. The nucleus contains a high proportion of hydrophilic glycosaminoglycans and functions as a cushion. The arches of the subaxial cervical vertebrae articulate with each other by horizontally oriented facet joints.

The anterior longitudinal ligament ascends along the anterior surface of the spine. It terminates over the anterior arch of the atlas inserting on the base of the skull. The posterior longitudinal ligament courses upward along the dorsal surface of the vertebral bodies, fans over the body of the axis and odontoid process, and terminates as a tectorial membrane, which also inserts into the skull. The ligamentum flavum connects the adjacent lamina; it is often a tenuous structure in the cervical spine. Coursing between spinous processes are the interspinous and supraspinous ligaments.

Anatomy of the aging spine

The aging spine undergoes considerable changes in anatomy [1]. The quantity of water present in the disk nucleus decreases and both spinal height and the cushioning effect previously described are reduced. Gaps and fissures may develop in the disks, and with time they may become desiccated and even ossified. As the spine decreases in length, there may be buckling of both anterior and posterior longitudinal ligaments. The buckling posterior ligament may project into the spinal canal, reducing the space available for the cord. Bony osteophytes and excrescences may develop in the region of the vertebral bodies; end plate osteophytes may grow across the disk spaces and merge with osteophytes of subjacent vertebra to form bridging osteophytes. If these bridging osteophytes involve the posterior end plates, they may also project into the spinal canal, narrowing the lumen.

Patients with congenitally narrow spinal canals are at greater risk for spinal cord compression as a result of these pathologic changes. Large bridging osteophytes on the anterior end plates may result in dysphagia, respiratory symptoms, or may lead to difficulties with airway management. The aperture of the foramen, which transmit the spinal nerves, may be reduced both with the loss of spinal length and ossification of these soft tissues around the vertebral column. These age-related changes account for the symptomatology in most patients presenting for cervical spine surgery.

Movement and stability of the cervical spine

Flexion-extension occurs in the upper cervical spine at both the atlanto-occipital and atlantoaxial articulations and a combined 24 degrees of motion may be achieved [2]. For the jaw to open wide, head extension must simultaneously occur [3]. Extension probably facilitates mouth opening by stretching the neck muscles responsible for jaw gape, allowing them to shorten by greater absolute lengths and increasing mouth opening. Head extension decreases the Mallampati class by an average of 0.5 for classes 2, 3, and 4 compared with when the examination is made with the head in a neutral position [4]. Significantly reduced extension limits mouth opening and Calder and colleagues [5] have reported that limited separation of the upper posterior spinal elements reduces both head extension and mouth opening resulting in more difficult direct laryngoscopy.

The ligaments contributing to the stability of the upper complex are the transverse, apical, and alar ligaments and the superior terminations of the anterior and posterior longitudinal ligaments. In adults, the transverse ligament limits separation of the odontoid process (dens) and the anterior arch of the atlas to less than or equal to 3 mm; this gap is termed the "anterior atlas-dens interval." Destruction of these ligaments is a common consequence of severe and long-standing rheumatoid arthritis and is also seen commonly in Down syndrome [6]. The interval between the posterior aspect of the odontoid process and the anterior aspect of the posterior ring of the atlas is termed the "posterior atlas-dens interval" and is also referred to as the "space available for the cord." A reduced posterior atlas-dens interval has been identified as being more predictive of increased potential for neurologic compromise than is an increased anterior atlas-dens interval [7]. The space available for the cord at C1 may be divided into one-half cord and one-half "space"; the space allows for some encroachment of the spinal lumen without cord compromise (Fig. 2). Progressive narrowing of the canal combined with widening of the cord diameter reduces the space available for the cord between the C4 and C7 levels such that at the lower levels, the spinal cord normally fills approximately 75% of the cross-sectional area of the canal [8].

In adults, the dimensions of the midcervical spinal cord remain relatively constant with the average midsagittal cord diameter being 8 to 9 mm but the vertebral canal at the same levels shows substantial individual variation [9].

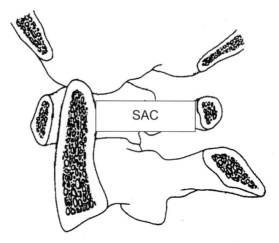

Fig. 2. Space available for the cord (SAC) at the C1 level. The odontoid process occupies about one third of the potential space, the spinal cord about one third, and the remainder is available as reserve; two thirds of the lumen is considered as SAC.

The canal is considered stenotic when its midsagittal dimension is less than 13 mm on a lateral radiograph or when the Torg-Pavlov ratio (calculated by comparing the sagittal diameter of the spinal canal with that of the corresponding vertebral body) is less than 0.8 [10]. A congenitally narrowed canal is hypothesized to increase the threat to the spinal cord with both acquired stenosis and following traumatic injury and is also an associated factor in transient cervical cord neuropraxia after injury [11].

A further 66 degrees of flexion-extension may be achieved in the lower cervical spine with the C5 to C7 segments contributing the largest component. There is an inverse relationship between age and range of motion (ie, as age increases, mobility decreases).

Biomechanics of the spinal cord and canal

For proper functioning of the spinal cord, a minimum canal lumen is required, both at rest and during movement, and cord compromise results if the canal space is less than that required; neurologic injury occurs if this reduction is persistent. The injury results from sustained mechanical pressure on the cord leading to both anatomic deformation and ischemia. Although neurologic deficits do not directly correlate with the degree of posttraumatic canal reduction, canal impingement is more commonly observed in patients with both spinal injury and neurologic deficit than in patients who do not have a deficit after spinal injury [12].

As the spine flexes, the posterior spinal elements, including the canal, transcribe an arc, but that of a larger circle than the anterior elements and the canal axially lengthens [13,14]. As it lengthens, its cross-sectional area is reduced, and as it shortens (in extension), its area is increased; this behavior is termed the "Poisson effect." With flexion, the cord is stretched and its diameter is also reduced and the converse effect occurs in extension. The shortening and folding of the cord when the spine is in extension may result in a relative increase in the ratio of cord size to canal lumen, despite the potential increase in the lumen. Posterior protrusion of the disk annulus and buckling of the ligamentum flavum occurs in extension, which may further reduce canal dimensions at any given level. A number of age-related pathologic processes, including osteophyte formation and ossification of the posterior longitudinal ligament, may lead to further impingement on the canal lumen; these typically manifest a greater impact during spinal extension and may result in canal occlusion (Fig. 3) [15]. The cord tolerates a degree of elastic deformation while still maintaining normal neurologic function [16]. It may be further stretched and deformed, however, if there is a local anomaly, such as an osteophyte, prolapsed disk, or subluxed vertebral body projecting into the canal. These deformations may, over time, result in the application of strain and shear forces to the cord and ultimately result in myelopathy [15].

Prone positioning is often associated with modest degrees of extension, and there is evidence that canal stenosis is increased in patients with cervical myelopathy who are positioned prone [17]. Again, this is likely a manifestation of the soft tissue encroachment on the spinal canal with extension and aggravated by the pre-existent canal compromise. The clinical relevance of these findings is that a persistent malposition of an abnormal neck may result in a degree of cord compression. If the abnormality is modest, it is likely that the malposition needs to be of greater magnitude and persistent

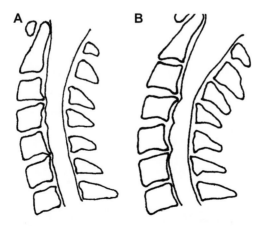

Fig. 3. Impact of extension on age-related changes. Posterior bridging osteophytes are diagrammed at the C3-C4 and C5-C6 levels and a buckling of the posterior longtitudinal ligament is shown at C4-C5 (*A*). With extension demonstrated in (*B*), the canal is shortened and the impact of the posterior changes on the lumenal space is increased; cord compression may occur or be aggravated.

to cause harm; as the anatomic derangement is increased, the duration of positional stress required to cause harm is shortened [18,19]. Prone positioning is also associated with increases in vena caval pressures, which may further reduce cord blood flow already compromised by cord compression by increasing resistance in the venous outflow channels [20].

Syndromes and disorders associated with cervical spinal pathology

Congenital syndromes with spinal pathology

The Chiari malformation is a congenital anomaly characterized by crowding of the posterior fossa by the neural elements and hindbrain herniation through the foramen magnum (Fig. 4) [21]. There is typically abnormal flow of cerebrospinal fluid across the foramen magnum and this may lead to the development of syringomyelia in the cervical cord. There are four types of the Chiari malformation described, and type I is the most common in adults, occurring in up to 0.5% of the population (Table 1) [21]. Type II malformations are more severe and associated with a myelomeningocele, and types III and IV are associated with high early mortality. Anomalies of the base of the skull and upper cervical spine are seen in many patients with type I and may include occipitalization of C1, fusion of C1 to C2, Klippel-Feil deformity, or cervical spina bifida occulta [22].

Although type I defects can be asymptomatic, patients may present with head and neck pain; occipital headache; gait disturbances; neurologic deficits of the upper extremities; and visual, co-ordination, and balance problems. The symptoms are thought to be related to either compression of the neural elements of the posterior fossa or spinal cord dysfunction

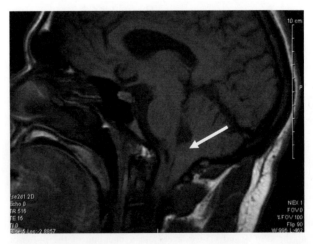

Fig. 4. Chiari type I malformation. Herniation of the cerebellar tonsils through the foramen magnum (*arrow*); crowding of the posterior fossa is also evident. This patient presented for suboccipital craniectomy.

Table 1
Chiari malformation types

Type	Characteristics
I	Displacement of cerebellar tonsils, crowding of posterior fossa, syringomyelia
II	Associated with myelomeningocele, displacement of medulla, fourth ventricle and cerebellum, elongation of pons and fourth ventricle, hydrocephalus common
III	Occipitocervical dysraphism with herniation of posterior fossa and brainstem
IV	Failed development of posterior fossa, malformations of brain and brainstem

related to the syrinx. In symptomatic patients, local decompression of the malformation, achieved by a suboccipital craniectomy, may relieve symptoms; more aggressive decompression with resection of cerebellar tissue and drainage of the syrinx with a syringosubarachnoid shunt may be necessary in some patients to provide relief.

Klippel-Feil syndrome is defined as a congenital fusion of two or more cervical vertebrae and three subtypes are described (Fig. 5, Table 2) [23]. Coexisting congenital defects of the spinal cord or brain are encountered in about a third of patients, consisting most commonly of cervical cord dysraphism or diastematomyelia and Chiari I malformations [24]. Although fused segments may directly limit the range of motion of the neck, more serious

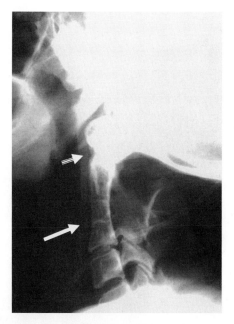

Fig. 5. Klippel-Feil syndrome type 1. Fused element comprising a number of contiguous vertebrae (*large arrow*); hypermobile C1-C2 articulation caused by the failed ossification of the tip of the odontoid process (*small arrow*).

Table 2
Klippel-Feil syndrome subtypes

Type	Characteristics
1	Cervical and upper thoracic fusion, typically of three or more levels
2	Multiple noncontiguous cervical fusions, associated hemivertebrae or atlanto-occipital fusion
3	Multiple contiguous, congenitally fused cervical segments

complications including instability, hypermobility, and symptomatic stenosis arise at the interspaces between fused segments [25]. Patients with progressive symptomatic segmental instability or neurologic compromise are candidates for surgical stabilization of the abnormal region of the cervical spine.

Inflammatory arthropathy and the cervical spine

Diffuse idiopathic skeletal hyperostosis is an ossifying disorder leading to new bone formation in spinal and extraspinal sites, paravertebral osteophyte formation, and ligamentous calcification with ossification (Fig. 6) [26]. The thoracolumbar spine is more frequently involved, although isolated or predominant cervical spine involvement is reported. Cervical spine involvement

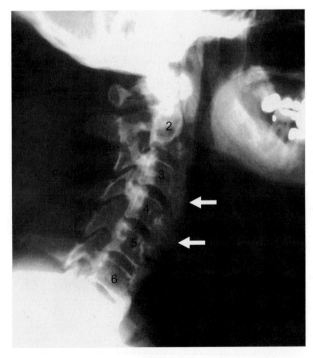

Fig. 6. Diffuse idiopathic skeletal hyperostosis (DISH). Multiple large anterior osteophytes characteristic of DISH (arrows).

in diffuse idiopathic skeletal hyperostosis is a recognized cause of various clinical manifestations involving the pharynx, larynx, and the esophagus resulting in such symptoms as dysphagia and airway symptoms, such as dyspnea or stridor; complications with endoscopy and intubation difficulties may also occur [26–28]. In patients with severe diffuse idiopathic skeletal hyperostosis, fractures of the cervical spine [29] may occur through the cervical body, and subsequent motion concentrates at the fracture site often leading to hematoma and cord compression; catastrophic neurologic sequelae may occur even after relatively minor trauma. Reduction and immobilization or instrumentation is advocated to restore spinal alignment and prevent neurologic injury.

Cervical spine involvement occurs in over half of patients with rheumatoid arthritis, usually in patients with severe, long-standing disease [6]. The most common abnormality is atlantoaxial subluxation, followed by atlanto-occipital arthritis with cranial settling and by lesions of the lower cervical spine [30]. Anterior atlantoaxial subluxation is the most prevalent form, accounting for about 80% of all types of subluxation. Vertical subluxation describes the upward migration of the odontoid process into the foramen magnum and results in inevitable neurologic compromise with myelopathy (Fig. 7). A large percentage of rheumatoid patients with cervical spine involvement progress toward complex instability patterns, including subaxial stepladder deformity, resulting in significant morbidity and

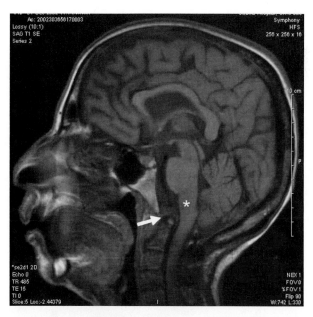

Fig. 7. Rheumatoid arthritis with vertical subluxation. Vertical subluxation of the odontoid process into the foramen magnum (*arrow*). There is considerable pannus surrounding the odontoid and the brainstem is elevated and compressed by the odontoid-pannus complex (*asterisk*).

mortality [31,32]. Once myelopathy occurs, the prognosis for neurologic recovery and long-term survival is poor. Surgery is indicated in patients with intractable pain and in those with progressive neurologic impairment and typically involves instrumentation and fusion.

Ankylosing spondylitis is a systemic inflammatory, progressive arthritic condition [33]. It mainly affects the sacroiliac joints and spine, and is characterized by inflammation or ossification of the disk, ligamentous structures, and facet joints (Fig. 8). With progression of the disease the spine frequently adopts a rigid fused kyphotic deformity. Atlantoaxial subluxation also occurs in up to 21% of patients with ankylosing spondylitis and may reflect a tendency toward hypermobility in spinal segments adjacent to fused elements. In advanced disease, a fixed cervical kyphosis may develop leading to a chin-on-chest deformity. The deformity prevents horizontal gaze; impedes activities of daily living, such as eating and drinking; and may induce severe pain. Cervicothoracic extension osteotomy with instrumentation (posterior or combined anterior and posterior) may be undertaken to return the spine to a more functional alignment [34].

Osteoporosis weakens the brittle ankylosing spondylitis spine and it is susceptible to fractures with minor or unrecognized trauma; they occur mainly in the lower cervical spine and are often displaced and unstable. Failure to immobilize the fracture may result in continuing movement at the fracture site, leading to a neurologic injury or rupture of the epidural veins

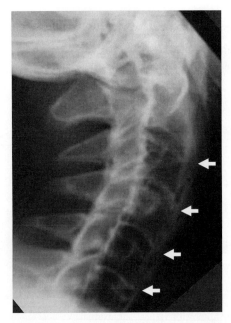

Fig. 8. Ankylosing spondylitis. Ossified anterior longitudinal ligament (*arrows*). Ossification of the posterior ligament is evident, and the vertebral bodies are significantly osteoporotic.

producing an epidural hematoma and subsequent cord compromise. A high rate of spinal cord injury is associated and mortality rates of 35% to 50% are associated with such fractures [35]. The onset of neurologic dysfunction may be delayed for weeks after the initial trauma [32]. In the presence of an unstable fracture, decompression and stabilization using internal fixation and bone graft, with or without laminectomy, is indicated.

Spondylomyelopathy and radiculopathy

The most common cause of radiculopathy is foraminal stenosis with encroachment of the spinal nerves primarily caused by decreased disk height and degenerative changes of the vertebral joints [36]. The final common pathway for cervical myelopathy is a decreased space available for the cord leading to spinal cord compression [37]. Many patients with cervical spondylotic myelopathy from purely degenerative changes also have some degree of congenital spinal stenosis. The age-related degenerative changes seen throughout the spine are the predominant pathology in cervical spondylotic myelopathy. Spinal cord compression resulting from these age-related degenerative changes is typically a slowly progressive process [38]. Cervical kyphosis is also common in patients with significant spondylotic changes, and this deformity aggravates the degree of compression as the spinal cord is stretched over the posterior aspects of the disks and vertebral bodies. Dynamic cord compression may occur with either extension or flexion in patients with severely compromised canal lumens [39]. Patients with chronic cervical spondylosis who suffer acute minor trauma, particularly a hyperextension injury, may sustain an acute spinal cord injury of varying severity superimposed on the long-standing myelopathy. Typically, this presents as a central cord syndrome with greater weakness in the upper extremities than in the lower extremities, and proximal rather than distal muscle involvement in each extremity.

For patients with foraminal stenosis and nerve compression or canal stenosis with cord compression and myelopathy, surgical decompression is indicated to alter the natural history of inevitable deterioration. Surgery can be expected to reduce pain and to slow or halt the progression of neurologic dysfunction, and may improve motor, sensory, and gait disturbances.

Cancer and metastasis to the cervical spine

The most common site of metastatic spread of tumors to the skeletal system occurs within the spine and metastatic tumors are the most frequent tumor involving the spinal column [40,41]. Metastases are more likely to be located within with the thoracic or lumbar regions than in the cervical spine; in particular, C1 and C2 are uncommonly involved. The tumors most likely to metastasize to the spine include lung, breast, prostate, and renal cell. The usual route of spread is hematogenous dissemination to the vertebral body with erosion back through the pedicles and extension into the epidural space; most lesions remain extradural [42]. Collapse of the vertebral body may occur and neurologic dysfunction may result either from the deformity or by invasion of the canal by tumor or bone. Patients with spinal metastases typically complain of pain but less commonly manifest signs and symptoms of nerve root or cord compression. Pain is initially localized but may be aggravated by movement and alleviated by immobility if instability develops. The average survival time is greater than 1 year if all metastatic spinal tumors are considered and ranges from 7 to 9 months with lung tumors to 30 months with breast carcinoma. Indications for surgery include spinal instability resulting from progressive deformity, progressive neurologic deficit, and intractable pain; the goal of surgery is to provide for pain palliation and maintain ambulatory status, and about half the patients are still alive 1 year after operation [43]. Because most lesions originate in the vertebral body, an anterior approach with corpectomy offers the most direct approach for tumor excision, canal decompression, and reconstruction of the load-bearing column; the intent is to decompress the canal at the site of the metastasis and to stabilize the spine across the involved segments [44]. Supplemental posterior instrumentation may be used if there is gross vertebral instability, a kyphotic deformity, or if the cervicothoracic junction is involved.

Cervical spine trauma

The incidence of cervical spine injuries in victims of blunt trauma is 1.8% [45,46]. There is a higher incidence of cervical injury in patients who have experienced head trauma, especially among those with severe injury as determined by a low Glasgow Coma Score [47–49]. Most patients with cervical spine injuries have stable injuries. The finding of a focal neurologic deficit has also been identified as an important clinical finding predicting spinal injury [50]. Most patients with cervical spine injuries also have other injuries; in only 20% of instances are traumatic injuries restricted to the cervical spine [51]. Missed or delayed diagnosis of cervical spine injuries is associated with a high incidence of secondary neurologic injury, and there is a clinical imperative to recognize unstable injury at the outset [52–54]. There is a consensus at this time that high-risk patients should be screened with a three-view series with CT of areas of concern; spiral CT has also been used to assess high-risk patients and the results are similar to those of the three-view plus CT method [55–58].

An unusual pattern of delayed secondary cervical cord injury has been described in spine-injured patients and is now named "subacute progressive ascending myelopathy" [59–61]. This syndrome typically occurs in patients with a serious cord injury at a lower spinal level who experience an ascending pattern of secondary injury involving multiple segments remote from the initial level after an uneventful early clinical course. T2-weighted MRI reveals a high signal intensity located centrally within the cord and extending rostral from the site of injury. Often no etiologic factors are identified and subacute progressive ascending myelopathy has been attributed to vascular perturbations (arterial hypotension or venous hypertension) or cord edema and inflammation.

Clinical management of the patient for cervical spine surgery

Diagnostic imaging of the cervical spine

Modern diagnostic imaging techniques are indispensable in the assessment and management of patients with cervical spinal or cord pathology and are used to diagnose and stage disorders, to facilitate treatment planning, and to evaluate the effect of treatment given.

Plain cervical radiography provides excellent screening imaging to assess bony anatomic characteristics and relationships and reveals many spinal pathologies and injuries. Unfortunately, not all injuries are revealed even with adequate plain imaging and a number of pathologic processes must be well advanced (eg, spinal metastasis) before they can be reliably detected. Both the occipitoatlantoaxial complex and the cervicothoracic junction may be difficult to assess with plain radiography; neural elements are poorly or not at all visualized. Tomograms may provide detailed assessments of osseous anatomy and relationships but are uncommonly used when CT is available. Myelography had been the gold standard for evaluating suspected cord compression but its status has been largely supplanted by MRI; it may still be useful if MRI is unavailable, contraindicated, or cannot be tolerated by the patient.

CT scanning provides detailed imaging of the osseous spinal axis and can be used either to evaluate areas of concern on plain radiography or as a primary imaging technique [62]. It provides useful information as to the degree of bony involvement by pathologic processes and can be used to assess both foraminal or canal compromise. Although it is not as useful to assess soft tissues and neural elements as is MRI, when combined with myelography, it can provide detailed assessment of the spinal axis.

MRI provides superb visualization of the neural elements and very good images of the osseous elements [63]. By varying the imaging techniques, various elements and pathologic states may be more critically evaluated. For example, T1 pulse sequences reveal the best anatomic detail, superior spatial resolution, and a good survey of marrow cavity (for assessing marrow replacement processes, such as metastasis), but demonstrate other pathologies poorly. T2 and fat-suppressed T2 images are very sensitive to pathologic changes in the neural and osseous elements and the paraspinal tissues and are superb for discriminating myelopathic changes in the cord. MRI can also be used to assess cerebrospinal fluid flow patterns to determine the patency of cerebrospinal fluid spaces and channels. Gadolinium enhancement increases the sensitivity of MRI investigations when used to evaluate disease processes that create enhancing lesions, such as metastatic cancer.

Surgery of the cervical spine: general principles

Generally speaking, surgeries on the cervical spine fall into one of two broad categories: decompression and fusion. Decompression of the canal or nerve foramen serves to provide greater functional space to the neural elements. The decompression may be limited or extensive, and more extensive decompressive operations tend to include fusion and immobilization. Simple decompression of the nerve foramen in the cervical region is typically done by diskectomy by way of an anterolateral approach, with the patient in the supine position. Small grafts, commonly anterior iliac crest bone or substitutes, are used to maintain anatomic relationships after diskectomy; placement of these grafts is facilitated by the use of small retractors used to spread the adjacent vertebral bodies.

Decompression of the canal is commonly done by a posterior approach with the patient in a prone position and the head fixed with surgical calipers. Most patients with cervical spondylosis and certainly those with ossification of the posterior longitudinal ligament have predominantly anterior compression of the cervical cord. Any posterior decompression procedure is an indirect technique that requires posterior shifting of the cord in the thecal sac to diminish the effect of the anterior compression. For this to occur, the preoperative sagittal alignment of the cervical spine must be at least straight and ideally lordotic. A kyphotic spine is less likely to allow sufficient posterior translation of the spinal cord to diminish symptoms. Multilevel anterior decompressions are indicated when the alignment of the cervical spine is kyphotic or when anterior bone elements are displaced into the canal compromising the lumen and they are also used in the surgical management of spinal metastases. Again, these procedures are done with the patient in a supine position and the head is typically fixed with surgical calipers.

The second broad category of cervical spine surgery is that of fusion and instrumentation. These operations may be combined with decompressive procedures to provide stability to a spine when the native stability has been compromised by the decompressive procedure or osteotomy (eg, ankylosing spondylitis) or may be done primarily to treat a spine rendered unstable by disease or injury. They may involve either an anterior or posterior approach. Modern instrumentation is typically segmental and the principal is to anchor the instrumentation to the stable segments adjacent to the injured or unstable segment and bridge the injury [64].

Airway management for cervical spine surgery

Patients with disorders of the cervical spine have a higher incidence of difficult intubation than is anticipated compared with matched controls, and the likelihood of these difficulties increases in patients with severe limitations of spinal movement [5]. In most patients presenting for limited procedures (eg, single level anterior discectomy) and in those patients with well-preserved spinal range of motion, however, the incidence of difficulties with airway management approach that of normal controls.

Patients with disease processes resulting in atlantoaxial instability require special consideration for airway management. When a patient with atlantoaxial instability is laying supine, passive movement of the head with either flexion or extension may result in separation of the atlas and the axis resulting in increased subluxation. In particular, the sniffing position may significantly increase subluxation [65]. Providing support of the upper cervical spine to affected patients while they are in the supine position shifts the odontoid process forward, closing the anterior atlas-dens interval and increasing the posterior atlas-dens interval [65]. This positioning may be achieved with the use of a small flat pillow on which is placed a dough-nut-shaped pillow. Care should be taken to minimize movement during airway interventions in these patients; consideration should be given to awake intubation in severely affected patients.

All airway maneuvers result in some degree of neck movement, both in general and specifically at the sites of injury or instability [66,67]. The amounts of movement are small, typically well within physiologic ranges, and their impact on secondary neurologic injury has not been defined. During laryngoscopy, in both awake and unconscious subjects, most cervical motion occurs at the craniocervical junction; the subaxial cervical segments including and subjacent to C4 are minimally displaced [68,69]. During laryngoscopy and intubation in a cadaver model with an unstable C1 to C2 segment, the space available for the cord was narrowed to a greater degree by preintubation maneuvers than it was by intubation techniques; both nasal and oral intubation techniques resulted in similar amounts of space available for the cord narrowing, and cricoid pressure produced no significant movement at the craniocervical junction [70]. Four authors have evaluated the impact of commonly used immobilization techniques, including manual in-line immobilization (MILI), in limiting spinal motion in unstable spine models [71–74]. All concluded that the amount of movement measured during airway interventions was small, although it was not uniformly reduced compared with movement registered when no immobilization was applied. Three authors have also assessed the influence of the type of laryngoscope blade on the spinal movements generated during direct laryngoscopy and overall, there seems to be little difference in the magnitudes of spinal movement relative to the type of blade used during direct laryngoscopy [73,75,76].

Cervical spine movements are generally less when rigid indirect laryngoscopes are used compared with the direct laryngoscope, with the notable exception of the Glidescope, which results in similar magnitudes of movement [76–81]. Visualization of the glottis is also improved with the use of the rigid laryngoscopes. The insertion of laryngeal mask airways results in little spinal movement, although insertion may exert high pressures against the upper cervical vertebrae [82,83]. The clinical relevance of these findings has yet to be clarified. Finally, spinal movements resulting from cricothyrotomy are small and similar to those recorded during other airway interventions [84].

Patients presenting for spinal surgery often arrive in the operating room wearing cervical collars. These collars reduce cervical movement somewhat and may afford a degree of comfort to patients with cervical pain aggravated by movement. Goutcher and Lochhead [85] concluded that the presence of a semirigid collar reduced mouth opening and interfered with airway management; removal of the anterior portion of the collar before attempts at tracheal intubation was encouraged. If it is believed that spinal immobilization is desirable during airway interventions, removal of the anterior portion should be undertaken only when it is feasible to replace it with another form of spinal immobilization, such as MILI.

The goal of MILI is to apply sufficient forces to the head and neck so as to limit the movement that might result during airway management. The intention is to apply forces that are equal in magnitude and opposite in direction to those being generated by the laryngoscopist to keep the head and neck in the neutral position. Avoiding traction forces during the application of MILI may be particularly important when there is gross spinal instability [71,86,87]. MILI reduces total spinal movement during the process of laryngoscopy and tracheal intubation [83], although Lennarson and colleagues [71,72] were unable to demonstrate that it resulted in reductions in movement at the site of instability in cadaver models.

Although MILI seems to have the least impact of all immobilization techniques on airway management, it may make direct laryngoscopy more difficult in some patients than if no immobilizing forces are being applied [73,88–90]. Anterior laryngeal or cricoid pressure often improves the view of the larynx when the neck is immobilized with MILI. Concern has been expressed in the past regarding the use of anterior cervical pressure in patients at risk for cervical instability, but Donaldson and colleagues [70] reported that application of cricoid pressure did not result in movement in a cadaver model of an injured upper cervical spine.

If the cervical spine is grossly unstable, consideration should be given to both intubating the trachea and positioning the patient while they are still awake. This can be accomplished with judicious sedation and generous application of local anesthesia to both the trachea and the skull before intubation and caliper placement. Although a prudent approach, it should be recognized that only a gross neurologic assessment is possible following positioning, and its accuracy may be diminished by the administered sedation.

The clinical practice of airway management in patients with cervical spine injury

A number of authors have reported their experiences and outcomes relating to airway management of cervical spine–injured patients; the most common management technique described has been the use of the direct laryngoscope [91–100]. These studies are limited by both their small sample size and their retrospective nature. They reveal, however, that neurologic deterioration in spine-injured patients is uncommon after airway management, even in high-risk patients undergoing urgent tracheal intubation facilitated by direct laryngoscopy. They are not sufficient to rule out the potential that airway management provided in isolation or as part of a more complex clinical intervention, even provided with the utmost care, may rarely result in neurologic injury.

McLeod and Calder [101] examined the association between the use of the direct laryngoscope in patients and subsequent spinal injury or pathology. Six reports dealing with 10 patients in whom it was alleged that direct laryngoscopy contributed to a neurologic injury were reviewed [102–107]. With the possible exception of one case, they concluded after review and analysis of the case reports that the reports failed to provide sufficient data to allow them to make the determination that the use of the direct laryngoscope was the cause of the neurologic injuries reported.

There is considerable enthusiasm, particularly among anesthesiologists, for the use of the fiberoptic bronchoscope in patients with cervical spine disease, injury, or instability. There is a report detailing the successful use of the bronchoscope to facilitate awake intubation in 327 consecutive patients presenting for elective cervical spine surgery; the bulk of the procedures were surgeries for cervical disk prolapse and there were no patients with traumatic injuries included in the review [108]. Although the procedure was well tolerated by most of the patients, 38 (12%) developed low oxygen saturations; in this group, the mean oxygen saturation measured by pulse oximetry was 84 ± 4 (range, 72%–89%).

Airway complications after cervical spine surgery

Airway complications are common after anterior cervical spine surgery and may range from acute airway obstruction to chronic vocal cord dysfunction [109]. Variables associated with postoperative airway complications are an exposure involving more than three vertebral bodies or involving C2, C3, or C4; a blood loss of greater than 300 mL; an operative time greater than 5 hours; and combined anteroposterior cervical spine surgery [109,110]. Vocal cord paralysis resulting from recurrent laryngeal nerve palsy is the most common otolaryngologic complication after anterior cervical spine surgery; the incidence is variable in the reports available [111,112]. The incidence of clinically symptomatic (hoarseness) postoperative recurrent laryngeal nerve palsy may be as high as 8% with prospective assessment, and that of asymptomatic palsy twice that rate. The nerve dysfunction is transient and most cases are resolved at 3 months. Airway complications may also occur after cervical spine surgery performed in the prone position and consist primarily of laryngeal edema and macroglossia [113]. Decreased venous return from the face and upper airway has been implicated as an etiologic factor; prolonged operations and extreme flexion positioning may increase the risk.

Postoperative visual loss after spinal surgery

Postoperative vision loss is a rare complication of spine surgery and more commonly associated with lumbar and thoracic procedures [114,115]. Only 4 (5%) of the 93 cases reported to the American Society of Anesthesiologists Postoperative Visual Loss Registry involved surgery at either the cervical or cervicothoracic levels [115]. The patients were generally healthy with a mean age of 50 years and most of the postoperative vision loss cases resulted from ischemic optic neuropathy. Surgery tended to be extensive, involving multiple levels in most patients; mean anesthetic durations were in excess of 9 hours and blood losses averaged 2 L.

Summary

Most patients presenting for cervical spine surgery do so because of age-related degenerative processes, which cause pain and usually minor degrees of neurologic compromise. The surgical procedures are usually limited in magnitude and the degree of difficulty anticipated with airway management is typically proportional to the biomechanical impact of the underlying disease process. A much smaller number present with severely degraded anatomy and the surgical procedures are far more invasive and high-risk and often intended to provide for a degree of pain palliation and to maintain ambulatory function. Some in this population have limited life prospects (eg, metastatic cancer), but many obtain substantial benefit from the surgery with improved quality of life. Careful preoperative evaluation, appropriate diagnostic imaging, and an approach to care formulated by collegial interaction between anesthesiologist and surgeon serves these patients well.

References

[1] Prescher A. Anatomy and pathology of the aging spine. Eur J Radiol 1998;27(3):181–95.
[2] Jofe MH, White AA, Panjabi MM. Clinically relevant kinematics of the cervical spine. In: The Cervical Spine Research Society. The cervical spine. 2nd edition. Philadelphia: JB Lippincott; 1989. p. 57–69.
[3] Koolstra JH, van Eijden TMGJ. Functional significance of the coupling between head and jaw movements. J Biomech 2004;37(9):1387–92.
[4] Mashour GA, Sandberg WS. Craniocervical extension improves the specificity and predictive value of the Mallampati airway evaluation. Anesth Analg 2006;103(5):1256–9.
[5] Calder I, Calder J, Crockard HA. Difficult direct laryngoscopy in patients with cervical spine disease. Anaesthesia 1995;50(9):756–63.
[6] Bouchard-Chabot A, Lioté F. Cervical spine involvement in rheumatoid arthritis: a review. Joint Bone Spine 2002;69(2):141–54.

[7] Boden S, Dodge L, Bohlman H, et al. Rheumatoid arthritis of the cervical spine. J Bone Joint Surg Am 1993;75(9):1282–97.

[8] Cusick JF, Yoganandan N. Biomechanics of the cervical spine 4: major injuries. Clin Biomech 2002;17(1):1–20.

[9] Banerjee R, Palumbo MA, Fadale PD. Catastrophic cervical spine injuries in the collision sport athlete, Part 1. Epidemiology, functional anatomy, and diagnosis. Am J Sports Med 2004;32(4):1077–87.

[10] Pavlov H, Torg JS, Robie B, et al. Cervical spinal stenosis: determination with vertebral body ratio method. Radiology 1987;164(3):771–5.

[11] Torg JS, Corcoran TA, Thibault LE, et al. Cervical cord neurapraxia: classifications, pathomechanics, morbidity, and management guidelines. J Neurosurg 1997;87(6): 843–50.

[12] Keene JS, Fischer SP, Vanderby R, et al. Significance of acute posttraumatic bony encroachment of the neural canal. Spine 1989;14(8):799–802.

[13] Panjabi MM, Yue JJ, Dvorak J, et al. Cervical spine kinematics and clinical instability. In: Clark CR, editor. The cervical spine. 4th edition. Philadelphia: Lippincott, Williams & Wilkins; 2005. p. 55–78.

[14] Paxinos O, Ghanayem AJ. Biomechanics of nonacute cervical spine trauma. In: Clark CR, editor. The cervical spine. 4th edition. Philadelphia: Lippincott, Williams & Wilkins; 2005. p. 102–9.

[15] Henderson FC, Geddes JF, Vaccaro AR, et al. Stretch-associated injury in cervical spondylotic myelopathy: new concept and review. Neurosurgery 2005;56(5):1101–13.

[16] Ching RP, Watson NA, Carter JW, et al. The effect of post-injury spinal position on canal occlusion in a cervical spine burst fracture model. Spine 1997;22(15):1710–5.

[17] Graham CB III, Wippold FJ, Bae KT, et al. Comparison of CT myelography performed in the prone positions in the detection of cervical spinal stenosis. Clin Radiol 2001;56(1): 35–9.

[18] Carlson GD, Gorden CD, Oliff HS, et al. Sustained spinal cord compression. Part I: time-dependent effect long-term pathophysiology. J Bone Joint Surg Am 2003;85(1):86–94.

[19] Benner BG. Etiology, pathogenesis, and natural history of discogenic neck pain, radiculopathy, and myelopathy. In: The Cervical Spine Research Society Editorial Committee. The cervical spine. 3rd edition. Philadelphia: Lippincott – Raven; 1998. p. 735–40.

[20] Lee TC, Yang LC, Chen HJ. Effect of patient position and hypotensive anesthesia on inferior vena caval pressure. Spine 1998;23(8):941–7.

[21] Bindal AK, Dunker SB, Tew JM Jr. Chiari 1 malformation: classification and management. Neurosurgery 1995;37(6):1069–74.

[22] Milhorat TH, Chou MW, Trinidad EM, et al. Chiari I malformations redefined: clinical and radiographic findings for 364 symptomatic patients. Neurosurgery 1999;44(5): 1005–17.

[23] Karasick D, Schweitzer ME, Vaccaro AR. The traumatized cervical spine in Klippel-Feil syndrome: imaging features. Am J Roentgenol 1998;170(1):85–8.

[24] Ulmer JL, Elster AD, Ginsberg LE, et al. Klippel-Feil syndrome: CT and MR of acquired and congenital abnormalities of cervical spine and cord. J Comput Assist Tomogr 1993; 17(2):215–24.

[25] Tracy MR, Dormans JP, Kusumi K. Klippel-Feil syndrome: clinical features and current understanding of etiology. Clin Orthop 2004;424:183–90.

[26] Crosby ET, Grahovac S. Diffuse idiopathic skeletal hyperostosis: an unusual cause of difficult intubation. Can J Anaesth 1993;40(1):54–8.

[27] Mader R. Clinical manifestations of diffuse idiopathic skeletal hyperostosis of the cervical spine. Semin Arthritis Rheum 2002;32(2):130–5.

[28] Naik B, Lobato EB, Sulek CA. Dysphagia, obstructive sleep apnea, and difficult fiberoptic intubation secondary to diffuse idiopathic skeletal hyperostosis. Anesthesiology 2004; 100(5):1311–2.

[29] Sreedharan S, Li YH. Diffuse idiopathic skeletal hyperostosis with cervical spinal cord injury: a report of 3 cases and a literature review. Ann Acad Med Singap 2005;34(3): 257–61.

[30] Takenaka I, Urakami Y, Aoyama K, et al. Severe subluxation in the sniffing position in a rheumatoid patient with anterior atlantoaxial subluxation. Anesthesiology 2004;101(5): 1235–7.

[31] Shen FH, Samartzis D, Jenis LG, et al. Rheumatoid arthritis: evaluation and surgical management of the cervical spine. Spine J 2004;4(6):689–700.

[32] Borenstein D. Inflammatory arthritides of the spine: surgical versus nonsurgical treatment. Clin Orthop 2006;443:208–21.

[33] Shen FH, Samartzis D. Surgical management of lower cervical spine fracture in ankylosing spondylitis. J Trauma 2006;61(4):1005–9.

[34] Belanger TA, Milam RA IV, Roh JS, et al. Cervicothoracic extension osteotomy for chin-on-chest deformity in ankylosing spondylitis. J Bone Joint Surg Am 2005;87(8):1732–8.

[35] Grisolia A, Bell RL, Peltier LF. Fractures and dislocations of the spine complicating ankylosing spondylitis: a report of six cases. Clin Orthop 2004;422:129–34.

[36] Carette S, Fehlings MG. Cervical radiculopathy. N Engl J Med 2005;353(4):392–9.

[37] Orr RD, Zdeblick TA. Cervical spondylotic myelopathy: approaches to surgical treatment. Clin Orthop 1999;359:58–66.

[38] Emery SE. Cervical spondylotic myelopathy: diagnosis and treatment. J Am Acad Orthop Surg 2001;9(6):376–88.

[39] Muhle C, Weinert D, Falliner A, et al. Dynamic changes of the spinal canal in patients with cervical spondylosis at flexion and extension using magnetic imaging. Invest Radiol 1998; 33(8):444–9.

[40] Simmons ED, Zheng Y. Vertebral tumours: surgical versus nonsurgical treatment. Clin Orthop 2006;443:233–47.

[41] Jenis LG, Dunn EJ, An HS. Metastatic disease of the cervical spine. Clin Orthop 1999;359: 89–103.

[42] Tasdemiroglu E, Kaya AH, Bek S, et al. Neurologic complications of cancer. Part 1: central nervous system metastasis. Neurosurgery Quarterly 2004;14(2):71–83.

[43] Vrionis FD, Small J. Surgical management of metastatic spinal neoplasms. Neurosurg Focus 2003;15(5):1–8.

[44] Liu JK, Apfelbaum RI, Chiles BW III, et al. Cervical spine metastasis: anterior reconstruction and stabilization techniques after tumor resection. Neurosurg Focus 2003;15(5):1–7.

[45] Crosby ET. Airway management in adults after cervical spine trauma. Anesthesiology 2006;104(6):1293–318.

[46] Goldberg W, Mueller C, Panacek E, et al. Distribution and patterns of blunt traumatic cervical spine injury. Ann Emerg Med 2001;38(1):17–21.

[47] Holly LT, Kelly DF, Counelis GJ, et al. Cervical spine trauma associated with moderate and severe head injury: incidence, risk factors, and injury characteristics. J Neurosurg 2002;96(Suppl 3):285–91.

[48] Demetriades D, Charalambides K, Chahwan S, et al. Nonskeletal cervical spine injuries: epidemiology and diagnostic pitfalls. J Trauma 2000;48(4):724–7.

[49] Hackl W, Hausberger K, Sailer R, et al. Prevalence of cervical spine injuries in patients with facial trauma. Oral Surg Oral Med Oral Pathol Oral Radiol Endod 2001;92(4):370–6.

[50] Blackmore CC, Emerson SS, Mann FA, et al. Cervical spine imaging in patients with trauma: determination of fracture risk to optimize use. Radiology 1999;211(3):759–65.

[51] Sekhon LHS, Fehlings MG. Epidemiology, demographics and pathophysiology of acute spinal cord injury. Spine 2001;26(Suppl):S2–12.

[52] Reid DC, Henderson R, Saboe L, et al. Etiology and clinical course of missed spine fractures. J Trauma 1987;27(9):980–6.

[53] Davis JW, Phreaner DL, Hoyt DB, et al. The etiology of missed cervical spine injuries. J Trauma 1993;34(3):342–6.

[54] Poonnoose PM, Ravichandran G, McClelland M. Missed and mismanaged injuries of the spinal cord. J Trauma 2002;53(2):314–20.

[55] Hadley MN. Guidelines of the American Association of neurologic surgeons and the congress of neurologic surgeons: radiographic assessment of the cervical spine in asymptomatic trauma patients. Neurosurgery 2002;50(Suppl):S30–5.

[56] Lindsey RW, Gugala Z. Clearing the cervical spine in trauma patients. In: Clark CR, editor. The cervical spine. 4th edition. Philadelphia: Lippincott, Williams & Wilkins; 2005. p. 375–86.

[57] Hadley MN. Guidelines of the American Association of Neurologic Surgeons and the Congress of Neurologic Surgeons. Radiographic spinal assessment in symptomatic trauma patients. Neurosurgery 2002;50(Suppl):S36–43.

[58] Morris CGT, McCoy E. Clearing the cervical spine in unconscious polytrauma victims, balancing risk and effective screening. Anaesthesia 2004;59(5):464–82.

[59] Yablon IG, Ordia J, Mortara R, et al. Acute ascending myelopathy of the spine. Spine 1989; 14(10):1084–9.

[60] Belanger E, Picard C, Lacerte D, et al. Subacute posttraumatic ascending myelopathy after spinal cord injury: report of three cases. J Neurosurg 2000;93(Suppl 2):294–9.

[61] Schmidt BJ. Subacute delayed ascending myelopathy after low spine injury: case report and evidence of a vascular mechanism. Spinal Cord 2006;44(5):322–5.

[62] Kaiser JA, Holland BA. Imaging of the cervical spine. Spine 1998;23(24):2701–12.

[63] Khanna AJ, Carbone JJ, Kebaish KM, et al. Magnetic resonance imaging of the cervical spine. J Bone Joint Surg Am 2002;84(Suppl 2):70–80.

[64] Foster MR. A functional classification of spinal instrumentation. Spine J 2005;5(6):682–94.

[65] Tokunaga D, Hase H, Mikami Y, et al. Atlanotaxial subluxation in different intraoperative head positions in patients with rheumatoid arthritis. Anesthesiology 2006;104(4):675–9.

[66] Aprahamian C, Thompson BM, Finger WA, et al. Experimental cervical spine injury model: evaluation of airway management and splinting techniques. Ann Emerg Med 1984;13(8):584–7.

[67] Hauswald M, Sklar DP, Tandberg D, et al. Cervical spine movement during airway management: cinefluoroscopic appraisal in human cadavers. Am J Emerg Med 1991;9(6): 535–8.

[68] Sawin PD, Todd MM, Traynelis VC, et al. Cervical spine motion with direct laryngoscopy and orotracheal intubation: an in vivo cinefluoroscopic study of subjects without cervical abnormality. Anesthesiology 1996;85(1):26–36.

[69] Horton WA, Fahy L, Charters P. Disposition of the cervical vertebrae, atlanto-axial joint, hyoid and mandible during x-ray laryngoscopy. Br J Anaesth 1989;63(4):435–8.

[70] Donaldson WF III, Heil BV, Donaldson VP, et al. The effect of airway maneuvers on the unstable C1-C2 segment: a cadaver study. Spine 1997;22(11):1215–8.

[71] Lennarson PJ, Smith DW, Sawin PD, et al. Cervical spinal motion during intubation: efficacy of stabilization maneuvers in the setting of complete segmental instability. J Neurosurg (Spine 2) 2001;94:265–70.

[72] Lennarson PJ, Smith D, Todd MM, et al. Segmental cervical spine motion during orotracheal intubation of the intact and injured spine with and without external stabilization. J Neurosurg (Spine 2) 2000;92:201–6.

[73] Gerling MC, Davis DP, Hamilton RS, et al. Effects of cervical spine immobilization technique and laryngoscope blade selection on an unstable cervical spine in a cadaver model of intubation. Ann Emerg Med 2000;36(4):293–300.

[74] Brimacombe J, Keller C, Kunzel KH, et al. Cervical spine motion during airway management: a cinefluoroscopic study of the posteriorly destabilized third cervical vertebrae in human cadavers. Anesth Analg 2000;91(5):1274–8.

[75] MacIntyre PR, McLeod ADM, Hurley R, et al. Cervical spine movements during laryngoscopy: comparison of the Macintosh and McCoy laryngoscope blades. Anaesthesia 1999; 54(10):413–8.

[76] Hastings RH, Vigil AC, Hanna R, et al. Cervical spine movement during laryngoscopy with the Bullard, Macintosh and Miller laryngoscopes. Anesthesiology 1995;82(4):859–69.

[77] Watts ADJ, Gelb AW, Bach DB, et al. Comparison of Bullard and Macintosh laryngoscopes for endotracheal intubation of patients with a potential cervical spine injury. Anesthesiology 1997;87(6):1335–42.

[78] Cooper SD, Benumof JL, Ozaki GT. Evaluation of the Bullard laryngoscope using the new intubating stylet: comparison with conventional laryngoscopy. Anesth Analg 1994;79(5): 965–70.

[79] Rudolph C, Schneider JP, Wallenborn J, et al. Movement of the upper cervical spine during laryngoscopy: a comparison of the Bonfils intubation fiberscope and the Macintosh laryngoscope. Anaesthesia 2005;60(7):668–72.

[80] Agro F, Barzoi G, Montechia F. Tracheal intubation using a Macintosh laryngoscope or a Glidescope in 15 patients with cervical spine immobilization. Br J Anaesth 2003;90(5): 705–6.

[81] Turkstra TP, Craen RA, Pelz DM, et al. Cervical spine motion: a fluoroscopic comparison during intubation with lighted stylet, Glidescope, and Macintosh laryngoscope. Anesth Analg 2005;101(3):910–5.

[82] Kihara S, Watanabe S, Brimacombe J, et al. Segmental cervical spine movement with the intubating laryngeal mask during manual in-line stabilization in patients with cervical pathology undergoing cervical spine surgery. Anesth Analg 2000;91(1):195–200.

[83] Keller C, Brimacombe J, Keller K. Pressures exerted against the cervical vertebrae by the standard and intubating laryngeal mask airways: a randomized, controlled, cross-over study in fresh cadavers. Anesth Analg 1999;89(5):1296–300.

[84] Gerling MC, Davis DP, Hamilton RS, et al. Effect of surgical cricothyrotomy on the unstable cervical spine in a cadaver model of intubation. J Emerg Med 2001;20(1):1–5.

[85] Goutcher CM, Lochhead V. Reduction in mouth opening with semi-rigid cervical collars. Br J Anaesth 2005;95(3):344–8.

[86] Bivins HG, Ford S, Bezmalinovic Z, et al. The effect of axial traction during orotracheal intubation of the trauma victim with an unstable cervical spine. Ann Emerg Med 1988; 17(1):25–9.

[87] Majernick TG, Bienek R, Houston JB, et al. Cervical spine movement during orotracheal intubation. Ann Emerg Med 1986;15(4):417–20.

[88] Heath KJ. The effect on laryngoscopy of different cervical spine immobilization techniques. Anaesthesia 1994;49(10):843–5.

[89] Nolan JP, Wilson ME. Orotracheal intubation in patients with potential cervical spine injuries. Anaesthesia 1993;48(7):630–3.

[90] Wood PR, Dresner M, Hayden Smith J, et al. Direct laryngoscopy and cervical spine stabilization. Anaesthesia 1994;49(1):77–8.

[91] Meschino A, Devitt JH, Koch JP, et al. The safety of awake tracheal intubation in cervical spine injury. Can J Anaesth 1992;39(2):114–7.

[92] Holley J, Jordan R. Airway management in patients with unstable cervical spine fractures. Ann Emerg Med 1989;18(11):1237–9.

[93] Rhee KJ, Green W, Holcroff JW, et al. Oral intubation in the multiply injured patient: the risk of exacerbating spinal cord damage. Ann Emerg Med 1990;19(5):511–4.

[94] Scanell G, Waxman K, Tommaga G, et al. Orotracheal intubations in trauma patients with cervical fractures. Arch Surg 1993;128(8):903–6.

[95] Shatney CH, Brunner RD, Nguyen TQ. The safety of orotracheal intubation in patients with unstable cervical spine fracture or high spinal cord injury. Am J Surg 1995;170(6): 676–80.

[96] Talucci RC, Shaikh KA, Schwab CW. Rapid sequence induction with oral endotracheal intubation in the multiply injured patient. Am Surg 1988;54(4):185–7.

[97] Suderman VS, Crosby ET, Lui A. Elective oral tracheal intubation in cervical spine-injured adults. Can J Anaesth 1991;38(6):785–9.

[98] McCrory C, Blunnie WP, Moriarty DC. Elective tracheal intubation in cervical spine injuries. Ir Med J 1999;90(6):234–5.

[99] Wright SW, Robinson GG II, Wright MB. Cervical spine injuries in blunt trauma patients requiring emergent endotracheal intubation. Am J Emerg Med 1992;10(2):104–9.

[100] Norwood S, Myers MB, Butler TJ. The safety of emergency neuromuscular blockade and orotracheal intubation in the acutely injured trauma patient. J Am Coll Surg 1994;179(6): 646–52.

[101] McLeod ADM, Calder I. Spinal cord injury and direct laryngoscopy: the legend lives on. Br J Anaesth 2000;84(6):705–8.

[102] Farmer J, Vaccaro A, Albert TJ, et al. Neurologic deterioration after cervical spinal cord injury. J Spinal Disord 1998;11(3):192–6.

[103] Muckart DJ, Bhagwanjee S, van der Merwe R. Spinal cord injury as a result of endotracheal intubation in patients with undiagnosed cervical spine fractures. Anesthesiology 1997; 87(2):418–20.

[104] Redl G. Massive pyramidal tract signs after endotracheal intubation: a case report of spondyloepiphyseal dysplasia congenital. Anesthesiology 1998;89(5):1262–4.

[105] Yan K, Diggan MF. A case of central cord syndrome caused by intubation: a case report. J Spinal Cord Med 1997;20(2):230–2.

[106] Yaszemski MJ, Shepler TR. Sudden death from cord compression associated with atlanto-axial instability in rheumatoid arthritis. Spine 1990;15(4):338–41.

[107] Hastings RH, Kelley SD. Neurologic deterioration associated with airway management in a cervical spine-injured patient. Anesthesiology 1993;78(3):580–3.

[108] Fuchs G, Schwarz G, Baumgartner A, et al. Fiberoptic intubation in 327 patients with lesions of the cervical spine. J Neurosurg Anesthesiol 1999;11(1):11–6.

[109] Sagi HC, Beutler W, Carroll E, et al. Airway complications associated with surgery on the anterior cervical spine. Spine 2002;27(9):949–53.

[110] Terao Y, Matsumoto S, Yamashita K, et al. Increased incidence of emergency airway management after combined anterior-posterior cervical spine surgery. J Neurosurg Anesthesiol 2004;16(4):282–6.

[111] Jung A, Schramm J, Lehnerdt K, et al. Recurrent laryngeal nerve palsy during anterior cervical spine surgery: a prospective study. J Neurosurg Spine 2005;2(2):123–7.

[112] Apfelbaum RI, Kriskovich MD, Haller JR. On the incidence, cause, and prevention of recurrent laryngeal nerve palsies during anterior cervical spine surgery. Spine 2000; 25(22):2906–12.

[113] Sinha A, Agarwal A, Gaur A, et al. Oropharyngeal swelling and macroglossia after cervical spine surgery in the prone position. J Neurosurg Anesthesiol 2001;13(3):237–9.

[114] Stevens WR, Glazer PA, Kelley SD, et al. Ophthalmic complications after spine surgery. Spine 1997;22(12):1319–24.

[115] Lee LA, Roth S, Posner KL, et al. The American Society of anesthesiologists postoperative visual loss registry: analysis of 93 spine surgery cases with postoperative visual losses. Anesthesiology 2006;105(4):652–9.

ELSEVIER
SAUNDERS

Anesthesiology Clin
25 (2007) 535–555

ANESTHESIOLOGY
CLINICS

Anesthetic Considerations for Awake Craniotomy for Epilepsy

Kirstin M. Erickson, MD[a],*, Daniel J. Cole, MD[b]

[a]*Department of Anesthesiology, Mayo Clinic College of Medicine,
200 First Street, SW, Rochester, MN 55901, USA*
[b]*Department of Anesthesiology, Mayo Clinic Hospital, 5777 East Mayo Boulevard,
Phoenix, AZ 85054, USA*

Awake craniotomy is the procedure of choice for patients when the area to be resected is immediately adjacent to eloquent cortex, such as that controlling language or motor function, and hence at risk of injury. Although the technique has other indications, including resection of tumors or vascular lesions impacting eloquent cortex, it was used initially to guide epileptogenic focus resection and this remains its primary role today. An awake brain procedure for the patient with epilepsy requires good patient cooperation, anticipation of specific problems, and clinical vigilance. The neuroanesthesiologist has a wide array of anesthetic options to achieve smooth management and high patient satisfaction.

Epilepsy affects approximately 0.55% to 1% of the population worldwide (between 2.3 and 2.7 million Americans), making it one of the most common neurologic diseases [1]. Of those treated with medications in the United States, 30% to 40% continue to have seizures [2]. Epilepsy is considered intractable when severe, frequent seizure activity cannot be adequately controlled by a reasonable trial of medications and prevents normal function or development. Many patients with intractable seizures may be candidates for surgical resection of their seizure focus. When the focus (either tumor or nonlesional focus) lies in or near eloquent brain (primary motor, sensory, memory, vision, and language cortex), an awake craniotomy may be the best intervention.

Eloquent brain near the central sulcus is so densely functional that it has proved to be intolerant to precise discrimination of the seizure foci and functional brain. Despite structural imaging and invasive intracranial monitoring,

---

* Corresponding author.
E-mail address: erickson.kirstin@mayo.edu (K.M. Erickson).

doi:10.1016/j.anclin.2007.06.001   *anesthesiology.theclinics.com*

devastating deficits may result from millimeter-sized errors during resection under general anesthesia. Such errors may result not only from assumptions about regional brain anatomy but also from the mechanical shifts in brain tissue that occurs during the resection itself [3]. Awake craniotomy with real-time neurocognitive testing is the most reliable method to preserve critical function. Although an awake resection still does not result in seizure freedom in every candidate, the technique has become widely considered the best balance of benefit and risk for patients with epileptic foci in eloquent brain.

Operation for elimination of seizures in modern medicine was first described by Victor Horsley in 1886. In the first half of the 20th century, electroencephalography (EEG) was developed and refined to detect seizures, and yet relatively few patients underwent operative treatment until the 1980s. This rather slow evolution in technique reflects both the development of reliable cortical language mapping and advancement in the understanding of epilepsy and its treatment [4–6]. In the late 1980s, a number of manuscripts on seizure resection began to appear in the neurosurgical literature and the procedure gained popularity [7–12]. Since then, advances in structural imaging, functional testing, and improved surgical methods including microsurgery and stereotaxis have allowed resection of lesions previously unidentified (cryptogenic epilepsy) with improved safety and accuracy [13]. Awake craniotomy with serial neurocognitive examinations to guide resection in eloquent areas is currently considered the gold standard for optimal focus resection.

Indications for awake operative resection of seizure focus

Although intracranial operation itself carries inherent risks, these risks do not outweigh the ongoing morbidity and mortality of uncontrolled epilepsy. These include accidental self-injury, depression, cognitive decline, social impairment, and sudden unexplained death. At least two retrospective trials and one prospective randomized controlled trial for mesial temporal lobe epilepsy (a common type of resectable epilepsy) showed that the morbidity and mortality associated with resection was less than that associated with the disorder [14–16].

The patient with epilepsy is considered a candidate for resection when two criteria are met: a sufficient trial of antiepileptic drugs has failed to attain adequate control, and when there is reasonable likelihood that an operation will benefit the patient. The first of these two criteria has evolved over recent years from earlier recommendations that a patient must have tried all combinations of antiepileptic drugs before becoming eligible for surgery. With the large number of available antiepileptic drugs, this process would take decades and it is no longer deemed necessary before considering operative intervention. Judging the adequacy of antiepileptic drug trials for a given patient must be done in the context of the prognosis and severity of the specific epileptic type [17]. In most centers, several members of an inter-disciplinary team including neurologists, neurophysiologists, social workers, radiologists, and neurosurgeons contribute expertise to decide whether a patient meets these criteria.

Surgical treatment is most beneficial for patients with partial epilepsy caused by discrete structural lesions (benign or neoplastic) and specific surgically remediable syndromes, including mesial temporal lobe epilepsy, which is described as the most common type of epilepsy and the most refrac-tory to pharmacotherapy [15,18,19]. Lesions or foci are commonly located in the temporal lobe and may be in or near functional cortex, depending on the hemisphere. Eloquent cortex includes Wernicke's speech area in the dominant temporal lobe, Broca's speech area in the dominant frontal lobe, and the motor strip. Areas associated with memory, both verbal and visuo-spatial, have also been mapped to the temporal lobes, although intraopera-tive testing of these functions has proved complex and time-consuming [20]. When intraoperative brain mapping requires neurologic assessment of speech or other function, an awake procedure is indicated to achieve max-imal resection of epileptic cortex with maximal preservation of function.

Compared with resection under general anesthesia, benefits of awake cra-niotomy have been reported to include (1) better preservation of language function [21]; (2) some prediction of seizure-free outcomes, based on corti-cography [21,22]; (3) shorter hospitalization [23,24], and thereby reduced cost [25]; (4) decreased use of invasive monitors [23,26,27]; and (5) decreased postoperative anesthetic complications including nausea and vomiting [28]. Data have not shown that seizure-free outcomes are any greater with resections done in awake resections with corticography versus those done under general anesthesia. An additional benefit gained from awake intrao-perative mapping has been a better understanding of human neuroanatomy and function.

Preoperative testing to localize seizure focus

A wide array of testing modalities is used to plan neurosurgical inter-vention accurately. Although these have shown great advancement in recent decades, none has obviated the need for intraoperative, awake patient monitoring when eloquent function near the central sulcus is involved.

When language function is potentially at stake, initial testing includes a Wada's test to determine hemispheric dominance. Unilateral intracarotid injection of a barbiturate (amobarbital) localizes language function by hemisphere and determines whether language neocortex is at risk.

Neuroradiologic imaging and electrophysiologic monitoring are the two pillars of seizure focus localization. MRI has largely replaced CT for its superior structural brain imaging and is used routinely. Functional MRI has further improved noninvasive identification of functional areas [29,30]. The sensitivity and specificity of MRI alone, however, is not great enough to guide resection in language neocortex accurately. Box 1 includes current diagnostic tests for localization of epileptogenic foci [31,32].

Radiologic adjuncts to MRI include positron emission tomography and single-photon emission CT. Positron emission tomography reflects brain glucose metabolism. If the scan is obtained during seizure activity hypermetabolism is found at a seizure focus, whereas interictally, hypometabolism is the typical finding in the region of a seizure focus. Single-photon emission CT, which demonstrates blood flow in the brain, is done within seconds of seizure initiation and requires immediate radionucleotide availability and intravenous access. A newer, more accurate way of using single-photon emission CT is subtraction ictal-interictal single-photon emission CT, which is then coregistered to MRI to indicate the cortical area of seizure initiation [31].

In addition to radiologic imaging, surgical candidates usually undergo invasive or noninvasive EEG localization. Diagnostic EEG is used in a variety of ways to localize epileptic activity and to test areas of normal cortical function (see Box 1). Precise surgical planning for seizure focus resection requires greater accuracy than scalp electrocorticography (ECoG) allows. Smaller strip electrodes and can be used to determine laterality of seizure initiation and may be placed by burr holes, whereas more specific localization of epileptic activity is done by subdural grid electrodes (arrays of recording electrodes more than one column wide), which are placed directly on the brain surface by open craniotomy. Inpatient continuous video-EEG, or outpatient EEG mapping, and intraoperative EEG can then be accomplished and the surgical approach planned.

Surgical procedure

Not all operations for epilepsy require an awake craniotomy. Temporal lobe operations may involve removal of only the structural lesion and associated epileptogenic cortex, cortical resection alone, excision of the amygdala and hippocampus, or removal of the entire anterior temporal lobe with the extent of posterior resection dependent on dominance. Only when intraoperative speech, motor, or other function (memory, vision) must be identified is an awake procedure required.

Details of neurosurgical technique and decision-making are beyond the scope of this article; however, several general points are of relevance to the anesthesiologist. Although craniotomy, surface, or depth ECoG, and resection may be done in one procedure, it is often performed in two separate operations. In this approach, a craniotomy for placement of subdural grid electrodes is usually done under general anesthesia, although awake craniotomy for grid placement guided by cortical stimulation (to identify the sensorimotor cortex and to reproduce the patient's aura) has been described [33]. Postoperatively, a period of ictal electrocorticographic recordings and cortical stimulation further delineate the site of seizure onset and

Box 1. Diagnostic tests used in evaluation for resection of epileptogenic foci

Tests of epileptic excitability
Noninvasive EEG
   Video EEG, long-term monitoring
   Outpatient long-term EEG monitoring
Invasive EEG
   Intraoperative electrocorticography
   Stereotactic depth-electrode, long-term recording
   Subdural grid or strip, long-term recording
Ictal single-photon emission CT
Subtraction ictal single-photon emission CT coregistered to MRI
Functional MRI*
Interictal and ictal magnetoencephalography*

Tests for structural abnormalities
X-ray films, CT, and other radiographic studies
MRI
Magnetic resonance spectroscopy

Tests for functional deficit
Interictal positron emission tomography
Interictal single-photon emission CT
Neuropsychologic batteries
Intracarotid amobarbital (Wada's test)
Interictal EEG
Magnetic resonance spectroscopy
Interictal magnetoencephalography*

Tests of normal cortical function (cortical mapping)
Intraoperative electrocorticography
Extraoperative subdural grid recording
Intracarotid amobarbital (Wada's test)
Positron emission tomography
Functional MRI
Magnetoencephalography*
Magnetic source imaging, or magnetoencephalography
   coregistered to MRI*

---

* Considered experimental for this indication.
Adapted from Engel J Jr. Surgery for seizures. N Engl J Med 1996;334:647–52.

functional anatomy. Return to the operating room occurs days to weeks later for grid removal and definitive resection of the epileptogenic center. This is when the awake technique is most often required. For a temporal lobe lesion, a temporal incision is made, a bone flap elevated, and the dura incised to expose up to 6 to 7 cm of the anterior temporal lobe. Stereotactic techniques correlating exposed brain to three-dimensional MRI may be used. A limited resection of epileptogenic brain is performed with guidance from cortical stimulation (ECoG) (Fig. 1). Function is continuously monitored during resection. When ECoG is used to reproduce a seizure aura, iced saline may be subsequently administered directly on the cortex to stop the epileptic activity. Usually, an operating microscope is used. Closure of the dura, bone flap, and scalp is routine. Surgical complications include injury to the brainstem, third and fourth cranial nerves, and either the middle cerebral or posterior cerebral arteries.

Pathologic diagnoses of identifiable seizure foci include mesial temporal sclerosis; neoplasm (glioma, ganglioma, hamartoma); and a wide variety of other epileptogenic lesions including glial scar caused by trauma or infarct, neurofibromatosis, tuberous sclerosis, cysts, and arteriovenous malformations. Outcomes are dependent on the type of epileptogenic lesion targeted, but in one large trial in patients with temporal lobe epilepsy, up to 60% were free of seizures 1 year [14].

Patient selection and preoperative evaluation

Attention should focus on issues critical for the awake patient, particularly mental maturity and the airway. Candidates for awake craniotomy

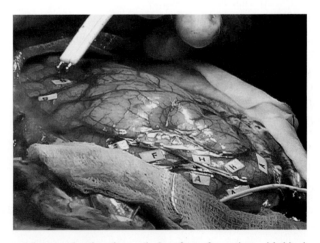

Fig. 1. Open craniotomy showing the cortical surface of a patient with bipolar stimulation using an Ojemann bipolar stimulator while testing appropriate neurologic function in an awake patient. Cortical labels shown include A (arm), F (face), and H (hand). (*Courtesy of* Fredric B. Meyer, MD.)

are initially selected by the neurosurgeon for both medical and psychologic readiness. The decision to proceed is then reached after careful preparation by neurologists and by the anesthesiologist and in discussion with the patient. Good rapport between patient and anesthesiologist, and among all members of the operating room team, cannot be overemphasized in making the procedure as safe and smooth as possible. Box 2 highlights considerations for preoperative evaluation.

The importance of selecting a motivated, mature patient who is able to cope in a strange and stressful environment for an extended period of time is crucial. It has been said that the only absolute contraindication to the awake technique is an uncooperative patient [34]. Anxiety disorder, low tolerance for pain, or such psychiatric disorders as schizophrenia may preclude candidacy because there is very little pharmacologic rescue that can be offered to the awake patient in pinion who has a psychologic crisis without sacrificing the entire awake technique. Screening may include tests of concentration or personality inventory aimed at discovering traits incompatible with cooperative performance in the operating room. Claustrophobia, if severe, may complicate positioning because usually surgical drapes must hang

---

Box 2. Considerations for preoperative anesthetic evaluation of the awake craniotomy patient

Patient cooperation
   Age and maturity
   Anxiety, claustrophobia, emotional stability
   Psychiatric disorders
Airway
   Intubation history
   Airway patency (obesity, obstructive sleep apnea, asthma or other pulmonary disease)
   Airway examination (ease of ability to mask ventilate, insert laryngeal mask airway, intubate)
   Gastroesophageal reflux
Epilepsy
   Form
   Frequency
   Treatment (medications taken)
Intracranial pressure
Nausea and vomiting
Hemodynamic stability

Adapted from Bonhomme V, Born JD, Hans P. Prise en charge anesthesique des craniotomies en état vigile. Ann Fr Anesth Reanim 2004;23:391.

very near the immobilized face and can cause a sense of smothering. Careful draping with a more open access to a patient's face, or perhaps the intermittent use of cool air blown over the face, may minimize this fearful sensation [35]. Movement disorders may also compromise a motionless surgical field, although one case report describes the use of regional blocks to eliminate involuntary extremity movements in a patient with unilateral spontaneous movements [36].

The airway and comorbidities affecting the airway must also be carefully considered. Ease of mask airway, Mallampati score, and other predictors of difficulty with laryngoscopy, and intubation history should be assessed with an eye to the potential for obstruction, wheezing, or other compromise. The anesthesiologist must plan for emergent laryngoscopy, perhaps in a difficult position because of surgical drapes or pinion, and ensure all necessary equipment is immediately at hand. Obstructive sleep apnea has been suggested as an absolute exclusion criterion [37]. Obesity, gastroesophageal reflux, and chronic cough or wheezing may be relative contraindications depending on severity.

Intracranial pressure must be adequately controlled because brain relaxation by hyperventilation is not attainable in a sedated, spontaneously breathing patient. Type and frequency of seizures, medication regimen, and serum levels, if applicable, may limit candidacy. Other factors including size of tumor, hemorrhagic risk, and hemodynamic stability are considered in conjunction with the surgeon. As with any type of anesthetic, anticipation of specific difficulties is a mainstay of care in the awake craniotomy.

Peripheral access sites should be assessed during the preoperative examination and the need for arterial cannulation and urinary catheter placement discussed with the patient if these are to be used.

Patient preparation

Patient preparation is usually extensive. The neurosurgeon first describes the procedure and explains the rationale for awake testing. As described by Jaskelainen and Randell [25], although awake brain surgery initially sounds frightening to a patient, once its purpose is carefully explained and reassurance given, the response is usually one of acceptance or even relief [34,38, 39]. After initial preparation with the surgeon, neurologists, neurophysiologists, and speech pathologists review specific language testing (naming, reading, repeating, responding) or motor testing (facial and extremity movement) that are done in the operating room. Reports of language mapping in bilingual patients suggest that with adequate preparation, testing both languages of fluency can be accomplished in a time-efficient way intraoperatively [40,41]. Likewise, children as young as 9 years are reported to tolerate awake craniotomy with good screening and preparation [42]. A developmentally delayed 16-year-old patient described as "very cooperative" also underwent an uneventful awake craniotomy for intractable seizure disorder [43] highlighting the importance of a motivated, cooperative patient. In some centers a test run of patient positioning and language testing in the operating room is done the day before surgery [37].

Positioning

Positioning of the awake patient is paramount. The anatomy of interest to all involved (anesthesiologist, surgeon, neurologist, and neurophysiologist) is the patient's head, and access to the surgical field, airway, speech, sight, and facial expression must all be made possible without causing the patient to feel smothered. The patient must remain in rigid pinion fixation, or at a minimum, lie motionless on an operating table for several hours. If pinion or epidural skull clamp fixation is not used (necessary for stereotactic techniques), the patient's head may rest in a donut-shaped gel pad or other conformed pillow, but must nonetheless remain immobile for several hours [44]. Both the supine and lateral positions are described, without report of difficulty. When the supine position is used, the head is turned to expose the temporal lobe and to allow gravity to aid frontal lobe retraction (Fig. 2). A reasonably soft mattress, padding of the extremities, and avoidance of extreme head rotation allow the patient to remain still, and provides protection from injuries of stretch and pressure. A wide open geometry of

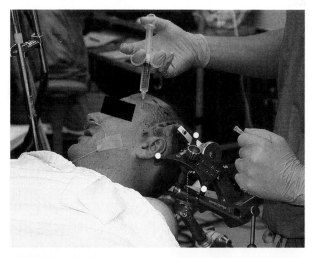

Fig. 2. A patient is positioned in pinion and Mayfield head holder with his head turned. The skin incision is marked and local infiltration of the scalp is in progress while patient is sedated. Nasal cannula for oxygen is taped to the face. The electrocorticography technician is in the background. (*Courtesy of* Fredric B. Meyer, MD.)

surgical drapes helps to minimize claustrophobia, whereas sufficient blanket coverage and forced air warming blanket maintains modesty and body temperature (Fig. 3). This arrangement also allows eye contact with the patient and provides a clear view for the patient to name objects or pictures. If motor testing is to be done, a clear view of the patient's arm, hand, and face is important. In some centers a microphone is placed near the patient's head or a video camera records the patient's face for viewing by the surgical team [45,46].

Monitoring

Little more than routine monitoring is often necessary. Because neither laboratory assessment nor beat-to-beat blood pressure monitoring is usually indicated intraoperatively, the presence of medical comorbidities should guide this determination. Certainly, end-expired carbon dioxide (CO_2) monitoring is essential both to airway vigilance and prevention of cerebral edema and increased brain volume. End-expired CO_2 is monitored during the awake portion if a nasal cannula with a CO_2 aspiration channel or face mask is used. When exhaled gas recordings are unreliable or difficult to measure, the arterial catheter may provide an ability to monitor blood gas CO_2 intermittently. Processed EEG monitoring, such as bispectral index, is reported as a guide for infusion anesthesia or total intravenous anesthesia [47–49], although the potential advantage seems rather minimal because it is only useful during the brief periods during general anesthesia when subdural grid recordings are not in use. A urinary catheter, if used, may be placed under sedation and prevents discomfort caused by bladder distention.

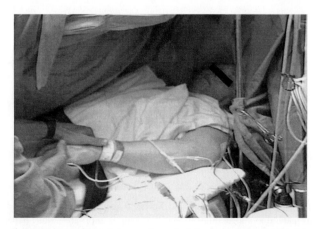

Fig. 3. A patient is positioned in pinion and surgical drapes awake and is undergoing motor testing of the left upper extremity. (*Courtesy of* Fredric B. Meyer, MD.)

Expanded role of the anesthesiologist

With any awake patient, and perhaps especially during an awake craniotomy, the role of the anesthesiologist broadens from clinician and physiologist to encompass the roles of coach, confidant, and interpreter. Unlike other cases in which the patient is awake or in which a wake-up test is used, the duration of required alertness is long (usually less than 1 hour but may be up to several hours); the head immobilized; the drapes large; and the options for managing unplanned events limited. The anesthesiologist must pay close attention to details of patient well-being. Beyond making frequent inquiries of the patient, the anesthesiologist must remain vigilant of the patient's rate and depth of breathing, skin color, and facial expression. The anesthesiologist may need to facilitate patient communication with the surgeon and give encouragement to ensure the patient continues to cope well emotionally. This type of anesthetic care is perhaps reminiscent of an earlier time in anesthetic history, but shifting emphasis to such bedside skills is exceptionally effective in managing the awake craniotomy.

Anesthetic management

A variety of anesthetic techniques have been described to safeguard the airway and to provide good operative conditions in an awake state during the critical portion of eloquent brain mapping. Currently, the two main themes in the literature are a technique known as "asleep-awake-asleep" (AAA) and monitored anesthetic care with conscious to moderate sedation. Although no generally accepted guidelines for managing such cases exist at this time, it has been suggested that monitored anesthetic care should be the standard approach [3]. Neuroleptic analgesia is also described but is no longer widely used for awake craniotomy, because the technique is associated with excessive sedation and a higher incidence of pain and seizures [26]. Newer medications, such as dexmedetomidine, propofol, and remifentanil, are shorter-acting, provide better pain control, result in fewer adverse effects, and affect neurocognitive testing comparatively little versus such drugs as droperidol [26,50–52].

Premedication

The goal of premedication is most often to achieve anxiolysis without oversedation. Other goals may include prevention of nausea, seizure, reflux, pain, hemodynamic instability, or other adverse effects. Oral clonidine, midazolam, alprazolam, and droperidol have all been used to provide anxiolysis and some amnesia of initial events, although oversedation may be a risk with even small doses of any of these. Clonidine, an α_2-agonist, provides blood pressure control and is less likely to induce cognitive impairment. Midazolam may help prevent nausea [53,54]. Benzodiazepines may occasionally produce paradoxical agitation. For this reason, and not to risk oversedation and compromise of the neurologic examination, most anesthesiologists do not routinely administer any sedative premedication [55,56]. Metoclopramide, ondansetron, ranitidine, and sodium bicitrate, or similar medications in these classes, may be administered for prevention of nausea, reflux, or aspiration pneumonia. Depending on the frequency of seizures, a patient may receive an oral loading dose of phenytoin or other antiepileptic drugs. Dexamethasone may be administered for elevated intracranial pressure or prevention of nausea [57]. Acetaminophen was administered routinely in one trial for mild analgesia [38]. If dexmedetomidine, a selective α_2-agonist, is chosen for intraoperative use and a loading dose is planned, glycopyrrolate may be helpful as a premedication to prevent bradycardia and hypotension. Further premedication should be tailored to a patient's comorbidities.

Local anesthetics

With any anesthetic technique for awake craniotomy, adequate local anesthesia is critical to minimizing opioid and sedative requirements and avoiding airway compromise. The neurosurgeon often depends on consultation with the anesthesiologist to determine maximal dose limits for the local anesthetic. Bupivacaine, levobupivacaine, and ropivacaine are chosen for their long duration, lasting approximately 6 to 8 hours. Levobupivacaine and ropivacaine are reported to have less cardiac and neurotoxicity in animals [58]. The maximum dose of bupivacaine should not exceed 3 mg/kg with or without epinephrine. Analgesia is used at the pinion sites (if three-point rigid pinion fixation is used); scalp; and dura. Reinfiltration at closure, although several hours later, is usually not necessary because of the duration of local anesthetic and institution of moderate sedation and analgesia or general anesthesia.

An alternative to local field block by the surgeon is the use of regional nerve block of the scalp. Girvin [59] described performing scalp blocks for awake craniotomy by targeting the six nerves supplying the scalp bilaterally at their most proximal points on the head. These include the greater and lesser occipital nerves, the greater auricular nerve, the auriculotemporal nerve, the zygomaticotemporal nerve, the supratrochlear nerve, and the supraorbital nerve. Recent reports of successful scalp blocks performed in this method for awake seizure focus resection describe the use of bupivacaine 0.25% [38,60], levobupivacaine 0.5%, and ropivacaine 0.75%, all with epinephrine [61,62]. In the descriptions of levobupivacaine and ropivacaine, volumes of 30 to 35 mL were used with additional infiltration of small volumes of the local anesthetic at the pinion sites, and at skin incision, 40 to 60 minutes after scalp block. Peak plasma concentration of these agents occurred at 15 minutes and no seizures or other signs of toxicity were reported [61,62].

Asleep-awake-asleep technique

The AAA technique calls for general anesthesia, with or without the use of an airway, during the opening and closing portions and emergence of the patient in the interim. This has also been described as a prolonged wake-up test with removal and replacement of an airway device. Most often the patient is induced with propofol and a short-acting opioid, pulses of fentanyl or a remifentanil infusion, and in some centers target-controlled infusions are used. Propofol infusion rates range from 75 to 250 µg/kg/min in reports. Sufentanil and alfentanil are cited less frequently, but are also easily managed opioids because of their short duration of action. Nitrous oxide may be added. A volatile anesthetic has been used by some for the initial craniotomy opening, although volatile anesthetic should be eliminated by the time ECoG testing is initiated. The rates of anesthetic infusion are adjusted to provide deep general anesthesia at beginning and end of the case, and a sleepy but responsive patient during testing. Propofol is turned off 15 minutes before ECoG recordings, because propofol has a predominantly suppressive effect at sedative doses and interferes with ECoG interpretation [51]. Rates as low as 10 µg/kg/min, however, are reported not to interfere with EcoG [63]. More often, only a low infusion of opioid is continued during the awake portion, such as remifentanil, 0.01 to 0.05 µg/kg/min [37,63]. The rate of opioid infusion can be adjusted independently of propofol to improve patient comfort or alter the rate of the patient's breathing during spontaneous ventilation.

A laryngeal mask airway is the airway device most often used for the asleep portions because of its ease of insertion, removal, and reinsertion without changing the position of a patient's head (and disruption of the surgical field). Controversy as to whether the laryngeal mask airway represents a secure airway is by no means settled, but in this arena, case reports and chart reviews report low complication rates for using the laryngeal mask airway as an airway device in the spontaneously breathing patient, and a backup for airway control in case of respiratory crisis [34]. One report describes the use of muscle relaxant (atracurium) and mechanical positive pressure ventilation by the laryngeal mask airway for cranial and dural opening following which the patient is allowed to breathe spontaneously [43]. Although this provides good patient comfort and satisfaction, even complete amnesia for the procedure, significant sedation can interfere with intraoperative testing.

In earlier reports, placement of a cuffed endotracheal tube is described, including the technique of extubation and reintubation over a tube exchanger [64], although this may interfere with language testing or, at a minimum, with patient comfort. Fiberoptic intubation is an option for replacement of a cuffed endotracheal tube in pinion fixation.

Monitored anesthesia care

The more commonly advocated technique (over AAA) is monitored anesthesia care, also called conscious sedation, for the opening and closing portions of the procedure. Pulses or infusions of many of the same medications (propofol, and fentanyl and its analogs) are used as for the AAA technique but at lower doses. Recently, the α_2-agonist dexmedetomidine has also become a popular choice for monitored anesthesia care during awake craniotomy.

Monitored anesthesia care perhaps better achieves the goal of providing a smooth transition to alertness, and obviates the difficulties of airway intervention. Oxygen by nasal cannula or face mask is used. The airway is not manipulated, although a nasal trumpet or oral airway can be helpful for the patient with obstructive breathing [27]. Target-controlled infusions or patient-controlled administration methods have been used [47,52]. Midazolam is a frequently reported adjunct. Suggested doses of remifentanil range from 0.03 to 0.09 μg/kg/min [39,63,65]. Propofol doses are often between 30 and 180 μg/kg/min [39,42,43,63,65]. When the dura is opened, some authors advocate continuing a low-dose infusion of remifentanil or dexmedetomidine throughout the awake portion to achieve a state in which the patient is relaxed but fully arousable to perform testing and respond to questions. Doses in the range of 0.005 to 0.01 μg/kg/min for remifentanil or 0.02 to 0.5 μg/kg/h for dexmedetomidine are described for use in manner [34,41,48,49,55,60,63,66,67]. This does not often interfere with cognitive testing or cortical mapping. Many anesthesiologists prefer to not administer any sedation during the period of testing, however, to prevent the possibility of any confounding variables. If propofol and remifentanil are used, propofol is turned off 10 to 15 minutes before testing or cortical mapping, and the remifentanil infusion is stopped (or decreased to the low rate above) about 2 minutes prior. Sedation is deepened again once all testing is completed, and is maintained until skin closure. Just before emergence a dose of longer-acting opioid is sometimes administered, such as 5 to 10 mg of morphine [34,63], for postoperative analgesia. Johnson and Egan [63] used pharmacokinetic simulations to show that rapid decreases in effect site concentration are achieved by such infusion management during awake craniotomy.

Medications

Several specific medication effects have been studied with regard to awake craniotomy for epilepsy. Although most data are from small or retrospective studies, such insight can provide some guidance in management of the awake craniotomy patient.

Propofol, although providing good patient satisfaction, and antiemetic and antiepileptic effects, may cause oversedation and poor operating conditions. Propofol is associated with hypoventilation (higher CO_2 and greater brain volume), although this is less of a problem when a target-controlled infusion is used or when opioids are not added [34,52].

Largely opioid-based techniques are associated with increased reports of seizures and nausea [56]. Among opioids, none of the short-acting fentanyl congeners, including the ultra short-acting remifentanil and alfentanil, used for awake craniotomy has been shown to be superior to its peers. Comparisons of fentanyl with sufentanil and alfentanil, and remifentanil with fentanyl, do not show any differences in complications and all provided good clinical conditions [39,56]. The desirable brevity of action common to these opioids may require the use of a longer-acting opioid for postoperative pain control. The problems of respiratory depression, increased brain volume, airway obstruction, and desaturation are common to all opioids.

Dexmedetomidine, the selective α_2-agonist with anesthetic-sparing effect, has been used for both monitored anesthesia care and AAA management of awake craniotomy since the first case report by Bekker and colleagues in 2001 [41,48,49,55,60,66–68]. Dexmedetomidine has been used as a rescue drug when a prolonged mapping interval (89 minutes) began to cause agitation in a patient receiving remifentanil [60]. The successful use of dexmedetomidine has even been reported in children as young as 12 years [41,49]. Dexmedetomidine is more titratable than clonidine, provides analgesia with minimal respiratory depression (little risk of hypocapnia), anxiolysis without agitation or hangover effect, and hemodynamic stability. Lower doses are suggested for awake craniotomy, because higher doses can impair patient responsiveness [69]. It may be used alone for sedation and analgesia, or with volatile, nitrous oxide, or total intravenous anesthesia as an adjunct to smooth induction, and emergence. The main disadvantages of dexmedetomidine include hypotension and bradycardia, which are reported to be dose-related and treatable, if not preventable [70].

A salient point regarding α_2-agonists for neuroanesthesia is the reduction in regional and global cerebral blood flow that results from cerebral vasoconstriction [71]. Although there is some evidence of cerebral protection in rabbits and rats by the drug [72,73], this report of sustained decreased cerebral blood flow suggests that dexmedetomidine may be detrimental to patients at risk of cerebral ischemia. Reduced cerebral perfusion pressure has also been reported in humans [74]. Although this has been cited as improving operating conditions (reducing brain edema) [67], it is recommended that α_2-agonists be used with caution in patients who have elevated intracerebral pressure (Table 1) [70,77–81].

Complications

Fortunately, complications are infrequent during and after awake craniotomy, because of the great amount of care taken with patient selection and preparation. Exact comparison with complications of craniotomy under general anesthesia is imperfect because of fewer, smaller studies of awake procedures. Nonetheless, less nausea and vomiting is reported in awake craniotomy, for tumors and for epileptic foci, likely related to use of propofol, lack of reversal medications, and lack of opioid use depending on the protocol used [27,28].

Table 1
Common anesthetic medications and adjuvants and their associated epileptogenicity
(anticonvulsant or proconvulsant activity)

Medication	Epileptogenicity
Propofol	Anticonvulsant at sedative doses
Dexmedetomidine	Possible anticonvulsant activity
Thiopental	Anticonvulsant and proconvulsant in low doses
Midazolam	Anticonvulsant
Diazepam	Anticonvulsant
Methohexital	Anticonvulsant and proconvulsant at low doses
Ketamine	Proconvulsant and anticonvulsant in doses used to treat status epilepticus
Etomidate	Proconvulsant and anticonvulsant in doses used to treat status epilepticus
Nitrous oxide	Likely no effect on EEG, possibly mildly proconvulsant
Isoflurane	Anticonvulsant, possibly mildly proconvulsant
Sevoflurane	Anticonvulsant, possibly mildly proconvulsant
Desflurane	Not proconvulsant
Local anesthetics	Anticonvulsant in low doses, proconvulsant in toxic doses
Opioids (fentanyl, remifentanil, alfentanil, sufentanil)	Proconvulsant in patients with epilepsy
Meperidine	Metabolite normeperidine is proconvulsant
Droperidol	No effect on EEG, although may lower seizure threshold
Metoclopramide	No effect on EEG
Ondansetron-granisetron	No effect on EEG
Succinylcholine	No effect on EEG
Vecuronium-Rocuronium	No effect on EEG
Atracurium-cisatracurium	Metabolite laudanosine is theoretically proconvulsant

Abbreviation: EEG, electroencephalography.

Airway complications and desaturation, not surprisingly, occur more frequently during awake craniotomy, because sedation is used in conjunction with an unprotected airway. In a recent large retrospective review, 0.6% of patients under AAA technique had airway complications (requiring intubation, laryngeal mask airway, or nasal airway), two thirds of whom were obese [27]. None had any adverse sequelae. Incidence of many of these complications has been shown to have decreased in recent years with increased experience [27,34,75]. Although some reports describe up to 16% of cases require intubation [37], others have found that the need for intubation during awake craniotomy to be very rare [76].

Likewise, hypoventilation and increased brain volume is a reported complication of awake craniotomy. Brain swelling may interfere with resection and dural and cranial closure. The large review of complications by Skucas and colleagues [27] reported two of 332 propofol-based AAA cases involved brain swelling caused by hypoventilation. It was thought that only one of the two (who sustained a significant hemorrhage with dural opening) suffered an adverse event as a result of increased brain volume. A prospective trial included 1 of 25 patients who required emergent intubation for brain swelling with no further sequelae after conversion to general anesthesia [37]. Others report hypoventilation but no detrimental increase in brain volume [34,52,75].

Intraoperative seizure is an expected risk in this population. Although reports suggest this occurs as frequently under general anesthesia [27], an unchecked seizure in an awake patient in pinion with an unsecured airway is potentially more detrimental. Fortunately, seizures stimulated by cortical mapping are usually aborted by the surgeon stopping the stimulation or delivering ice-cold saline directly onto the cortical surface. Seizures that are spontaneous or do not stop with these measures are treated with small doses of benzodiazepine, propofol, or barbiturate. Rarely do these require intubation. A postictal period may interfere with neurocognitive testing.

Hemodynamic changes including hypertension, hypotension, and tachycardia were found to be more frequent, albeit not harmful to any patient when promptly treated, with awake craniotomy by AAA technique than under general anesthesia [27]. Patient agitation and movement can be managed by altering sedation medication and making other small changes in the patient's immediate surroundings, such as temperature, amount of light, and padding, although occasionally more drastic measures including conversion to general anesthesia are necessary. The anesthesiology team must always be ready to treat emergence delirium quickly in patients being managed with AAA techniques. Rarely, there have been reports of violent emergence from anesthesia resulting in patient injury from struggling out of the head-holding device, and loss of intravenous access. Other reported intraoperative complications, including venous air embolism, in awake craniotomy patients are apparently no more frequent than in craniotomy under general anesthesia [77–82]. Complications are managed best if anticipated and prevented through patient selection, preparation, and appropriate premedication.

Summary

A variety of anesthetic methods, with and without airway manipulation, are available to facilitate awake intraoperative examinations and cortical stimulation, which allow more aggressive resection of epileptogenic foci in functionally important brain regions. Currently, dexmedetomidine or alternatively propofol with fentanyl or remifentanil are the most commonly chosen regimens for seamless transition from the asleep or sedated state to alertness and back during craniotomy. Careful patient selection and preparation combined with attentive cooperation of the medical team are the foundation for a smooth awake procedure. With improved pharmacologic agents and variety of techniques at the neuroanesthesiologist's disposal, awake craniotomy has become an elegant approach to epileptic focus resection in functional cortex.

References

[1] CDC & Epilepsy foundation websites. Accessed December, 2006.
[2] Kwan P, Brodie MJ. Early identification of refractory epilepsy. N Engl J Med 2000;342(5): 314–9.
[3] Meyer FB, Bates LM, Goerss SJ, et al. Awake craniotomy for aggressive resection of primary gliomas located in eloquent brain. Mayo Clin Proc 2001;76(7):677–87.
[4] Penfield W, Roberts L. Speech and brain mechanism. Princeton (NJ): University Press; 1951.
[5] Ojemann G, Ojemann J, Lettich E, et al. Cortical language localization in left, dominant hemisphere: an electrical stimulation mapping investigation in 117 patients. J Neurosurg 1989;71(3):316–26.
[6] Ojemann G, Mateer C. Human language cortex: localization of memory, syntax, and sequential motor-phoneme identification systems. Science 1979;205(4413):1401–3.
[7] Engel J Jr. Surgical treatment of the epilepsies. New York: Raven Press; 1987.
[8] Wieser HG, Elger CE, Hess RM. Presurgical evaluation of epileptics: basics, techniques, implications. Berlin: Springer-Verlag; 1987.
[9] Dam M, Andersen AR, a Rogvi-Hansen B, et al. Epilepsy surgery: non-invasive versus invasive focus localization. Acta Neurol Scand Suppl 1994;89:891–218.
[10] Duchowny M, Resnick R, Alvarez L, editors. Pediatric epilepsy surgery. J Epilepsy 1990;3(Suppl 1).
[11] Apuzzo MLJ. Neurosurgical aspects of epilepsy. Park Ridge (IL): American association of neurological surgeons; 1991.
[12] Spencer SS, Spencer DD. Surgery for epilepsy. Boston: Blackwell Scientific; 1991.
[13] Pilcher WH, Rusyniak WG. Complications of epilepsy surgery. Neurosurg Clin N Am 1993; 4(2):311–25.
[14] Wiebe S, Blume WT, Girvin JP, et al. A randomized, controlled trial of surgery for temporal-lobe epilepsy. N Engl J Med 2001;345(5):311–8.
[15] Engel J Jr, Wiebe S, French J, et al. Practice parameter: temporal lobe and localized neocortical resections for epilepsy. Epilepsia 2003;44(6):741–51.
[16] Spencer SS, Berg AT, Vickrey BG, et al. Initial outcomes in the multicenter study of epilepsy surgery. Neurology 2003;61(12):1680–5.
[17] Engel J Jr. Surgery for seizures. N Engl J Med 1996;334(10):647–52.
[18] Engel J Jr. Etiology as a risk factor for medically refractory epilepsy: a case for early surgical intervention. Neurology 1998;51(5):1243–4.
[19] Langfitt JT. Cost-effectiveness of anterotemporal lobectomy in medically intractable complex partial epilepsy. Epilepsia 1997;38(2):154–63.
[20] Ojemann GA, Schoenfield-McNeill J. Activity of neurons in human temporal cortex during identification and memory for names and words. J Neurosci 1999;19(13):5674–82.
[21] Sahjpaul RL. Awake craniotomy: controversies, indications and techniques in the surgical treatment of temporal lobe epilepsy. Can J Neurol Sci 2000;(27 Suppl 1):S55–63, [discussion: S92–6].
[22] Kanazawa O, Blume WT, Girvin JP. Significance of spikes at temporal lobe electrocorticography. Epilepsia 1996;37(1):50–5.
[23] Taylor MD, Bernstein M. Awake craniotomy with brain mapping as the routine surgical approach to treating patients with supratentorial intraaxial tumors: a prospective trial of 200 cases. J Neurosurg 1999;90(1):35–41.
[24] Blanshard HJ, Chung F, Manninen PH, et al. Awake craniotomy for removal of intracranial tumor: considerations for early discharge. Anesth Analg 2001;92(1):89–94.

[25] Jaaskelainen J, Randell T. Awake craniotomy in glioma surgery. Acta Neurochir Suppl 2003;8831–5.

[26] Danks RA, Rogers M, Aglio LS, et al. Patient tolerance of craniotomy performed with the patient under local anesthesia and monitored conscious sedation. Neurosurgery 1998;42(1): 28–34, [discussion: 34–6].

[27] Skucas AP, Artru AA. Anesthetic complications of awake craniotomies for epilepsy surgery. Anesth Analg 2006;102(3):882–7.

[28] Manninen PH, Tan TK. Postoperative nausea and vomiting after craniotomy for tumor surgery: a comparison between awake craniotomy and general anesthesia. J Clin Anesth 2002;14(4):279–83.

[29] Lehericy S, Duffau H, Cornu P, et al. Correspondence between functional magnetic resonance imaging somatotopy and individual brain anatomy of the central region: comparison with intraoperative stimulation in patients with brain tumors. J Neurosurg 2000;92(4): 589–98.

[30] Vlieger EJ, Majoie CB, Leenstra S, et al. Functional magnetic resonance imaging for neurosurgical planning in neurooncology. Eur Radiol 2004;14(7):1143–53.

[31] So EL. Role of neuroimaging in the management of seizure disorders. Mayo Clin Proc 2002; 77:1251–64.

[32] Schiffbauer H, Berger MS, Ferrari P, et al. Preoperative magnetic source imaging for brain tumor surgery: a quantitative comparison with intraoperative sensory and motor mapping. Neurosurg Focus 2003;15:E7.

[33] Cohen-Gadol AA, Britton JW, Collignon FP, et al. Nonlesional central lobule seizures: use of awake cortical mapping and subdural grid monitoring for resection of seizure focus. J Neurosurg 2003;98(6):1255–62.

[34] Sarang A, Dinsmore J. Anaesthesia for awake craniotomy: evolution of a technique that facilitates awake neurological testing. Br J Anaesth 2003;90(2):161–5.

[35] Brock-Utne JG. Awake craniotomy. Anaesth Intensive Care 2001;29(6):669.

[36] Gebhard RE, Berry J, Maggio WW, et al. The successful use of regional anesthesia to prevent involuntary movements in a patient undergoing awake craniotomy. Anesth Analg 2000; 91(5):1230–1.

[37] Picht T, Kombos T, Gramm HJ, et al. Multimodal protocol for awake craniotomy in language cortex tumour surgery. Acta Neurochir 2006;148(2):127–37, [discussion: 137–8].

[38] Whittle IR, Midgley S, Georges H, et al. Patient perceptions of awake brain tumour surgery. Acta Neurochir 2005;147(3):275–7, [discussion: 277].

[39] Manninen PH, Balki M, Lukitto K, et al. Patient satisfaction with awake craniotomy for tumor surgery: a comparison of remifentanil and fentanyl in conjunction with propofol. Anesth Analg 2006;102(1):237–42.

[40] Lucas TH II, McKhann GM II, Ojemann GA, et al. Functional separation of languages in the bilingual brain: a comparison of electrical stimulation language mapping in 25 bilingual patients and 117 monolingual control patients. J Neurosurg 2004;101(3):449–57.

[41] Everett LL, van Rooyen IF, Warner MH, et al. Use of dexmedetomidine in awake craniotomy in adolescents: report of two cases. Paediatr Anaesth 2006;16(3):338–42.

[42] Klimek M, Verbrugge SJ, Roubos S, et al. Awake craniotomy for glioblastoma in a 9-year-old child. Anaesthesia 2004;59(6):607–9.

[43] Hagberg CA, Gollas A, Berry JM. The laryngeal mask airway for awake craniotomy in the pediatric patient: report of three cases. J Clin Anesth 2004;16(1):43–7.

[44] Leuthardt EC, Fox D, Ojemann GA, et al. Frameless stereotaxy without rigid pin fixation during awake craniotomies. Stereotact Funct Neurosurg 2002;79(3–4):256–61.

[45] Bernstein M. Outpatient craniotomy for brain tumor: a pilot feasibility study in 46 patients. Can J Neurol Sci 2001;28(2):120–4.

[46] Costello TG, Cormack JR. Anaesthesia for awake craniotomy: a modern approach. J Clin Neurosci 2004;11(1):16–9.

[47] Hans P, Bonhomme V, Born JD, et al. Target-controlled infusion of propofol and remifentanil combined with bispectral index monitoring for awake craniotomy. Anaesthesia 2000; 55(3):255–9.

[48] Bekker AY, Kaufman B, Samir H, et al. The use of dexmedetomidine infusion for awake craniotomy. Anesth Analg 2001;92(5):1251–3.

[49] Ard J, Doyle W, Bekker A. Awake craniotomy with dexmedetomidine in pediatric patients. J Neurosurg Anesthesiol 2003;15(3):263–6.

[50] Archer DP, McKenna JM, Morin L, et al. Conscious-sedation analgesia during craniotomy for intractable epilepsy: a review of 354 consecutive cases. Can J Anaesth 1988;35(4): 338–44.

[51] Herrick IA, Craen RA, Gelb AW, et al. Propofol sedation during awake craniotomy for seizures: electrocorticographic and epileptogenic effects. Anesth Analg 1997;84(6):1280–4.

[52] Herrick IA, Craen RA, Gelb AW, et al. Propofol sedation during awake craniotomy for seizures: patient-controlled administration versus neurolept analgesia. Anesth Analg 1997; 84(6):1285–91.

[53] Bauer KP, Dom PM, Ramirez AM, et al. Preoperative intravenous midazolam: benefits beyond anxiolysis. J Clin Anesth 2004;16(3):177–83.

[54] Heidari SM, Saryazdi H, Saghaei M. Effect of intravenous midazolam premedication on postoperative nausea and vomiting after cholecystectomy. Acta Anaesthesiol Taiwan 2004;42(2):77–80.

[55] Almeida AN, Tavares C, Tibano A, et al. Dexmedetomidine for awake craniotomy without laryngeal mask. Arq Neuropsiquiatr 2005;63(3B):748–50.

[56] Gignac E, Manninen PH, Gelb AW. Comparison of fentanyl, sufentanil and alfentanil during awake craniotomy for epilepsy. Can J Anaesth 1993;40(5 Pt 1):421–4.

[57] Chen MS, Hong CL, Chung HS, et al. Dexamethasone effectively reduces postoperative nausea and vomiting in a general surgical adult patient population. Chang Gung Med J 2006;29(2):175–81.

[58] Ohmura S, Kawada M, Ohta T, et al. Systemic toxicity and resuscitation in bupivacaine-, levobupivacaine-, or ropivacaine-infused rats. Anesth Analg 2001;93(3):743–8.

[59] Girvin JP. Resection of intracranial lesions under local anesthesia. Int Anesthesiol Clin 1986; 24(3):133–55.

[60] Moore TA II, Markert JM, Knowlton RC. Dexmedetomidine as rescue drug during awake craniotomy for cortical motor mapping and tumor resection. Anesth Analg 2006;102(5): 1556–8.

[61] Costello TG, Cormack JR, Mather LE, et al. Plasma levobupivacaine concentrations following scalp block in patients undergoing awake craniotomy. Br J Anaesth 2005;94(6):848–51.

[62] Costello TG, Cormack JR, Hoy C, et al. Plasma ropivacaine levels following scalp block for awake craniotomy. J Neurosurg Anesthesiol 2004;16(2):147–50.

[63] Johnson KB, Egan TD. Remifentanil and propofol combination for awake craniotomy: case report with pharmacokinetic simulations. J Neurosurg Anesthesiol 1998;10(1):25–9.

[64] Shuer LM. Epilepsy surgery: surgical considerations, anesthesiologist's manual of surgical procedures. In: Jaffe RA, Samuels SI, editors. Anesthesiologist's Manual of Surgical Procedures. 2nd edition. Philadelphia: Lippincott Williams & Wilkins; 1999. p. 54–5.

[65] Keifer JC, Dentchev D, Little K, et al. A retrospective analysis of a remifentanil/propofol general anesthetic for craniotomy before awake functional brain mapping. Anesth Analg 2005;101(2):502–8, [table of contents].

[66] Mack PF, Perrine K, Kobylarz E, et al. Dexmedetomidine and neurocognitive testing in awake craniotomy. J Neurosurg Anesthesiol 2004;16(1):20–5.

[67] Ard JL Jr, Bekker AY, Doyle WK. Dexmedetomidine in awake craniotomy: a technical note. Surg Neurol 2005;63(2):114–6, [discussion: 116–7].

[68] Souter MJ, Rozet I, Ojemann JG, et al. Dexmedetomidine sedation during awake craniotomy for seizure resection: effects on electrocorticography. J Neurosurg Anesthesiol 2007; 19(1):38–44.

[69] Bustillo MA, Lazar RM, Finck AD, et al. Dexmedetomidine may impair cognitive testing during endovascular embolization of cerebral arteriovenous malformations: a retrospective case report series. J Neurosurg Anesthesiol 2002;14(3):209–12.

[70] Cormack JR, Orme RM, Costello TG. The role of alpha2-agonists in neurosurgery. J Clin Neurosci 2005;12(4):375–8.

[71] Prielipp RC, Wall MH, Tobin JR, et al. Dexmedetomidine-induced sedation in volunteers decreases regional and global cerebral blood flow. Anesth Analg 2002;95(4):1052–9, [table of contents].

[72] Hoffman WE, Kochs E, Werner C, et al. Dexmedetomidine improves neurologic outcome from incomplete ischemia in the rat: reversal by the alpha 2-adrenergic antagonist atipamezole. Anesthesiology 1991;75(2):328–32.

[73] Maier C, Steinberg GK, Sun GH, et al. Neuroprotection by the alpha 2-adrenoreceptor agonist dexmedetomidine in a focal model of cerebral ischemia. Anesthesiology 1993; 79(2):306–12.

[74] Talke P, Tong C, Lee HW, et al. Effect of dexmedetomidine on lumbar cerebrospinal fluid pressure in humans. Anesth Analg 1997;85(2):358–64.

[75] Berkenstadt H, Perel A, Hadani M, et al. Monitored anesthesia care using remifentanil and propofol for awake craniotomy. J Neurosurg Anesthesiol 2001;13(3):246–9.

[76] Duffau H, Capelle L, Denvil D, et al. Usefulness of intraoperative electrical subcortical mapping during surgery for low-grade gliomas located within eloquent brain regions: functional results in a consecutive series of 103 patients. J Neurosurg 2003;98(4):764–78.

[77] Bonhomme V, Born JD, Hans P. Prise en charge anesthésique des craniotomies en état vigile [Anaesthetic management of awake craniotomy]. Ann Fr Anesth Reanim 2004;23(4): 389–94, [in French].

[78] Roper SN, Alphin RS. Epilepsy surgery. In: Cucchiara RF, Black S, Michenfelder JD, editors. Clinical neuroanesthesia. 2nd edition. New York: Churchill Livingstone; 1998. p. 367–88.

[79] Kofke WA, Tempelhoff R, Dasheiff RM. Anesthetic implications of epilepsy, status epilepticus, and epilepsy surgery. J Neurosurg Anes 1997;9(4):349–72.

[80] Tanaka K, Oda Y, Funao T, et al. Dexmedetomidine decreases the convulsive potency of bupivacaine and levobupivacaine in rats: involvement of α_2-adrenoceptor for controlling convulsions. Anesth Analg 2005;100:687–96.

[81] Stoelting RK. Pharmacology and physiology in anesthetic practice. Philadelphia: Lippincott-Raven; 1999. p. 40, 41, 92, 96, 144, 168.

[82] Cascino GD, So EL, Sharbrough FW. Alfentanil-induced epileptiform activity in patients with partial epilepsy. J Clini Neurophysiol 1993;10(4):520–5.

ELSEVIER
SAUNDERS

Anesthesiology Clin
25 (2007) 557–577

ANESTHESIOLOGY
CLINICS

Perioperative Uses of Transcranial Perfusion Monitoring

Martin Smith, MBBS, FRCA

*Department of Neuroanaesthesia and Neurocritical Care, The National Hospital
for Neurology and Neurosurgery, University College London Hospitals NHS Trust
and Centre for Anaesthesia, University College London,
Box 30, Queen Square, London, WC1N 3BG, UK*

The most important goals of neuroanesthesia are to maintain cerebral perfusion to meet the tissue demands of oxygen and glucose and, under circumstances of reduced perfusion, to protect the brain. Perioperative transcranial perfusion monitoring provides early warning of impending brain ischemia to steer the neurosurgeon and guide the neuroanesthesiologist to optimize cerebral perfusion and oxygenation. The monitoring options include measurement of cerebral blood flow (CBF), intracranial pressure (ICP), and cerebral perfusion pressure (CPP), and assessment of the adequacy of perfusion by measurement of cerebral oxygenation and brain tissue biochemistry. Some monitoring techniques are well established, whereas others are relatively new to the clinical arena and their indications are still being evaluated (Table 1).

There are few widely accepted indications for specific perioperative neuromonitoring techniques. This article reviews currently available monitors and discusses their application in the perioperative period.

Intracranial pressure monitoring

ICP is usually monitored by an intraventricular catheter or intraparenchymal microsensor. Other available techniques are rarely used and have a substantially lower accuracy (Table 2) [1]. Intraventricular catheters provide the gold standard technique for ICP monitoring. This method measures global ICP and has the additional advantages of allowing in vivo calibration and therapeutic drainage of cerebrospinal fluid [1,2]. Placement of the

---

E-mail address: martin.smith@uclh.nhs.uk

1932-2275/07/$ - see front matter © 2007 Elsevier Inc. All rights reserved.
doi:10.1016/j.anclin.2007.05.002   *anesthesiology.theclinics.com*

Table 1
Applications of neuromonitoring techniques

Neuromonitoring technique	Established Neuro ICU applications	Established perioperative applications
Intracranial pressure	Yes	Yes
Quantitative cerebral blood flow	Yes	Research
Transcranial Doppler	Yes	Yes
Cerebrovascular reactivity	Yes	Research
Jugular venous oximetry	Yes	Yes
Brain tissue oxygenation	Yes	Yes
Near infrared spectroscopy	Research	Research
Cerebral microdialysis	Yes	Research

ventricular catheter can be difficult, however, in the presence of severe brain swelling or of an intracranial mass lesion. There is also significant risk of catheter-related ventriculitis during prolonged monitoring [3]. Modern microtransducer systems can be placed directly in the brain parenchyma through a cranial access device, or in the subdural space by a burr hole or craniotomy. The complication rates, including infection risk, are minimal [4]. Measured ICP may not be representative of global pressure, however, because transtentorial and interhemispheric pressure gradients may be present [5]. Microtransducer systems perform well [6] but may drift during long-term monitoring and in vivo recalibration is not possible [2]. ICP monitoring allows measurement of absolute ICP levels, calculation of CPP, and identification and analysis of pathologic ICP waveforms. Cerebrovascular pressure reactivity (CVR) and pressure-volume compensatory reserve may also be calculated [7].

Table 2
Comparison of intracranial pressure monitoring devices

Method	Advantages	Disadvantages
Intraventricular catheter	• Gold standard • Measures global pressure • Allows therapeutic drainage of CSF • In vivo calibration possible	• Insertion may be difficult • Most invasive method • Risk of hematoma • Risk of ventriculitis
Microtransducer sensor	• Robust technology • Intraparenchymal or subdural placement • Low procedure complication rate • Low infection risk	• Small zero drift over time • No in vivo calibration • Measures local pressure
Epidural catheter	• Easy to insert • No penetration of dura • Low infection rate	• Limited accuracy • Rarely used
Lumbar CSF pressure	• Extracranial procedure	• Does not reflect ICP • Dangerous if ICP elevated

Abbreviations: CSF, cerebrospinal fluid; ICP, intracranial pressure.

Indications for perioperative ICP monitoring include patients with traumatic brain injury (TBI), surgery for large brain tumors with mass effect, hydrocephalus, intracranial and subarachnoid hemorrhage (SAH), and the presence of significant cerebral edema from whatever cause.

After dural opening the ICP is virtually zero but brain swelling may impair neurosurgical access and result in regional ischemia. In a prospective study of almost 700 patients undergoing craniotomy for supratentorial brain tumor, elevated subdural ICP at the start of surgery was an independent risk factor for intraoperative brain swelling and ICP greater than 13 mm Hg indicated that brain swelling was highly probable [8]. Intraoperative ICP monitoring can also be used to identify, prevent, and treat posture-related intracranial hypertension during surgery. In patients with SAH, 10-degree reverse Trendelenburg position decreased ICP in 25 of 28 patients regardless of anesthetic agent, whereas CPP was unchanged [9]. The effect of preoperative ICP and intraoperative CPP on outcome after TBI has also been examined [10]. Mean ICP was higher in patients with unfavorable compared with favorable outcome (47.4 versus 26.4 mm Hg), although intraoperative CPP was a better overall predictor of outcome. Neuroendoscopy results in intracranial hypertension in up to 50% of patients and this may be associated with postoperative morbidity, including new neurologic deficits [11].

Postoperative ICP monitoring is indicated in patients in whom there is a risk of intracranial hypertension, particularly if the patient remains sedated. The need for postoperative ICP monitoring should be identified and instituted early. ICP monitoring is commonly used after surgery for TBI to guide postoperative ICP and CPP-directed therapy on the neurocritical care unit and is recommended by expert consensus guidelines [12].

Cerebral blood flow

Modern imaging techniques provide sophisticated and detailed hemodynamic and metabolic information over multiple regions of interest in the brain. They are only able, however, to provide snapshot images, require transfer of patients to specialized imaging facilities, and have limited availability. Their use in the perioperative period is generally limited to research applications. Positron emission tomography (PET) is widely used as a diagnostic and clinical research tool and is increasing the understanding of cerebral pathophysiology. It also allows data from bedside monitors of perfusion and oxygenation to be compared with actual measures of CBF and oxygen consumption [13,14].

Kety-Schmidt method

The first practical method of measuring CBF was described by Kety and Schmidt [15] in 1945. The methodology has been described in detail [15] but, in brief, it uses nitrous oxide (N_2O) as an inert tracer gas and calculates CBF from the arteriovenous difference of N_2O concentration based on application of the Fick principle. It measures global CBF and is unable to discriminate between gray and white matter flow. The technique as originally described has many disadvantages, including the requirement for timely and repeated arterial and venous blood sampling. The Kety-Schmidt method forms the basis of many CBF measurement techniques in use today, however, and remains the gold standard against which new methods of measurement are validated.

Radioactive tracer techniques

A modification of the Kety-Schmidt technique using inhalation or injection of [133]xenon (^{133}Xe) is the most widely used bedside technique for measuring absolute CBF [16]. CBF is calculated by analysis of the exponential clearance of the radioisotope from the brain, measured by scintillation counters placed over the scalp and producing two-dimensional maps of cortical blood flow. [133]Xe is rapidly cleared so repeat studies can be undertaken within 30 minutes. The accuracy and specificity of the method depends on the number of detectors, but it is possible to achieve high spatial resolution. Although this method can be relatively easily applied at the bedside, it has limited clinical applications in the perioperative period, although it is a useful research tool.

Continuous quantitative cerebral blood flow monitoring

Laser Doppler flowmetry and thermal diffusion flowmetry offer the potential for continuous CBF monitoring. Laser Doppler flowmetry provides reliable measurement of local cortical blood flow based on assessment of the Doppler shift of laser light by moving red blood cells [17]. The technique requires the cortex to be exposed by a burr hole, so it cannot be used to follow changes during induction of anesthesia or in the early stages of surgery. Laser Doppler flowmetry has been used postoperatively to detect ischemia after SAH [18], although arbitrary units and the extremely localized measurement of CBF limit the usefulness of the technique. Thermal diffusion flowmetry differs from laser Doppler flowmetry in offering a quantitative assessment of regional tissue perfusion in terms of absolute flow values. The thermal diffusion flowmetry catheter consists of a thermistor heated to a few degrees above tissue temperature and a second, more proximal, temperature probe. The temperature difference between thermistor and temperature probe is a reflection of heat transfer and can be translated into a measurement of CBF. Thermal diffusion flowmetry provides a sensitive, real-time assessment of local CBF [19] but there are currently limited clinical data and questions about accuracy and reliability have been raised [20].

Double-indicator dilution technique

An intriguing bedside method of assessing CBF, the transcerebral double-indicator dilution technique, has been described by Wietasch and

colleagues [21]. Bolus injections of ice-cold indocyanine green are administered via a central venous line and the resulting thermo-dye curves are
recorded simultaneously in the aorta and jugular venous bulb using combined fiberoptic thermistor catheters. CBF is calculated from the mean transit times of the indicators through the brain. The authors claim that
transcerebral double-indicator dilution technique is less time consuming
and less cumbersome than alternative methods.

Transcranial Doppler ultrasonography

Transcranial Doppler (TCD) was introduced in 1982 and has become
established as a noninvasive, real-time technique for the examination of
cerebral hemodynamics [22]. It is the only method that can be used with relative ease in the operating room [23]. TCD uses ultrasound waves to measure the velocity of blood flow through large cerebral vessels from the
Doppler shift caused by red blood cells moving through the field of view.
TCD does not determine actual blood flow but is a technique for measuring
relative changes in CBF.

A low frequency (2 MHz) pulsed wave probe is used to insonate a basal
cerebral vessel through an acoustic cranial window, an area of the skull with
sparse or no cancellous bone that causes little attenuation and scattering of
the signal. The TCD flow velocity waveform resembles an arterial pulse
wave and may be quantified into peak systolic, end diastolic, and mean
flow velocities, and pulsatility index. If the angle of insonation and the
diameter of the insonated vessel remain constant, changes in measured
blood flow velocity reflect changes in CBF [24]. Pulsatility index reflects distal cerebrovascular resistance and, because it is dimensionless, is not affected
by angle of insonation. Providing the limitations are recognized, it is possible to use TCD to monitor the cerebral circulation and guide the perioperative care of patients with TBI, SAH, and others at risk of cerebral ischemia
[23]. The probe can be fixed in place to ensure a constant angle of insonation
and artifact-free recordings during and after surgery (Fig. 1).

TCD is widely used during carotid endarterectomy and can quantify the
risk of cerebral ischemia during carotid cross clamping [25]. TCD indices
during carotid endarterectomy correlate well with subsequent EEG changes
and have been used as an indication for shunt placement [26]. Emboli can be
detected as characteristic short-duration, high-intensity "chirps," and waveform analysis allows differentiation between air and particulate emboli [27].

TCD also has a role in the diagnosis and management of cerebral vasospasm after SAH and has become routine in the perioperative care of
patients during surgical or neuroradiologic treatment of intracranial aneurysms [28]. Because changes in CBF itself affect flow velocity, the assessment
of vasospasm from measurement of flow velocity alone may be insufficient.
Lindegaard and coworkers [29] described the use of a hemispheric index,
comparing flow velocity in the middle cerebral artery and internal carotid

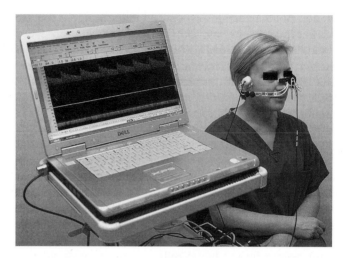

Fig. 1. PC-based transcranial Doppler system (Doppler-Box, Compumedics Germany Gmbh, Hamburg, Germany) and probe fixation device suitable for perioperative use.

artery on the same side, that is unaffected by changes in CBF. An index of greater than 3 is indicative of vasospasm and values greater than 6 suggest severe spasm. The sensitivity and specificity of TCD for the diagnosis of vasospasm is generally high, although there is considerable interindividual variation. High flow velocities may be tolerated in some patients, whereas in others vasospasm may be present despite normal flow velocity. Treatment decisions are not usually based on TCD findings alone. Mascia and colleagues [30] assessed the accuracy of TCD using receiver-operator characteristic analysis and found that mean flow velocity thresholds of 100 and 160 cm/s were most accurate for the detection of angiographic and clinical vasospasm, respectively, in the middle cerebral artery. Consecutive TCD examinations should be performed after SAH and flow velocity greater than 140 cm/s, or flow velocity increases greater than 50 cm/s/d from baseline, are generally accepted to be indicative of developing or established vasospasm [31].

TCD may be used to monitor the integrity of pressure autoregulation and CO_2 reactivity [32] in the perioperative period to guide management of CBF and minimize the risk of ischemia. TCD has also been used to estimate ICP noninvasively with an absolute accuracy of $\pm$ 10 to 15 mm Hg [33].

Measurement of cerebrovascular reactivity

The loss of CVR renders the brain more susceptible to ischemic insults. Because CVR may be disturbed or abolished by intracranial pathology and some anesthetic agents, the ability to monitor CVR in the perioperative period is an attractive proposition.

Methods of testing static and dynamic autoregulation are well established [32] but most are interventional, intermittent, and are not practical options in the perioperative period. More recently, methods for the continuous assessment of CVR that require no intervention have been described. The ICP response to changes in arterial blood pressure depends on the pressure-reactivity of cerebral vessels. This is a key component of pressure autoregulation and disturbed pressure reactivity implies disturbed pressure autoregulation. A pressure-reactivity index can be derived from continuous monitoring and analysis of slow waves in arterial blood pressure and ICP [7,34]. Under normal circumstances, an increase in arterial blood pressure leads to cerebral vasoconstriction within 5 to 15 seconds and a secondary reduction of cerebral blood volume and ICP. When CVR is impaired, cerebral blood volume and ICP increase passively with arterial blood pressure. Opposite effects occur when arterial blood pressure is reduced. Pressure-reactivity index is determined by calculating the correlation coefficient of consecutive time averaged data points of ICP and arterial blood pressure recorded over a 4-minute period [33]. A negative value for pressure-reactivity index, when arterial blood pressure is inversely correlated with ICP, indicates a normal CVR, and a positive value indicates a nonreactive cerebrovascular circulation. Pressure-reactivity index correlates with standard measures of cerebral autoregulation [34] and abnormal values are predictive of poor outcome after TBI [35]. Oxygen reactivity, measured using brain tissue oxygen monitoring (intraparenchymal brain tissue oxygenation [$Ptio_2$]), provides additional information about cerebrovascular autoregulation, and has been correlated with pressure-reactivity index [36]. CVR can also be assessed continuously using TCD. The moving correlation coefficient between arterial blood pressure and mean and systolic flow velocities during spontaneous fluctuations in arterial blood pressure is calculated over 3-minute epochs, yielding a mean and systolic index of autoregulation [37].

The potential value of CVR assessment in the perioperative period was demonstrated in a recent study when pressure-reactivity index was used to monitor changes in CVR in patients undergoing decompressive craniectomy [38]. Dynamic pressure autoregulation has also been measured during acute aneurysm surgery and can be used to optimize intraoperative blood pressure management [39].

Measurement of cerebral oxygenation

Jugular venous oximetry

Jugular venous oxygen saturation ($Sjvo_2$) provides information about the balance between global cerebral oxygen delivery and metabolic demand and can be used as a nonquantitative assessment of the adequacy of CBF [40]. The normal $Sjvo_2$ is 55% to 75%, which is lower than mixed venous saturation reflecting the high oxygen requirement of the normal brain. Derived variables, such as the arterial to jugular venous oxygen concentration difference

(AjvDO$_2$), have also been extensively used in the study of cerebral metabolism [41]. Normal AjvDO$_2$ is 4 to 8 mL O$_2$/100 mL blood.

The technique of jugular venous oximetry is relatively straightforward. A catheter is inserted into an internal jugular vein and advanced to the jugular bulb. The position of the catheter is crucial to minimize the risk of extracranial contamination, which is around 3% if the catheter is correctly placed. Typically, around two thirds of the sampled blood is drained from the ipsilateral hemisphere, although there is large interindividual variability and it is impossible to predict in an individual patient which side gives more relevant information [42]. Sjvo$_2$ monitoring accurately reflects global cerebral oxygenation only if the dominant jugular bulb is cannulated [43]. The right side is often chosen because it is usually dominant [44]. The correct side can be identified more accurately, however, by ultrasound examination of the internal jugular vein, by identifying the largest ICP rise caused by manual compression of each internal jugular vein, or by identification of the larger jugular foramen on CT scan. Once the catheter position has been checked on a lateral cervical spine radiograph, measurement of Sjvo$_2$ can be made continuously using a fiberoptic catheter or directly by aspirating blood samples. Blood should be withdrawn at a rate of less than 2 mL/min to minimize the risk of falsely elevated values caused by aspiration of extracranial blood [45]. Fiberoptic catheters require regular recalibration and, even under stable conditions, less than half of total monitoring time produces high-quality data. Notwithstanding these practical difficulties, Sjvo$_2$ is widely used for perioperative oxygenation monitoring [46].

Sjvo$_2$ levels less than 55% suggest cerebral hypoperfusion with oxygen demand exceeding supply, whereas levels greater than 80% indicate relative hyperemia, caused either by raised CBF or reduced oxygen demand (Fig. 2) [44,47]. Because Sjvo$_2$ is a global, hemispheric measure it cannot detect regional ischemia [48]. PET evidence suggests that Sjvo$_2$ does not fall below 50% until approximately 13% of the brain becomes ischemic [49].

Calculation of the AjvDO$_2$ can serve as an indirect measure of relative changes in CBF [44]: CBF = CMRO$_2$/AjvDO$_2$, where CMRO$_2$ is the cerebral

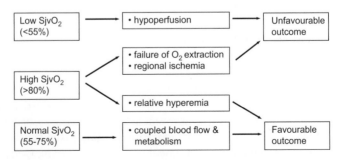

Fig. 2. Interpretation of jugular venous oxygen saturation values.

metabolic rate for oxygen. If $CMRO_2$ remains constant, changes in $AjvDO_2$ reflect changes in CBF, but such estimates of CBF are often inaccurate because of the anatomic limitations of the technique. Jugular bulb catheters are most commonly used to measure trends in oxygenation indices.

In 1994, Matta and colleagues [46] reported the intraoperative use of $Sjvo_2$ monitoring in 100 consecutive patients undergoing craniotomy. They found that the jugular catheter could be placed quickly and detected frequent episodes of jugular venous desaturation that would otherwise have been undiagnosed and untreated. The benefits of $Sjvo_2$ monitoring to assess cerebral hypoperfusion and guide intraoperative blood pressure management have been confirmed in a study of patients undergoing intracranial aneurysm surgery [50]. $Sjvo_2$ monitoring has also been extensively investigated in patients undergoing cardiopulmonary bypass when episodes of jugular desaturation occur frequently, particularly during rewarming, and are correlated with higher incidence of severe postoperative cognitive dysfunction and higher mortality [51].

Most of the literature regarding $Sjvo_2$ monitoring has focused on the monitoring and management of TBI [52]. There is a significant association between jugular venous desaturation and poor neurologic outcome, with poor outcome occurring in 55% of patients with no episodes of desaturation, 74% of those with one episode, and 90% of those with multiple episodes [53]. There is some evidence that $Sjvo_2$ monitoring can be used to guide hyperventilation after TBI and that treatment of desaturation may improve outcome [47]. This is controversial, however, because of the lack of sensitivity of this technique to regional ischemia.

Brain tissue oxygen tension

$Ptio_2$ is increasingly being measured whenever ICP monitoring is indicated and is becoming established as the gold standard bedside monitor of cerebral oxygenation [54]. Currently, only one $Ptio_2$ monitor is commercially available for use in humans (Licox, GMS, Kiel-Mielkendorf, Germany) (Fig. 3). This sensor uses a closed polarographic (Clark-type) cell with reversible electrochemical electrodes. Oxygen diffuses from the brain tissue across a semipermeable membrane and is reduced by a gold polarographic cathode. This produces a flow of electrical current proportional to the oxygen concentration in a temperature-dependent manner [55]. A sensor-specific smart card allows straightforward and rapid calibration. A run-in time of around 1 hour is required following insertion of a brain $Ptio_2$ probe and this has implications for intraoperative monitoring. $Ptio_2$ provides a highly focal measurement of cerebral oxygenation and, although this offers the potential of selective monitoring of critically perfused tissue, accurate placement of the probe is crucial and global changes may be missed [48].

Brain $Ptio_2$ is related to other physiologic variables and these relationships have been examined to understand the physiologic basis for critical

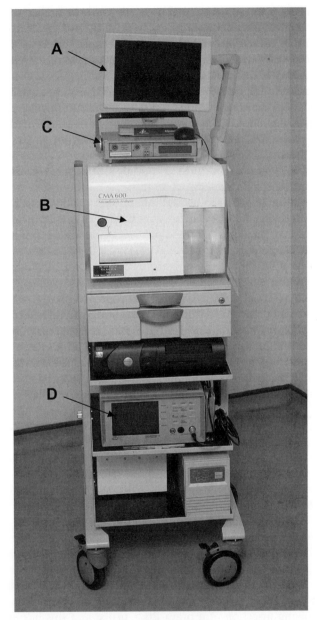

Fig. 3. Multimodality monitoring stack. (*A*) Microdialysis data display. (*B*) Microdialysis bed-side analyzer (CMA 700, Solna, Sweden). (*C*) Brain tissue oxygen monitor (Licox, GMS, Kiel-Mielkendorf, Germany). (*D*) Continuous jugular venous oxygen saturation monitor (Abbott Oximetrix SO2 Monitor, Abbott, UK, Maidenhead, UK).

oxygenation thresholds. PET studies have shown correlation between $Ptio_2$ and regional CBF [56] and also between changes in $Ptio_2$ and changes in regional venous oxygen saturation [13]. Brain $Ptio_2$ is increased by an increase in fraction of inspired oxygen (and in Pao_2) [57], red cell transfusion [58], and increases in MAP and CPP [59] and is most likely to represent a balance between CBF, oxygen extraction fraction, and Pao_2. Normal brain $Ptio_2$ values are in the region of 35 to 50 mm Hg [60]. Under normoxic conditions, a high brain $Ptio_2$ reflects increased tissue perfusion, whereas low $Ptio_2$ reflects low or inadequate perfusion. Low $Ptio_2$ does not always represent ischemia, however, because it may occur as a result of cerebral hypometabolism (eg, related to sedative agents or hypothermia) in the presence of stable oxygen extraction and coupled hypoperfusion.

$Ptio_2$ monitoring allows rapid detection of intraoperative cerebral ischemia and the possibility that therapy may be initiated before irreversible neuronal damage occurs. It has been recommended during aneurysm surgery and may identify patients at risk for procedure-related ischemia [61]. Using a threshold of 15 mm Hg, brain $Ptio_2$ is more effective than somatosensory evoked potential monitoring at predicting ischemia [62]. Hoffman and colleagues [63] compared $Ptio_2$ of cortex adjacent to arteriovenous malformations with control (nonischemic) areas of brain in patients undergoing elective aneurysm surgery. Brain $Ptio_2$ in control patients did not change during surgery. In the arteriovenous malformations patients, $Ptio_2$ was low before arteriovenous malformation resection, suggesting reduced perfusion and chronic hypoxia, and increased markedly postresection suggesting hyperperfusion. The effect of dural opening and tumor resection on $Ptio_2$ has also been investigated. In patients with intraoperative brain swelling, low peritumoral $Ptio_2$ increased dramatically on dural opening and following tumor resection, suggesting the presence of significant hypoxia in peritumoral edema [64]. This emphasizes the importance of maintaining CPP during brain tumor surgery and suggests that $Ptio_2$ monitoring might be used to guide intraoperative blood pressure management. Reduced brain $Ptio_2$ has also been shown to improve in association with reductions in ICP and increases in CPP following decompressive craniectomy [65]. Furthermore, patients with severe brain hypoxia before surgery were more likely to have poorer outcome, raising the possibility that $Ptio_2$ monitoring may be used to select patients who might benefit from surgical decompression.

Most clinical data on $Ptio_2$ monitoring come from studies after TBI. Reduced $Ptio_2$ is associated with poor outcome [66], but a threshold for cerebral hypoxia has not been clearly identified. It is likely, however, that such a threshold would relate to both duration and depth of hypoxia. In a recent PET study of TBI, brain regions with $Ptio_2$ values less than 10 mm Hg had significantly lower hyperventilation-induced increases in mean oxygen extraction fraction [14]. In another study, when CPP was augmented from 70 to 90 mm Hg, the $Ptio_2$ value associated with normal oxygen extraction fraction was 14 mm Hg [59]. These data suggest that the ischemic threshold lies below 14 mm Hg, but critical values for $Ptio_2$ are best considered within a range as opposed to a precise threshold [54]. The ceiling of $Ptio_2$ during augmentation of CPP is highest in areas of focal ischemia [67], suggesting that beneficial effects are occurring in at-risk tissue. What is less clear is whether manipulation of $Ptio_2$ is able to affect outcome. In a recent study of 28 patients, however, standard ICP- and CPP-guided therapy combined with interventions to maintain $Ptio_2$ greater than 25 mm Hg resulted in lower mortality than that in a group of 25 historical controls receiving ICP- and CPP-guided therapy alone [68].

Regional and global oxygenation monitoring techniques are not competitive or mutually exclusive. Neither $Sjvo_2$ nor $Ptio_2$ monitoring alone identifies all episodes of ischemia and they should be considered complementary with monitoring strategies taking advantage of the unique features of each technique [48].

Near infrared spectroscopy

Near infrared spectroscopy (NIRS) is a noninvasive technique based on the transmission and absorption of near infrared light (700–1000 nm) as it passes through tissue. Oxygenated and deoxygenated hemoglobin have different absorption spectra and cerebral oxygenation and hemodynamic status can be determined by their relative absorption of near infrared light. Earlier NIRS methodology was limited to measuring changes in tissue chromophore concentration, but recent advances have allowed measurement of absolute hemoglobin oxygen saturation [69] and absolute concentrations of oxyhemoglobin and deoxyhemoglobin [70]. NIRS interrogates arterial, venous, and capillary blood within the field of view and the derived saturation represents a tissue oxygen saturation measured from these three compartments. In addition to monitoring oxygenation variables, NIRS has been used to measure regional CBF [71] and cerebral blood volume [72], but these techniques have not been validated. More recently, it has become possible to measure changes in the concentration of the terminal complex of the electron transfer chain, cytochrome-c oxidase, in adults [73]. This measurement has been validated in animal studies as a measure of changes in cellular energy status [74] and offers the potential to assess intramitochondrial redox state after human brain injury. Two types of NIRS instrumentation are available for clinical use: the INVOS series (Somanetics Corporation, Troy, Michigan) and the NIRO series (Hamamatsu Photonics, Hamamatsu City, Japan) (Fig. 4). The INVOS presents a single numerical value for regional cerebral saturation (rSO_2), whereas the NIRO provides a tissue oxygenation index in percentage terms and changes in oxyhemoglobin and deoxyhemoglobin variables and oxidized cytochrome-c oxidase.

Trends in NIRS variables may detect ischemic events and rSO_2 has been used to monitor ischemia during interventional radiologic procedures [75]

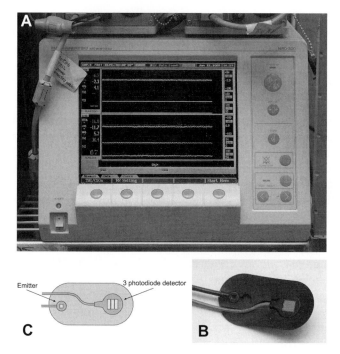

Fig. 4. Near infrared spectroscopy system. (*A*) NIRO 300 spectrometer (Hamamatsu Photonics, Hamamatsu City, Japan). (*B*) Transcranial optodes. (*C*) Schematic of optodes.

and carotid cross clamping [76,77]. NIRS has also been used to detect intraoperative increases in cortical oxygen saturation and blood volume, indicative of a hyperemic state, after arteriovenous malformation resection [78]. NIRS-measured cerebral oxygenation has been compared with $SjvO_2$ and brain $PtiO_2$ in patients with TBI [57] and tentative ischemic thresholds for NIRS variables have recently been described [79]. Monitoring and treatment of rSO_2 during cardiopulmonary bypass has been shown to minimize the incidence of cerebral desaturation and is associated with a lower incidence of postoperative systemic organ dysfunction [80].

NIRS has the potential to provide continuous, noninvasive measurement of cerebral hemodynamic, oxygenation, and metabolic variables over multiple regions of interest with high temporal resolution. There is lack of standardization of the technology for clinical use, however, and in some cases the algorithms are not published [81]. It is difficult to translate data between studies using different technologies. Another concern is the potential contamination of the NIRS signal from extracranial sources, although the wider application of spatially resolved spectroscopy, which has high sensitivity and specificity to intracranial changes, helps in resolving this issue [77]. Modern broadband spectroscopy systems also allow improved temporal and spatial resolution and the opportunity for multisite, real-time measurement [73]. NIRS has many potential advantages over other techniques but further technologic advances are necessary before it can become a reliable clinical monitor.

Cerebral microdialysis

Cerebral microdialysis (MD) is a well-established laboratory tool that is being increasingly used as a bedside monitor to provide on-line analysis of brain tissue biochemistry during neurointensive care. The principles and clinical applications of cerebral MD have recently been reviewed [82,83]. The MD catheter consists of a fine double-lumen probe, lined at its tip with a semipermeable dialysis membrane that is placed in brain tissue (Fig. 5). The probe is perfused by an inlet tube with fluid isotonic to the tissue interstitium and the perfusate passes along the membrane before exiting by outlet tubing into a collecting chamber. Diffusion drives the passage of molecules across the membrane along their concentration gradient (Fig. 6). The MD catheter acts as an artificial blood capillary and the concentration of substrate in the collected fluid (the microdialysate) depends in part on the balance between substrate delivery to, and uptake and excretion from, the brain extracellular fluid. A commercially available MD analyzer (CMA, Solna, Sweden) measures microdialysate concentrations of glucose, lactate, pyruvate, glycerol, and glutamate on-line (see Fig. 3). The concentration of these substances in the microdialysate does not correspond to their true extracellular fluid concentration and the proportion of the extracellular fluid concentration in the microdialysate is termed the "relative recovery." This is dependent on membrane pore size, membrane area, perfusate flow rate, and diffusion speed of the substance.

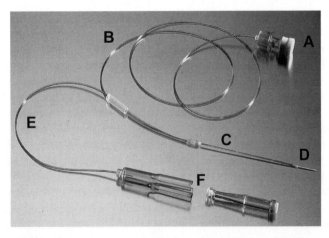

Fig. 5. Components of clinical microdialysis catheter. (*A*) Perfusate pump connector. (*B*) Inlet tube. (*C*) Microdialysis catheter. (*D*) Microdialysis membrane. (*E*) Outlet tube. (*F*) Collecting vial and holder.

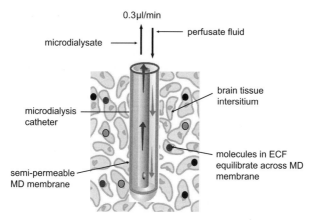

Fig. 6. Schematic of microdialysis catheter located in brain tissue. Isotonic fluid is pumped through the microdialysis catheter at a rate of 0.3 μL min⁻¹. Molecules at high concentration in the brain extracellular fluid equilibrate across the semipermeable microdialysis membrane and can be analyzed in the microdialysate. ECF, extracellular fluid; MD, microdialysis.

In clinical practice the most commonly used system comprises a catheter that is 10 mm in length with a 20- or 100-kd molecular weight cutoff, perfused with commercially available perfusate solution (Perfusion Fluid CNS, CMA Microdialysis) at a rate of 0.3 $\mu L/min^{-1}$ [82]. Samples are usually collected and analyzed at hourly intervals. It is recommended that the MD catheter be placed in at-risk tissue (ie, adjacent to a mass lesion or, in the case of an aneurysm, in the territory of the parent vessel) [84]. This allows biochemical changes to be measured in the area of brain most vulnerable to ischemic insult.

Most clinical experience with cerebral MD relates to monitoring patients with TBI and SAH in the neurocritical care unit [82,83]. Severe cerebral hypoxia or ischemia is typically associated with marked increases in the lactate-pyruvate ratio [85], and lactate-pyruvate ratio greater than 20 to 25 is associated with poor outcome after TBI [86]. It has traditionally been assumed that increases in lactate-pyruvate ratio are caused only by tissue ischemia and, although increases in lactate-pyruvate ratio correlate with PET-measured oxygen extraction fraction [59], it has not been possible to establish a hypoxic threshold associated with raised lactate-pyruvate ratio [87]. It is now apparent that anaerobic glycolysis may occur not only because of hypoxia and ischemia but also because of mitochondrial failure and failure of effective use of delivered oxygen [88]. Cerebral MD offers a unique opportunity to monitor such cellular dysfunction. Glycerol is a marker of ischemic cell damage and increased MD glycerol concentrations are associated with poor outcome after TBI [89]. Increased levels of excitatory amino acids [90] and reduced brain extracellular fluid glucose levels [91] may also predict or be associated with metabolic catastrophes occurring after acute brain injury. MD is becoming established as a tool to assist clinical decision making during neurointensive care [82,83].

Because cerebral MD measures changes at the cellular level, it has the potential to detect hypoxia and ischemia before changes can be detected by more conventional monitoring techniques or before a change in clinical status. In one study, a rise in lactate-pyruvate ratio and glycerol predicted the occurrence of a delayed ischemic deficit related to cerebral vasospasm 11 to 23 hours before its clinical appearance [92]. Such predictive value of MD might offer substantial advantages over other monitoring techniques in the perioperative period.

MD is an attractive technique to monitor impending ischemia during neurovascular surgery when early detection may prevent or minimize damage by prompting a change in operative or anesthetic management. In one study, increases in lactate, lactate-pyruvate ratio, and glutamate were associated with reductions in brain Ptio$_2$ during aneurysm surgery, although, unlike Ptio$_2$, were not predictive of subsequent infarction [93]. Changes in glutamate have also been demonstrated to be an excellent marker of neuronal damage and subsequent neurologic deficit after extracranial-intracranial bypass surgery [94].

The intraoperative applications of cerebral MD are currently limited by technology. The usual hourly sampling rate is unlikely to offer adequate time resolution in the operative setting. Increased perfusate flow rate allows sufficient volume of sample to be retrieved at 15-minute intervals, albeit at the expense of lower relative recovery of measured variables. For clinically useful detection of metabolic changes during surgery, however, more rapid sampling is likely to be required. A continuous cerebral MD technique has been described, although such technology is currently not available commercially [95]. The future success of cerebral MD as a perioperative monitor depends on the choice of biomarkers; their sensitivity, specificity, and predictive value for secondary neurochemical events; and the availability of practical methods for analysis of biomarkers.

Summary

Given the physiologic complexity of the human brain it is not surprising that a single variable or a single device is unable to provide adequate monitoring of cerebral well-being during surgery or of the multiple pathophysiologic processes that occur after brain injury. It is for this reason that multimodality monitoring, including combined measures of cerebral perfusion, oxygenation, and metabolic status, is often recommended [96,97]. Most neuromonitors have been developed and tested in the neurocritical care unit and, although some translate well into the operating room, others are less suited to this environment because of incompatibility or inadequate temporal resolution. Multiparameter probes that measure ICP, Ptio$_2$ and CBF are likely to be available for clinical use in the near future. It is also likely that technical advances will lead to the development of monitors that deliver noninvasive, continuous, multisite measurement of cerebral hemodynamics, oxygenation, and metabolic status and that will be suited to the perioperative period. Currently, every monitor of cerebral perfusion and oxygenation has its own specific shortcomings and none is a standard of care in the perioperative period.

References

[1] Zhong J, Dujovny M, Park HK, et al. Advances in ICP monitoring techniques. Neurol Res 2003;25:339–50.

[2] Steiner LA, Andrews PJD. Monitoring the injured brain: ICP and CBF. Br J Anaesth 2006; 97:26–38.

[3] Lozier AP, Sciacca RR, Romagnoli MF, et al. Ventriculostomy-related infections: a critical review of the literature. Neurosurgery 2002;51:170–81.

[4] Martinez-Manas RM, Santamarta D, de Campos JM, et al. Camino intracranial pressure monitor: prospective study of accuracy and complications. J Neurol Neurosurg Psychiatr 2000;69:82–6.

[5] Sahuquillo J, Poca MA, Arribas M, et al. Interhemispheric supratentorial intracranial pressure gradients in head-injured patients: are they clinically important? J Neurosurg 1999;90:16–26.

[6] Czosnyka M, Czosnyka Z, Pickard JD. Laboratory testing of three intracranial pressure microtransducers: technical report. Neurosurgery 1996;38:219–24.

[7] Czosnyka M, Pickard JD. Monitoring and interpretation of intracranial pressure. J Neurol Neurosurg Psychiatr 2004;75:813–21.

[8] Rasmussen M, Bundgaard H, Cold HE. Craniotomy for supratentorial brain tumors: risk factors for brain swelling after opening the dura mater. J Neurosurg 2004;101:621–6.

[9] Tanski A, Rasmussen M, Juul N, et al. Effects of reverse 10° Trendelenburg on subdural intracranial pressure and cerebral perfusion pressure in patients subjected to craniotomy for cerebral aneurysm. J Neurosurg Anesthesiol 2006;18:11–7.

[10] Kuo JR, Yeh TC, Sung KC, et al. Intraoperative applications of intracranial pressure monitoring in patients with severe head injury. J Clin Neurosci 2006;13:218–23.

[11] Fabregas N, Lopez A, Valero R, et al. Anesthetic management of surgical neuroendoscopies: usefulness of monitoring the pressure inside the neuroendoscope. J Neurosurg Anesthesiol 2000;12:21–8.

[12] Brain Trauma Foundation. Guidelines for the management of severe traumatic brain injury. J Neurotrauma 2007;24(Suppl 1):S37–44.

[13] Gupta AK, Hutchinson PJ, Fryer T, et al. Measurement of brain tissue oxygenation performed using positron emission tomography scanning to validate a novel monitoring method. J Neurosurg 2002;96:263–8.

[14] Menon DK, Coles JP, Gupta AK, et al. Diffusion limited oxygen delivery following head injury. Crit Care Med 2004;32:1384–90.

[15] Kety SS, Schmidt CF. The determination of cerebral blood flow in man by the use of nitrous oxide in low concentrations. Am J Physiol 1945;143:53–5.

[16] Anderson RE. Cerebral blood flow xenon-133. Neurosurg Clin N Am 1996;7:703–8.

[17] Bolgnese P, Miller JI, Heger IM, et al. Laser-Doppler flowmetry in neurosurgery. J Neurosurg Anesthesiol 1993;5:151–8.

[18] Johnson WD, Bolognese P, Miller JI, et al. Continuous postoperative ICBF monitoring in aneurismal SAH patients using a combined ICP-laser Doppler fibreoptic probe. J Neurosurg Anesthesiol 1996;8:199–207.

[19] Jaeger M, Soehle M, Schuhmann MU, et al. Correlation of continuously monitored regional cerebral blood flow and brain tissue oxygen. Acta Neurochir (Wien) 2005;147:51–6.

[20] Vajkoczy P, Horn P, Thorne C, et al. Regional cerebral blood flow monitoring in the diagnosis of cerebral vasospasm following aneurismal subarachnoid hemorrhage. J Neurosurg 2003;98:1227–34.

[21] Wietasch GJK, Mielck F, Scholz M, et al. Bedside assessment of cerebral blood flow by double-indicator dilution technique. Anesthesiology 2000;92:367–75.

[22] Aaslid R, Markwalder TM, Nornes H. Non-invasive transcranial Doppler ultrasound recording of flow velocity in basal cerebral arteries. J Neurosurg 1982;57:769–74.

[23] Lam AM, Newell DW. Intraoperative use of transcranial Doppler ultrasonography. Neurosurg Clin N Am 1996;7:709–22.

[24] Valdueza JM, Balzer JO, Villringer A, et al. Changes in blood flow velocity and diameter of the middle cerebral artery during hyperventilation: assessment with MR and transcranial Doppler sonography. AJNR Am J Neuroradiol 1997;18:1929–34.

[25] Dunne VG, Besser M, Ma WJ. Transcranial Doppler in carotid endarterectomy. J Clin Neurosci 2001;8:140–5.

[26] Jansen C, Vriens EM, Eikelboom BC, et al. Carotid endarterectomy with transcranial Doppler and electroencephalographic monitoring: a prospective study in 130 operations. Stroke 1993;24:665–9.

[27] Ringelstein EB, Droste DW, Babikan VL, et al. Consensus on microembolus detection by TCD. International consensus group on microemboli detection. Stroke 1998;29:725–9.

[28] Spingborg JB, Frederksen H-J, Eskesen V, et al. Trends in monitoring patients with aneurysmal subarachnoid haemorrhage. Br J Anaesth 2005;94:259–70.

[29] Lindegaard KF, Nornes H, Bakke SJ, et al. Cerebral vasospasm diagnosis by means of angiography and blood velocity measurements. Acta Neurochir (Wien) 1989;100:12–24.

[30] Mascia L, Fedorko L, TerBrigge K, et al. The accuracy of transcranial Doppler to detect vasospasm in patients with aneurismal subarachnoid haemorrhage. Intensive Care Med 2003;29:1088–94.

[31] Lerch C, Yonekawa Y, Muroi C, et al. Specialised neurocritical care, severity grade and outcome of patients with aneurismal subarachnoid hemorrhage. Neurocrit Care 2006;5:85–92.

[32] Rasulo FA, Balestreri M, Matta B. Assessment of cerebral pressure autoregulation. Curr Opin Anaesthesiol 2002;15:483–8.

[33] Czosnyka M, Matta B, Smielewski P, et al. Cerebral perfusion pressure in head-injured patients: a non-invasive assessment using transcranial Doppler ultrasonography. J Neurosurg 1998;88:802–8.

[34] Czosnyka M, Smielewski P, Kirkpatrick P, et al. Continuous assessment of the cerebral vasomotor reactivity in head injury. Neurosurgery 1997;41:11–7.

[35] Steiner LA, Czosnyka M, Piechnik SK, et al. Continuous monitoring of cerebrovascular pressure reactivity allows determination of optimal cerebral perfusion pressure in patients with traumatic brain injury. Crit Care Med 2002;30:733–8.

[36] Jaeger M, Scuhmann MU, Soehle M, et al. Continuous assessment of cerebrovascular autoregulation after traumatic brain injury using brain tissue oxygen pressure reactivity. Crit Care Med 2006;34:1783–8.

[37] Piechnik SK, Yang X, Czosnyka M, et al. The continuous assessment of cerebrovascular reactivity: a validation of the method in healthy volunteers. Anesth Analg 1999;89:944–9.

[38] Wang EC, Ang BT, Wong J, et al. Characterisation of cerebrovascular reactivity after craniectomy for acute brain injury. Br J Neurosurg 2006;20:24–30.

[39] Schmieder K, Moller F, Engelhardt M, et al. Dynamic cerebral autoregulation in patients with ruptured and unruptured aneurysms after induction of general anaesthesia. Zentralbl Neurochir 2006;67:81–7.

[40] Schell RM, Cole DJ. Cerebral monitoring: jugular vein oximetry. Anesth Analg 2000;90:559–66.

[41] Macmillan CSA, Andrews PJD. Cerebrovenous oxygen saturation monitoring: practical considerations and clinical relevance. Intensive Care Med 2000;26:1028–36.

[42] Stocchetti N, Paparella A, Bridelli F, et al. Cerebral venous oxygen saturation studied with bilateral samples in the internal jugular vein. Neurosurgery 1994;34:38–43.

[43] Lam JM, Chan MS, Poon WS. Cerebral venous oxygen saturation monitoring: is dominant jugular bulb cannulation enough? Br J Neurosurg 1996;10:357–64.

[44] Robertson CS, Narayan RK, Gokaslan ZL, et al. Cerebral arterio-venous oxygen difference as an estimate of cerebral blood flow in comatose patients. J Neurosurg 1989;70:222–30.

[45] Matta B, Lam AM. The rate of blood withdrawal affects the accuracy of jugular venous bulb oxygen saturation measurements. Anesthesiology 1997;86:806–8.

[46] Mata BF, Lam AM, Mayberg TS, et al. A critique of the intraoperative use of jugular venous bulb catheters during neurosurgical procedures. Anesth Analg 1994;79:745–50.

[47] Cruz J. The first decade of continuous monitoring of jugular bulb oxyhemoglobin saturation: management strategies and clinical outcome. Crit Care Med 1998;26:344–51.

[48] Gupta AK, Hutchinson PJ, Al-Rawi P, et al. Measuring brain tissue oxygenation compared with jugular venous oxygen saturation for monitoring cerebral oxygenation after traumatic brain injury. Anesth Analg 1999;88:549–533.

[49] Coles JP, Fryer TD, Smielewski P, et al. Incidence and mechanisms of cerebral ischemia in early clinical head injury. J Cereb Blood Flow Metab 2004;24:202–11.

[50] Moss E, Dearden NM, Berridge I. Effects of changes in mean arterial pressure on SjO2 during cerebral aneurysm surgery. Br J Anaesth 1995;75:527–30.

[51] Croughwell ND, Newman MF, Blumenthal JA, et al. Jugular bulb saturation and cognitive dysfunction after cardiopulmonary bypass. Ann Thorac Surg 1994;58:1702–8.

[52] Robertson CS, Gopinath SP, Goodman JC, et al. SjvO2 monitoring in head-injured patients. J Neurotrauma 1995;12:891–6.

[53] Gopinath SP, Robertson CS, Contant CF, et al. Jugular venous desaturation and outcome after head injury. J Neurol Neurosurg Psychiatr 1994;57:717–23.

[54] Rose JC, Neill TA, Hemphill JC. Continuous monitoring of the microcirculation in neurocritical care: an update on brain tissue oxygenation. Curr Opin Crit Care 2006;12:97–102.

[55] Nortje J, Gupta AK. The role of tissue oxygen monitoring in patients with acute brain injury. Br J Anaesth 2006;97:95–106.

[56] Scheufler KM, Rohrborn HJ, Zentner J. Does tissue oxygen-tension reliably reflect cerebral oxygen delivery and consumption? Anesth Analg 2002;95:1042–8.

[57] McLeod AD, Igielman F, Elwell C, et al. Measuring cerebral oxygenation during normobaric hyperoxia: a comparison of tissue microprobes, near-infrared spectroscopy and jugular venous oximetry. Anesth Analg 2003;97:851–6.

[58] Smith MJ, Stiefel MF, Magge S, et al. Packed red blood cell transfusion increases local cerebral oxygenation. Crit Care Med 2005;33:1104–8.

[59] Johnston AJ, Steiner LA, Coles JP, et al. Effect of cerebral perfusion pressure augmentation on regional oxygenation and metabolism after head injury. Crit Care Med 2005;33:189–95.

[60] Hoffman WE, Charbel FT, Edelman G. Brain tissue oxygen, carbon dioxide, and pH in neurosurgical patients at risk for ischemia. Anesth Analg 1996;82:582–6.

[61] Doppenberg EMR, Watson JC, Broaddus WC, et al. Intraoperative monitoring of substrate delivery during aneurysm and haematoma surgery: initial experience in 16 patients. J Neurosurg 1997;87:809–16.

[62] Jodicke A, Hubner F, Boker DK. Monitoring of brain tissue oxygenation during aneurysm surgery: prediction of procedure-related ischemic events. J Neurosurg 2003;98:515–23.

[63] Hoffman WE, Charbel FT, Edelman G, et al. Brain tissue gases and pH during arteriovenous malformation resection. Neurosurgery 1997;40:294–301.

[64] Pennings FA, Bouma GJ, Kedaria M, et al. Intraoperative monitoring of brain tissue and carbon dioxide pressures reveals low oxygenation in peritumoral brain edema. J Neurosurg Anesthesiol 2003;15:1–5.

[65] Stiefel MF, Heuer GG, Smith MJ, et al. Cerebral oxygenation following decompressive hemicraniectomy for the treatment of refractory intracranial hypertension. J Neurosurg 2004;101:241–7.

[66] Valadka AB, Gopinath SP, Contant CF, et al. Relationship of brain tissue PO2 to outcome after severe head injury. Crit Care Med 1998;26:1576–81.

[67] Stocchetti N, Chieregato A, De MM, et al. High cerebral perfusion pressure improves low values of local brain tissue O2 tension (PtiO2) in focal lesions. Acta Neurochir 1998; 71(Suppl):162–5.

[68] Stiefel MF, Spiotta A, Gracias VH, et al. Reduced mortality rate in patients with severe traumatic brain injury treated with brain tissue oxygen monitoring. J Neurosurg 2005;103: 805–11.

[69] Suzuki S, Takasaki S, Ozaki T, et al. A tissue oxygenation monitor using NIR spatially resolved spectroscopy. SPIE Proc 1999;3597:582–92.

[70] Fantini S, Hueber D, Franceschini MA, et al. Non-invasive optical monitoring of the newborn piglet brain using continuous-wave and frequency-domain spectroscopy. Phys Med Biol 1999;44:1543–63.

[71] Gora F, Shinde S, Elwell CE, et al. Noninvasive measurement of cerebral blood flow in adults using near-infrared spectroscopy and indocyanine green: a pilot study. J Neurosurg Anesthesiol 2002;14:218–22.

[72] Hopton P, Walsh TS, Lee A. Measurement of cerebral blood volume using near-infrared spectroscopy and indocyanine green elimination. J Appl Physiol 1999;87:1981–7.

[73] Tisdall M, Tachtsidis I, Leung TS, et al. Near infrared spectroscopic quantification of changes in the concentration of oxidized cytochrome oxidase in the healthy human brain during hypoxemia. J Biomed Optics 2007;12:024002.

[74] Springett RJ, Wylezinska M, Cady EB, et al. The oxygen dependency of cerebral oxidative metabolism in the newborn piglet studied with 31P NMRS and NIRS. Adv Exp Med Biol 2003;530:555–63.

[75] Luer MS, Pharm D, Dujovnt M, et al. Regional cerebral oxygen saturation during intra-arterial papaverine therapy for vasospasm. Neurosurgery 1995;36:1033–6.

[76] Samra SK, Dy EA, Welch K, et al. Evaluation of a cerebral oximeter as a monitor of cerebral ischemia during carotid endarterectomy. Anesthesiology 2000;93:964–70.

[77] Al-Rawi PG, Smielewski P, Kirkpatrick PJ. Evaluation of a near-infrared spectrometer (NIRO 300) for the detection of intracranial oxygenation changes in the adult head. Stroke 2001;32:2492–500.

[78] Asgari S, Rohrborn HJ, Engelhorn T, et al. Intraoperative measurement of cortical oxygen saturation and blood volume adjacent to cerebral arteriovenous malformation using near-infrared spectroscopy. Neurosurgery 2003;52:1298–304.

[79] Al-Rawi PG, Kirkpatrick PJ. Tissue oxygen index: thresholds for cerebral ischemia using near-infrared spectroscopy. Stroke 2006;37:2720–5.

[80] Murkin JM, Adams SJ, Novick RJ, et al. Monitoring brain oxygen saturation during coronary bypass surgery: a randomized, prospective study. Anesth Analg 2007;104: 51–8.

[81] Owen-Reece H, Smith M, Elwell CE, et al. Near infrared spectroscopy. Br J Anaesth 1999; 82:418–26.

[82] Tisdall MM, Smith M. Cerebral microdialysis: research technique or clinical tool. Br J Anaesth 2006;97:18–25.

[83] Hillered L, Vespa PM, Hovda DA. Translational neurochemical research in acute human brain injury: the current status and potential future for cerebral microdialysis. J Neurotrauma 2005;22:3–41.

[84] Bellander BM, Cantais E, Enblad P, et al. Consensus meeting on microdialysis in neurointensive care. Intensive Care Med 2004;30:2166–9.

[85] Hutchinson PJ, Gupta AK, Frywe TF, et al. Correlation between cerebral blood flow, substrate delivery, and metabolism in head injury: a combined microdialysis and triple oxygen positron emission tomography study. J Cereb Blood Flow Metab 2002;22: 735–45.

[86] Zauner A, Doppenberg E, Woodward J, et al. Continuous monitoring of cerebral substrate delivery and clearance: initial experience in 24 patients with severe acute brain injuries. Neurosurgery 1997;41:1082–93.

[87] Stahl N, Mellergard P, Hallstrom A, et al. Intracerebral microdialysis and bedside biochemical analysis in patients with fatal traumatic brain lesions. Acta Anaesthesiol Scand 2001;45: 977–85.

[88] Vespa P, Bergsneider M, Hattori N, et al. Metabolic crisis without brain ischemia is common after traumatic brain injury: a combined microdialysis and positron emission tomography study. J Cereb Blood Flow Metab 2005;25:763–74.

[89] Clausen T, Alves OL, Reinert M, et al. Association between elevated tissue glycerol levels and poor outcome following severe traumatic brain injury. J Neurosurg 2005;103:233–8.

[90] Kett-White R, Hutchinson PJ, Al-Rawi PG, et al. Adverse cerebral events detected after subarachnoid hemorrhage using brain oxygen and microdialysis probes. Neurosurgery 2002;50: 1213–21.

[91] Vespa PM, McArthur D, O'Phelan K, et al. Persistently low extracellular glucose correlates with poor outcome 6 months after human traumatic brain injury despite a lack of increased lactate: a microdialysis study. J Cereb Blood Flow Metab 2003;23:865–77.

[92] Skjoth-Rasmussen J, Schulz M, Kristensen SR, et al. Delayed neurological deficit detected by an ischemic pattern in the extracellular metabolites in patients with aneurismal subarachnoid hemorrhage. J Neurosurg 2004;100:8–15.

[93] Kett-White R, Hutchinson PJ, Czosnyka M, et al. Effects of variation in cerebral haemodynamics during aneurysm surgery on brain tissue oxygen and metabolism. Acta Neurochir 2002;81(Suppl):327–9.

[94] Mendelowitsch A, Sekhar LN, Wright DC, et al. An increase in extracellular glutamate is a sensitive method of detecting ischaemic neuronal damage during cranial base and cerebrovascular surgery: an in vivo microdialysis study. Acta Neurochir (Wien) 1998;140:349–50.

[95] Bhatia R, Hashemi P, Razzaq A, et al. Application of rapid-sampling, online microdialysis to the monitoring of brain metabolism during aneurysm surgery. Neurosurgery 2006;58: 313–20.

[96] Armonda RA, Vo AH, Bell R, et al. Multimodal monitoring during emergency hemicraniectomy for vein of Labbe thrombosis. Neurocrit Care 2006;4:241–4.

[97] DeGeorgia MA, Deogaonkar A. Multimodal monitoring in the neurological intensive care unit. Neurologist 2005;11:45–54.

ANESTHESIOLOGY
CLINICS

ELSEVIER
SAUNDERS

Anesthesiology Clin
25 (2007) 579–603

Monitoring and Intraoperative Management of Elevated Intracranial Pressure and Decompressive Craniectomy

W. Andrew Kofke, MD, MBA, FCCM[a],*,
Michael Stiefel, MD, PhD[b]

[a]*Department of Anesthesia and Critical Care, University of Pennsylvania, 3400 Spruce St., Dulles 7, Philadelphia, PA 19104, USA*
[b]*Department of Neurosurgery, University of Pennsylvania, Philadelphia, PA*

There are numerous clinical scenarios wherein a critically ill patient may present with neurologic dysfunction. In a general sense these scenarios often involve ischemia, trauma, or neuroexcitation. Each of these may include a period of decreased cerebral perfusion pressure (CPP), usually due to elevated intracranial pressure (ICP), eventually compromising cerebral blood flow (CBF) sufficiently to produce permanent neuronal loss, infarction, and possibly brain death. Elevated ICP is thus a common pathway for neural demise and it may arise from a variety of causes, many of which may result in a neurosurgical procedure intended to ameliorate the impact or etiology of elevated ICP.

Intracranial hypertension

The brain, spinal cord, cerebrospinal fluid (CSF), and blood are encased in the skull and vertebral canal, thus constituting a nearly incompressible system. In a totally incompressible system, pressure would vary linearly with increased volume. However, there is capacitance in the system, thought to be provided by the intervertebral spaces and the vasculature. Once this capacitance is exhausted the ICP increases dramatically with increased intracranial volume (Fig. 1). This is based on the relation:

---

* Corresponding author.
E-mail address: andrew.kofke@uphs.upenn.edu (W.A. Kofke).

1932-2275/07/$ - see front matter © 2007 Elsevier Inc. All rights reserved.
doi:10.1016/j.anclin.2007.05.007   *anesthesiology.theclinics.com*

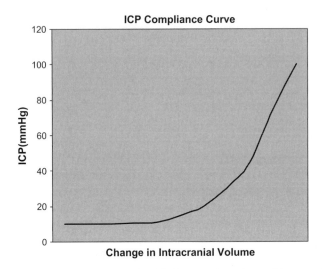

Fig. 1. Conceptual depiction of the relationship between the volume of intracranial contents and pressure. Initial increases in volume have little effect on ICP until a threshold of capacitive exhaustion is reached, after which pressure rises abruptly.

CBF = (MAP−ICP)/CVR, where CBF is Cerebral Blood Flow, MAP is Mean Arterial Pressure, ICP is Intracranial Pressure, and CVR is Cerebrovascular Resistance.

Although increasing ICP may be associated with decrements in CBF, the effect of increasing ICP on CBF is not straightforward, as MAP may increase with ICP elevations [1], and CVR adjusts with decreasing CPP (increasing cerebral blood volume) to maintain CBF until maximal vasodilatation occurs (Fig. 2) [2–5]. This maximum vasodilation, with increased cerebral blood volume, is thought to occur when CPP is less than or equal to 50 mm Hg, although considerable interindividual heterogeneity in this value exists [6]. Thus, increasing ICP is often associated with cerebral vasodilatation or increasing MAP to maintain CBF, making assessment a relatively complex process.

Normal ICP is less than 10 mm Hg, while ICP greater than 20 mm Hg is generally associated with a need for escalation of ICP-reducing therapy [7,8]. However, this is an epidemiologically derived number. Head trauma studies have indicated that patients with ICP greater than 20 mm Hg generally do not do well [7]. Still, physiologically, simply elevating ICP to greater than 20 mm Hg is not necessarily associated with decrements in CBF, provided the above-noted compensatory mechanisms occur [9]. Nonetheless, increasing ICP because of mass lesions or obstruction of CSF outflow can exhaust compensatory mechanisms. When this occurs, compromise of CBF does eventually occur. Initially, abnormality arises in distal runoff of the cerebral circulation. As the process continues, compromise of diastolic perfusion arises. With this the normally continuous (through systole and

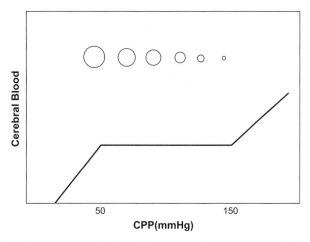

Fig. 2. Relationship between cerebral blood flow and perfusion pressure. Cerebral blood flow stays relatively constant between cerebral perfusion pressures of approximately 50 mm Hg to 150 mm Hg. The changing vascular caliber required to accomplish this (with associated change in cerebral blood volume) is schematically depicted across the top.

diastole) cerebral perfusion becomes discontinuous (Fig. 3) [10]. Further compromise of CBF results in anaerobic metabolism, exacerbation of edema, and ultimately intracranial circulatory arrest [10,11]. Thus, when ICP increases it is important to detect it and ascertain whether this lethal sequence of events may be occurring.

Two types of intracranial hypertension

In a general sense there are two types of intracranial hypertension, categorized according to CBF as hyperemic or oligemic (Fig. 4). Although conceptualized here as a dichotomous process, undoubtedly the real physiology is more of a continuum between the two. In the normal state, increases in CBF are not associated with increased ICP, as the normal capacitive mechanisms absorb the increased intracranial blood volume. However, in the situation of disordered intracranial compliance, small increases in intracranial volume due to increased CBF produce increases in ICP [3,12].

This raises an important issue: elevated ICP has traditionally been considered to be a concern because it indicates that cerebral perfusion might be jeopardized. It is, however, unclear whether it is appropriate to be concerned about high ICP-inducing intracranial oligemia when the cause of the high ICP is intracranial hyperemia. There have been no detailed examinations of this question, although there have been some studies which allow reasonable inferences about the significance of hyperemic intracranial hypertension.

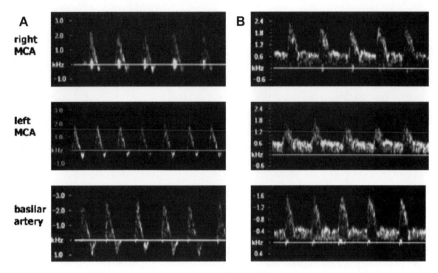

Fig. 3. Transcranial Doppler depiction of the effects of decreasing cerebral perfusion pressure on blood flow velocity. Initally, at normal perfusion pressure, a normal waveform is evident with blood flow present during systole and diastole. Increasing intracranial pressure with associated decreased cerebral perfusion pressure encroaches on diastolic flow until intracranial pressure exceeds diastolic blood pressure, at which point diastolic flow stops. Continued increase in intracranial pressure to exceed systolic blood pressure produces total intracranial circulatory arrest throughout systole and diastole, producing the to and fro waveform on the right indicating blood pumping against the swollen brain and bouncing backward within the basal arteries of the brain. (*From* Reinhard M, Petrick M, Steinfurth G, et al. Acute increase in intracranial pressure revealed by transcranial Doppler sonography. J Clin Ultrasound 2003;31:326; with permission.)

For many years it has been known that brief noxious stimuli briefly increase ICP in the setting of decreased intracranial compliance. Recent studies have reported that such situations are associated with hyperemia [13], strongly suggesting that hyperemic intracranial hypertension is not a dangerous situation [14]. However, it is reasonable to be concerned, at least theoretically, about such hyperemia for three reasons. First, elevated ICP due to hyperemia in one portion of the brain may increase ICP to compromise CBF in other areas of the brain in which regional CBF (rCBF) is marginal. Second, increased pressure in one area of the brain may produce gradients leading to a herniation syndrome. Third, inappropriate hyperemia may predispose the brain to worsened edema or hemorrhage, as occurs with other hyperperfusion syndromes [12,15]. Thus, hyperemic intracranial hypertension has a theoretical potential to be deleterious, but this has yet to be conclusively demonstrated. For brief periods, as may occur during intubation or other limited noxious stimuli, it is suggested that it may not be problematic [16].

In contrast, oligemic intracranial hypertension is associated with compromised cerebral perfusion [17]. This is supported by the high mortality

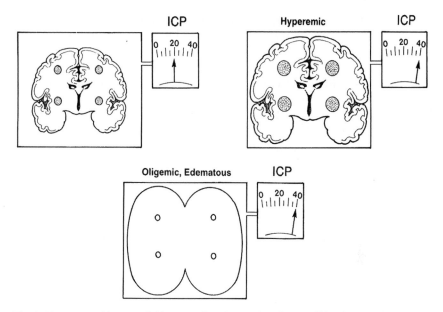

Fig. 4. Two types of intracranial hypertension. From a baseline condition intracranial pressure can increase in two ways. One is via an increase in cerebral blood volume, associated with reflex vasodilation due to moderate blood pressure decreases or due to hyperemia. The second mecahnism of intracranial hypertension is via malignant brain edema or other expanding masses encroaching on the vascular bed, to produce intracranial ischemia. (*From* Kofke WA, Wechsler L. Neurointensive care. In: Albin M, editor. Textbook of neurosanesthesia. New York: McGraw-Hill; 1997. p. 1247–348; with permission.)

observed in head trauma patients in whom ICP rises because of brain edema after head injury, with decrements in CBF [7,18]. Transcranial Doppler (TCD) and CBF studies on these patients have demonstrated that CBF is low and perfusion is discontinuous during the cardiac cycle (see Fig. 3) [10,18]. Moreover, jugular venous bulb data indicates that O_2 extraction is markedly increased [19], suggesting anaerobic metabolism [18]. In this setting noxious stimuli can further increase the ICP, thus producing the situation of hyperemic on oligemic intracranial hypertension. Presumably, in this setting the hyperemic rise in ICP acts to further compromise rCBF in areas of brain edema.

Blood pressure interactions with intracranial pressure: plateau waves

In a pioneering 1960 study, Lundberg [20] monitored ICP in hundreds of patients, identifying characteristic pressure waves. One category of these waves has been identified as plateau waves, which are known to be associated with increased cerebral blood volume (CBV) [2]. Such waves occur when the ICP abruptly increases to systemic blood pressure levels, occasionally accompanied by neurologic deterioration. Rosner and Becker [3] have synthesized the data and convincingly suggest that CBV dysautoregulation is responsible for plateau waves. They induced mild head trauma in cats and subsequently intensively monitored the animals after the insult. With normal fluctuations in blood pressure, while in the normal range, Rosner and Becker observed that mild blood pressure decrements to a mean of approximately 70 mm Hg to 80 mm Hg preceded the development of plateau waves (Fig. 5). Cerebral blood volume in normally autoregulating brain tissue increases with decreasing blood pressure. However, the increase in CBV is nonlinear. There is an exponential increase in CBV as perfusion pressure decreases to levels of approximately 80 mm Hg and below (Fig. 6) [3,21]. A small decrease in blood pressure, although in the normotensive range, produces exponential increases in CBV in a setting of abnormal intracranial compliance, with the ICP at the elbow of the ICP-intracranial volume curve. Thus, a small decrease in blood pressure introduces an exponential CBV change upon an exponential ICP relation such that ICP will increase abruptly and to a significant extent. Plateau waves spontaneously resolve with a hypertensive response or with hyperventilation, which will act to oppose the increase in CBV. Clearly, to develop a plateau wave there must be a portion of the brain with normally reactive vasculature in the presence of other brain areas with a mass effect and elevated ICP: a situation of heterogeneous autoregulation (Fig. 7). Such data indicate that, in addition to preventing and treating plateau waves, it is probably important to maintain MAP in the 80 mm Hg to 100 mm Hg range in patients with high ICP.

Conversely, hypertension can also increase ICP, with animal models showing increased brain water with dopamine-induced increased blood pressure [22]. Typically, within the normal autoregulatory range, changes in blood pressure have no effect on ICP. However, with brain injury, and associated vasoparalysis, blood pressure increases mechanically produce cerebral vasodilatation, increasing ICP (Fig. 8) [23]. It appears that both

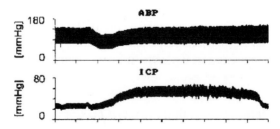

Fig. 5. In an animal head trauma model, a trivial-appearing and transient decrease in systemic arterial blood pressure in the setting of borderline cerebral perfusion pressure, precipitates sufficient cerebral vasodilatation to markedly increase the intracranial pressure. Restoration of cerebral perfusion pressure is associated with abolition of the plateau wave. Reprinted from reference. (*Adapted from* Schmidt B, Czosnyka M, Schwarze JJ, et al. Cerebral vasodilatation causing acute intracranial hypertension: a method for noninvasive assessment. J Cereb Blood Flow Metab 1999;19:990–6; with permission.)

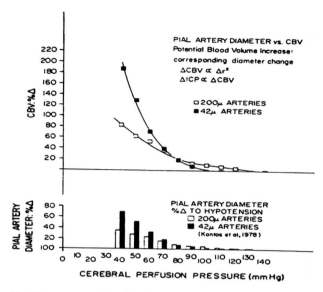

Fig. 6. Vasodilatation occurs at a logarithmic rate as cerebral perfusion pressure is reduced. Intracranial pressure will increase at a proportional rate within each pressure range, with the most rapid increase occurring below a cerebral perfusion pressure of 80 mm Hg. (*From* Rosner M, Becker D, The etiology of plateau waves: a theoretical model and experimental observations. In: Is, Nagai H, Brock M, editors. Intracranial pressure. New York: Springer-Verlag. 1983, p. 301; with kind permission of Springer Science and Business Media.)

increasing and decreasing blood pressure can increase ICP, suggesting the presence of a CPP optimum for ICP, probably 80 mm Hg to 100 mm Hg, although this has not been definitively determined experimentally. This concept is summarized in Fig. 9.

Treatment of intracranial hypertension

The general goal in treating intracranial hypertension is to promote adequate oxygen and nutrient supply by maintaining adequate CPP, oxygenation, and glucose supply (without hyperglycemia). The clinical strategy is to diagnose and treat the underlying causes, avoid exacerbating factors, and reduce ICP. Underlying causes include masses (tumors and hematomas), hydrocephalus, cerebral edema, and cerebrovascular dilatation.

Therapy of intracranial hypertension is primarily directed at removing the cause. When this is not possible, therapy is aimed at controlling ICP, with the hope that the primary cause of the intracranial hypertension will resolve. Controlling ICP is thus a supportive maneuver, intended to preserve viable neuronal tissue until the high ICP situation resolves. Therapeutic maneuvers involve one or more of six classes of therapy: (1) decrease cerebral blood volume, (2) decrease CSF volume, (3) induce serum hyperosmolarity, (4) resect dead or injured brain tissue or resect viable but less important

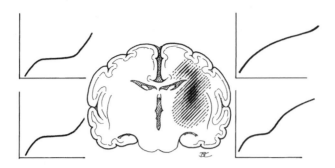

Fig. 7. Heterogeneous injury with some areas of retained autoregulation provides physiologic conditions conducive to the development of plateau waves. (*From* Kofke WA, Wechsler L. Neurointensive care. In: Albin M, editor. Textbook of neurosanesthesia. New York: McGraw-Hill; 1997. p. 1247–348; with permission.)

brain tissue (eg, anterior temporal lobe), (5) resect nonneural masses or hematomas, and (6) remove the calvarium (decompressive craniectomy) to permit unopposed outward brain swelling. Recent advances in the use of brain tissue oxygen (PbrO$_2$) monitors occasionally affect the manner in which these maneuvers are employed, to ensure continued optimal PbrO$_2$.

Cerebral blood volume reduction

Cerebral blood volume can be decreased with hyperventilation, CBF-decreasing drugs, mannitol, or hypothermia.

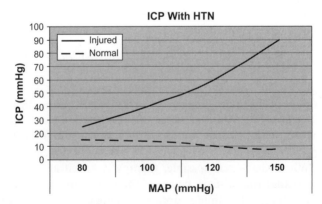

Fig. 8. In the context of a significant amount of injured brain with accompanying dysautoregulation, systemic hypertension produces intracranial hypertension, presumable from distension of injured, poorly autoregulating blood vessels. (*Adapted from* Matakas F, et al. Increase in cerebral perfusion pressure by arterial hypertension in brain swelling. A mathematical model of the volume-pressure relationship. J Neurosurg 1975;42(3):282–9.)

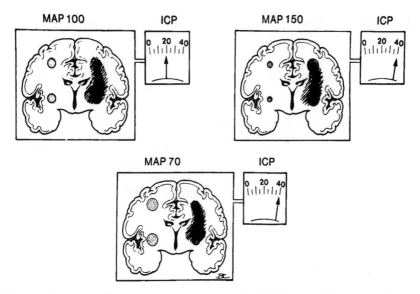

Fig. 9. In the setting of heterogeneous autoregulation in the brain, conditions may predispose to cerebral blood volume-mediated increases in intracranial pressure, with either increases or decreases in blood pressure. (*From* Kofke WA, Wechsler L. Neurointensive care. In: Albin M, editor. Textbook of neurosanesthesia. New York: McGraw-Hill; 1997. p. 1247–348; with permission.)

Hyperventilation

Hyperventilation can acutely reduce CBF and CBV to reduce ICP [24–28]. However, CBF returns to its original state within hours in a normal situation [24,28]. It is thus unclear why sustained decreases in ICP can be achieved with hyperventilation. There are several adverse effects of hyperventilation. Hyperventilation introduces a risk of decreasing CBF to a dangerous level (Fig. 10) [29,30]. In a recent study of trauma patients, routine hyperventilation was associated with worse neurologic outcome at 3 and 6 months after the injury [31], but the mechanism for this finding is unclear. Nonetheless, it can be an effective means to decrease ICP if the patient has hyperemic intracranial hypertension or is in an emergent herniation syndrome. The presence of hyperemia can be determined by the use of direct brain CBF determination or via jugular bulb oximetry [13,32]. Brain tissue $PbrO_2$ may be helpful in this determination but this remains to be definitively demonstrated. High ICP associated with a low arteriovenous oxygen content difference ($AVDO_2$) across the brain (3 vol%–4 vol%) is thought to indicate that hyperventilation can be safely used. In an emergent situation, even if the nature of the high ICP (oligemic versus hyperemic) is not known, acutely administered hyperventilation should be employed to keep ICP down, or to reverse a herniation syndrome or plateau wave, until more definitive diagnosis or therapy can be performed.

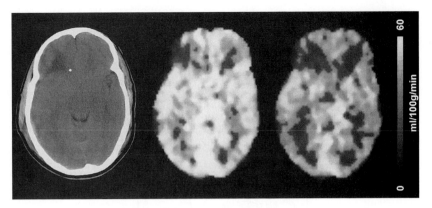

Fig. 10. Effect of hyperventilation on the burden of hypoperfusion. Radiographic computed tomography (left) and gray scale positron emission tomographic imaging of cerebral blood flow obtained from a 31-year-old man 7 days after injury at relative normocapnia (middle), Paco$_2$ 35 torr (4.7 kPa), and hypocapnia (right), 26 torr (3.5 kPa). Voxels with a cerebral blood flow of less than 10 mL$\times$100g^{-1}$\times$min^{-1} are shaded in black. Note the right frontal contusion and small pariet al. subdural hematoma. Baseline ICP was 21 mm Hg and baseline CPP was 74 mm Hg. Baseline Sjvo$_2$ values of 70% and AVDO$_2$ of 3.7 mL/dL are consistent with hyperemia and support the use of hyperventilation for ICP control. Hyperventilation did result in a reduction in ICP to 17 mm Hg and an increase in CPP to 76 mm Hg, with maintenance of Sjvo$_2$ and AVDO$_2$ within desirable ranges (58% and 5.5 mL/mL respectively). However, despite these Sjvo$_2$ and AVDO$_2$ figures, baseline HypoBV was 141 mL and increased to 428 mL with hyperventilation. These increases were observed in both perilesional and normal regions of brain tissue. (*From* Coles, J, et al. Effect of hyperventilation on cerebral blood flow in traumatic head injury: clinical relevance and monitoring correlates. Crit Care Med 2002;30(9):1950–9.)

Cerebral blood volume-decreasing drugs

Cerebral blood flow-decreasing (and therefore CBV decreasing) drugs which can decrease ICP include barbiturates [33–35], benzodiazepines [36], etomidate [37,38] and propofol [35,39]. Notably, all are central nervous system depressants. Therefore, their use indicates acceptance on the part of the clinician to lose a reliable neurologic examination. Unlike hyperventilation, these agents decrease CBF coupled to cerebral metabolic rate (CMR). Thus, the CBF decreases should not provide a milieu for anaerobic metabolism. Lidocaine also decreases CBF and CMR to decrease ICP, although with a less pronounced decrement in neurologic function [40,41]. Mannitol's immediate effects are also thought to be mediated by reduction in CBV (25), although this is undoubtedly minor and temporary as a mechanism.

Cerebrospinal fluid drainage

Cerebrospinal fluid volume is reduced by removal via ventricular drain (Fig. 11). Leaving a drain open risks excessive CSF drainage when the patient coughs, or with drain manipulation in the course of routine nursing procedures, and can contribute to collapse of the ventricles or bleeding.

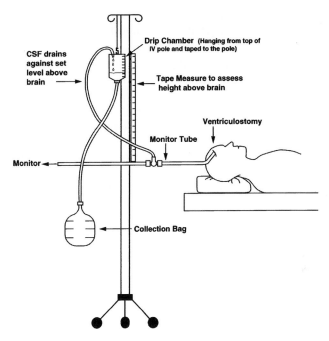

Fig. 11. External ventricular drainage system. (*From* Coles J, et al. Effect of hyperventilation on cerebral blood flow in traumatic head injury: clinical relevance and monitoring correlates. Crit Care Med 2002;30(9):1950–9.)

Excessive and abrupt decrease in local pressure around the drain can produce intracranial gradients, leading to a herniation syndrome. Leaving the drain clamped and monitored, however, risks the development of untreated intracranial hypertension.

Hyperosmolar therapy

Mannitol has become the traditional mainstay of hyperosmolar therapy. After initial hypoviscosity-mediated autoregulatory vasoconstricution [42], it may induce a further decrease in ICP through brain dehydration in areas with an intact blood brain barrier [43–45]. However, this may be limited through generation of intracellular idiogenic osmoles [46,47], equalizing transmembrane osmolar gradients. Theoretically, this effect might be limited through concomitant administration of a loop diuretic [48].

Unfortunately, mannitol can have delayed effects to increase ICP. This can occur by four mechanisms. First, as a potent diuretic, mannitol can have a secondary effect to decrease blood volume, thus decreasing cardiac output and blood pressure. This can result in normal reflex autoregulatory increases in CBV, which can increase ICP [3]. Second, the increased urine output, if not replaced with commensurate intravenous fluid therapy, can elevate hematocrit, thus opposing the initial mannitol-induced decrease in viscosity [49]. Third, mannitol can cross the blood brain barrier in an unpredictable manner, with the possibility introduced of rebound increase in ICP, similar to that observed with urea [49,50]. This is partly related to the reflection coefficient of 0.9, indicating that even in a normal brain it can slowly diffuse into the brain [51]. Fourth, there is a theoretical possibility of generation of increased intracellular osmolarity, via so-called "idiogenic osmoles," which may predispose to rebound increase in brain volume with discontinuation of mannitol [46,47]. These complications of mannitol are probably lessened if urine output is replaced with balanced crystalloid infusion and if, once blood osmolarity is increased, it is not allowed to decrease to the prior level unless clinical improvement indicates that weaning of ICP-reducing therapy is appropriate. This certainly should be considered in any patient demonstrating periodic abrupt increases in ICP.

Hypertonic saline

Hypertonic saline (HTS) is a recently revisited alternative to mannitol. With a reflection coefficient of 1.0 [51] and no potential to produce deleterious diuresis and undesired hypovolemia, it has properties that make it an attractive hyperosmolar agent. Moreover, clinical reports indicate that it is an effective ICP-reducing drug, finding a very useful niche in the group of patients who are refractory to mannitol.

Hypertonic saline has undergone scrutiny in many laboratory and clinical studies, with virtually all indicating a beneficial effect to decrease ICP. Notably, this is not a particularly new observation, having been initially reported in 1919 by McKesson [52]. Studies generally have employed 3%, 7.5%, or 23.4% saline with or without a colloid, typically dextran or hetastarch.

In human beings, the effect of HTS has been reported in ischemic stroke, intracerebral hemorrhage (ICH), subarachnoid hemorrhage (SAH), traumatic brain injury (TBI), and hepatic encephalopathy. All studies show that HTS effectively and reproducibly reduces ICP with concomitant improvement in CPP. Early case reports by Worthley and colleagues [53], in patients with refractory ICP elevations, supported the therapeutic potential for this therapy and supported the many studies that followed. A retrospective study by Qureshi and colleagues [54] showed that HTS decreases ICP in head trauma and in postoperative brain edema, but not in nontraumatic ICH or ischemic stroke. Schatzman and colleagues [55] performed a prospective nonrandomized evaluation of HTS in severe head injury, also finding that it effectively reduced ICP. A subsequent prospective randomized study by Vialet and colleagues [56] in TBI patients found better ICP control compared with mannitol. Another prospective randomized study did not show better ICP control with HTS compared with standard therapy. However, in that study the sample size was relatively small and the HTS subjects had more comorbidites than the control group on entry into the study

[57]. Three studies report that HTS can be safely and effectively used in children to decrease ICP after TBI [58–60], Tseng and colleagues [61], studying severe SAH patients, reported that HTS therapy effectively decreased ICP while concomitantly increasing CBF. Schwartz and colleagues [62] evaluated HTS/hetastarch therapy in ischemic stroke patients with high ICP, compared with mannitol. Both therapies decreased ICP but the HTS group had better control. Indeed, Suarez and colleagues [63] showed one important effect of 23.4% HTS in eight patients, as a therapy that effectively decreases ICP when all other medical therapies do not work. Similar observations in patients with refractory intracranial hypertension were reported by Horn and colleagues [64].

Hypertonic saline clearly has the potential to exert a positive impact in the management of intracranial hypertension. However, there are concerns expressed about possible occasional deleterious effects, which have been reviewed by Suarez [65].

Optimizing brain oxygenation

The advent of brain tissue pO_2 monitoring is making optimizing brain oxygenation an additional area of concern in the management of elevated ICP. Hypoxemia, usually below PaO_2 approximately 50 mm Hg to 60 mmHg, is associated with vasodilatio [66]. At the opposite extreme, Floyd and colleagues [67], in a group of healthy volunteers, have demonstrated the vasonstrictive effect of hyperoxemia and its accompanying hypocapnea. Nakajima and colleagues [68] evaluated this phenomenon in patients with cerebrovascular disease, finding that areas of the brain with impaired cerebrovascular reserve were not adversely affected by hyperoxia.

The optimal PaO_2 to seek in a brain-injured patient is presently unclear. There is data to support hyperoxic therapy, along with data to suggest that such an approach is deleterious. In addition, the bedside decision about PaO_2 management is further coupled to cerebrovascular reserve issues. Thus, a low PaO_2 that would normally be tolerated through vasodilation may not be so well tolerated if vasodilatory reserve is compromised with, for example, carotid occlusion, brain edema, or anemia.

Fiskum et al [69], among others, have reported in laboratory studies that hyperoxic therapy promotes generation of free radicals, and that such oxidative stress causes mitochondrial injury which will act to impair neurologic recovery. This notion from in vitro considerations is supported by in vivo studies in rodents and dogs, which have demonstrated worse neurologic outcome when hyperoxia is employed before or after an ischemic insult [70–72].

Conversely, brain tissue PO_2 monitoring [73] demonstrates that brain hypoxia, which may occur in the presence of whole body normoxia, results in poor neurologic outcome in patients who have either suffered traumatic or SAH brain injury [73–78]. Although the risks associated with brain hyperoxia in patients with underlying brain injury have not been clearly defined, brain tissue oxygen monitoring allows one to provide that minimal fraction of inspired oxygen (FiO_2)—to avoid lung toxicity from hyperoxia— that permits the optimal (not too high not too low) brain tissue oxygen level ($PbrO_2$ greater than 20 mm Hg). This may entail use of FiO_2 greater than 60% with concomitant risk of pulmonary oxygen toxicity [79]. In the absence of a $PbrO_2$ monitor, the clinician is left basing therapy on assumptions about brain oxygenation. In patients with mild brain injury, the clinician should provide high enough FiO_2 to produce oxygen saturation (SaO_2) greater than 95%. Conversely, if there is elevated ICP or areas of brain hypoperfusion, then a reasonable empiric approach would be to use an FiO_2 of 60%. This will maximize PaO_2 and $PbrO_2$, but without significant risk of acute pulmonary injury.

Resection of brain tissue

Resection of brain tissue is occasionally employed for malignant intracranial hypertension. Because of its proximity to the brainstem, one approach is to resect part of the temporal lobe in an effort to avert a herniation syndrome [80]. An alternative approach, suggested specifically for malignant intracranial hypertension due to stroke, is to resect dead and swelling infarcted tissue, leaving noninfarcted tissue intact [81]. However, difficulties identifying such tissue intraoperatively risk inadvertant resection of viable tissue.

Resection of nonneural masses or hematomas

When clinical examination indicates a global decrement in level of consciousness, indicating elevated ICP, and imaging studies indicate the presence of a mass lesion, then urgent surgical removal of the mass is thought to be indicated [80]. Nonetheless, there is some controversy about this. With intracerebral hematomas, the literature does not demonstrate improved outcomes following aggressive surgical intervention [82]. However, surgical intervention can be life-saving in patients suffering acute epidural hematoma with abrupt neurologic deterioration or for cerebellar hematomas [82]. Efficacy of surgery for patients with subdural hematomas is less clear, although surgical intervention in patients with acute subdural hematomas in the context of a recent injury and neurologic deterioration seems appropriate.

Surgical removal of skull and dura

The failure of medical therapy and the continued deterioration of the patient mandate the consideration of alternate means of therapy. In patients with persistent cerebral swelling or increased ICP, in the absence of a mass lesion, decompressive craniectomy (DCH) has been advocated to prevent transtentorial herniation. Surgical decompression has been tested in patients with severe TBI or stroke with varying results [83–86]. It is hypothesized that through decompressive surgery, the vicious cycle of extensive edema caused by elevated ICP, resulting in ischemia of neighboring brain tissue and further infarction, may be interrupted [87]. Decompressive surgery may then increase CPP and optimize perfusion, thus allowing a functionally compromised but viable brain to survive [88].

The concept of wide bone removal for treatment of intracranial hypertension has existed since the dawn of neurosurgery. The use of DCH to control elevated ICP has a long history. In 1901 Kocher wrote, "If there is no cerebrospinal fluid pressure, but brain pressure does exist, pressure relief must be obtained by opening the skull. . . . In the early stage it is not easy to diagnose increased brain pressure; in the late stage, the performance of the procedure alone will be of no use [89]" As early as 1905, Cushing [90] performed a subtemporal decompression for relief of elevated ICP related to neoplastic growth, and later reported the application of this operation to wartime trauma [91]. In 1971, Kjellberg and Prieto (1971) reported the results of 73 patients undergoing extensive bifrontal craniectomies and ligation of the sagittal sinus for posttraumatic injury. Overall, only 18% of the patients survived, including 11 of 50 (22%) with nonpenetrating head trauma.

Two forms of decompressive surgery exist: hemicraniectomy and bifrontal craniectomy. A hemicraniectomy is often performed in situations when there is unilateral injury or focal pathology. In brief, decompressive hemicraniectomy is performed by removing a large bone flap with a diameter of at least 12 cm (including the frontal, parietal, temporal, and parts of the occipital squama). The skull is removed so that the floor of the middle cerebral fossa can be exposed. The dura is opened in a cruciate fashion and left widely open. Dural substitutes may be applied over the dural defect. The bone is either placed into the patient's abdomen or stored in a bone freezer. The temporalis muscle is reapproximated and the skin closed.

Decompressive bifrontal craniectomy is effective for patients with bifrontal injury, or in those patients with diffuse swelling with no focal pathology. A bifrontal craniectomy is performed with a bicoronal skin incision and reflection of the temporalis muscle. Burr holes are located at either side of the sagittal sinus at the posterior extent, bilaterally at the keyhole, and bilaterally at the root of the zygoma. Bitemporal burr holes are also created. A large bifrontal craniectomy is created, extending posteriorly into the parietal bones approximately 3 cm to 5 cm posterior to the coronal sutures. A bone cut is made anteriorly over the sagittal sinus. The sagittal sinus is ligated and divided anteriorly to allow for further anterior expansion. Dural substitutes may be placed or affixed in a watertight fashion to the dural openings.

Regardless of the type of decompressive surgery, there continues to be controversy concerning the usefulness of DCH for intractable intracranial hypertension. While DCH has been shown to be effective in reducing ICP, its effect on patient outcome is less certain and studies differ on whether DCH improves overall outcome [84,85,92–94]. One reason for this dilemma is that there is no single reliable monitor of brain function in sedated or comatose patients who have elevated ICP. Furthermore the optimal time to perform DCH has not yet been defined.

Unfortunately, all of the reports on DCH use are in non randomized case series, having never undergone prospective randomized investigation with a recent Cochrane review, suggesting that the procedure remains without firm supportive evidence [95]. Nonetheless, hemicraniectomy or bifrontal craniectomy remain an attractive approach that seems to improve survival in those who are moribund [96,97]. Obviously this aggressive approach is in need of a prospective randomized trial. Current trials are ongoing for trauma (http://clinicaltrials.gov/show/NCT00155987) and for stroke (http://clinicaltrials.gov/ct/show/NCT00190203). Anesthetic management issues relate to management of intracranial hypertension before the decompression. In addition, careful control of blood pressure may be needed. In the context of elevated ICP and worsening neurologic condition, blood pressure control with ICP reducing anesthetics (eg, thiopental, propofol) is most appropriate.

Anesthetic effects with intracranial hypertension

A patient presenting for surgery with intracranial hypertension, or for decompressive craniectomy, requires consideration of the effects of anesthetic drugs on the neuropathophysiologic processes. There is little data on the impact of anesthetic management on patient outcomes in this situation. However, there is ample information on the effects of anesthetics on CBF and ICP. In the absence of better information, it becomes most appropriate to use anesthetic drugs associated with lower ICP. Such drugs usually decrease cerebral metabolic rate with a coupled decrease in CBF and ICP. This presupposes the presence of appropriately reactive cerebral vasculature, even if heterogeneously present. In the presence of diffusely nonreactive cerebral blood vessels, it probably does not matter which anesthetic drug is employed.

Another consideration is whether hypnosis or analgesia are needed in the context of a patient who is unconscious from an underlying disease that is producing the elevated ICP. There are numerous reports that indicate the effect of noxious stimuli to increase ICP [41], clearly causing a hyperemic ICP increase [13,14]. There is thus a good argument for judicious opioid use. The extent of hypnotic or amnestic drugs to administer becomes a matter of judgment. Given that there are situations where a patient can appear to be unconscious and yet have awareness would indicate that such drugs generally should be used unless contraindicated by other physiologic concerns. Certainly, the anesthetic drugs most associated with decreased ICP are in the hypnotic class, such that meaningful doses may need to be given anyway, although not specifically to produce hypnosis but with hypnosis as a useful side effect.

Volatile anesthetics all have a dose-related tendency to increase CBF or induce cerebral vasodilation [98], probably most pronounced with halothane [99,100] but also reported with isoflurane [99,101], sevoflurane [100–103], and desflurane [104]. Notably there are some reports of metabolically coupled decreases in CBF with sevoflurane [105]. Based on potential increased blood flow and blood volume it is expected that their use, at least in higher doses, around the minimum alveolar anesthetic concentration (MAC) dose or higher, will increase ICP. Nonetheless, several reports indicate that ICP does not rise appreciably in brain tumor patients with isoflurane and desflurane [106] and that CO_2 reactivity is retained in patients being anesthetized with these agents [104,107,108], such that any hyperemia can be treated with hyperventilation. In addition, all of these drugs have, in various contexts, been shown to have neuroprotective qualities that might support their use, perhaps in lower doses. Compared with opioids, propofol, and ketamine in an animal model of traumatic brain injury, isoflurane produced the best histological outcome [109]. Notably, isoflurane has been described to be neuroprotective in animal models of brain ischemia, although not preventing apoptosis [110,111]. Indeed, Wei and colleagues [112] suggest isoflurane may primarily produce apoptosis, whereas sevoflurane appears to prevent apoptosis. Such studies of course do not address the potentially negative effect of preventing programmed cell death of cells that have become dysfunctional from a prior injury. Desflurane has been reported to increase brain tissue partial pressure of oxygen (pO_2) [113]. Given increased attention to this measure and suggestions of a positive correlation between brain tissue oxygen pressure (pbO_2) and good outcome, desflurane, after more study, may have a larger role in anesthetic management of patients with elevated ICP and TBI [114].

There is little support for the use of nitrous oxide (N_2O) in patients who suffer from elevated ICP or brain injury. This drug clearly can increase ICP and CBF [115–117]. In one case report, ICP rises were clearly temporally associated with N_2O on and off, but the effect was blocked by prior benzodiazepine use [118]. However, this effect is complicated by the presence of associated surgical stress and the N_2O dose. Given to human beings at a hyperbaric 1 MAC, in the absence of surgery, it produced severe systemic excitation with opisthotonos that one would certainly expect to be associated with neuroexcitation, increased CBF, and increased ICP [119]. Given to human beings in the context of pre-existing high dose isoflurane and a flat electroencephalogram (EEG), it produced increased CBF velocity suggesting a direct vasodilatory neurovascular effect [98]. Given to rodents at approximately 0.5 MAC, in the context of postsurgery, it was associated with increased extracellular dopamine [120], suggesting neuroexcitation. However, given to unstressed, unaware mice, a consistent neuroexciation could not be found on evaluation of metabolic rate by autoradiography [121]. In terms of neurotoxicity in rodents, N_2O appears to have a biphasic effect, being neuroprotective at doses less than 0.5 MAC, but is increasingly neurotoxic as doses are increased to approach a hyperbaric 1-MAC dose [122]. Therefore, there is little support for the use of N_2O in patients with elevated ICP and brain injury.

On the contrary, barbiturates have been used for decades for the management of intracranial hypertension [34,123]. Although there is little doubt that they effectively reduce ICP, there remains controversy regarding their role in improving outcome. Nonetheless, in the context of this discussion on anesthetics for patients with elevated ICP, this category of drugs (eg, barbiturates, propofol, etomidate) [35], should be an integral component of the anesthetic for patients with brain swelling, due to ICP-decreasing qualities [124]. When choosing which drug, amongst this group, to use for a particular patient, the physician should take into consideration their differences in the extent of hemodynamic depression (barbiturates and propofol are stronger than etomidate) [124], duration (barbiturates last longer than etomidate, which lasts longer than propofol), and adrenal suppression (etomidate) [125]. Moreover, there can be issues with the preservative with etomidate if used for a prolonged time at high doses [126].

Opioids are often used as the analgesic component of a general anesthetic. Mu opioids are the mainstay of antinociception during surgery. In patients with elevated ICP, preventing the systemic response to noxious stimuli can effectively prevent associated ICP spikes arising there from [13,127,128]. Thus opioids have an important place in perioperative management of the patient with elevated ICP. Opioids have the additional advantage of producing relatively minor direct hemodynamic depression and can be reversed with a specific antagonist, naloxone. However, there are some possible adverse effects based mostly on observations in animals [129–133], but with enough human correlation to be a bit worrisome [129]. In rodents mu opioids have been conclusively demonstrated to produce limbic system seizure, activation, and injury at high doses [129,131–133] with exacerbation of ischemic [134] and traumatic injury [135]. Congruent limbic activation has been observed in human beings at both high and low doses [129], with occasional idiosyncratic reports of opioid-induced seizure and support for electroconvulsive seizure [136]. Nonetheless, there is so far no evidence that opioid use can produce neural injury in human beings. There is evidence in animals that opioid neurotoxicity is attenuated with gabaergic therapy [137], suggesting that opioids used in the context of such concomitant therapy would be most unlikely to exacerbate the brain damage associated with high ICP. Certainly any theoretical risk of opioid neurotoxicity is easily outweighed by the well-documented risk of ICP spikes associated with nociception.

Summary

Intracranial hypertension can arise due to a complex interplay of numerous factors. The elevated ICP can be due to either hyperemia, in the context of abnormal intracranial compliance, or as edema, or other masses with attendant oligoemia. Both increased and decreased blood pressure can contribute to ICP elevations, but with significantly different causes. Moreover, several other physiologic and pharmacologic factors can exert a significant impact on ICP, largely due to effects on cerebral blood volume. Therapeutic maneuvers to treat intracranial hypertension involve one or more of six classes of therapy: (1) decrease cerebral blood volume, (2) decrease CSF volume, (3) induce serum hyperosmolarity, (4) resect dead or injured brain tissue or resect viable but less important brain tissue (eg, anterior temporal lobe), (5) resect nonneural masses or hematomas, and (6) remove the calvarium (decompressive craniectomy) to permit unopposed outward brain swelling. These therapies can be introduced through a variety of physiologic, pharmacologic, and surgical approaches. Anesthetic management of patients with intracranial hypertension is basically superimposed on the above-noted considerations. In general, the most suitable anesthetic is one which produces decrements in cerebral blood flow and volume with matched decreases in cerebral metabolic rate, with careful attention to interactions with any other ongoing ICP reducing therapies and avoidance of factors which may exacerbate the primary problem or ICP.

References

[1] Cushing H. Concerning a definite regulatory mechanism of the vaso-motor centre which controls blood pressure during cerebral compression. Johns Hopkins Hospital Bulletin 1901;12:290–2.

[2] Risberg J, Lundberg N, Ingvar D. Regional cerebral blood volume during acute rises in the intracranial pressure (plateau waves). J Neurosurg 1969;31:303–10.

[3] Rosner M, Becker D. Origin and evolution of plateau waves. Experimental observations and a theoretical model. J Neurosurg 1984;50:312–24.

[4] Greenberg JH, Alavi A, Reivich M, et al. Local cerebral blood volume response to carbon dioxide in man. Circ Res 1978;43:324–31.

[5] Sakai F, Nakazawa K, Tazaki Y, et al. Regional cerebral blood volume and hematocrit measured in normal human volunteers by single photon emission computed tomography. J Cereb Blood Flow Metab 1985;5:207–13.

[6] Strandgaard S, Olesen J, Skinhoj E, et al. Autoregulation of brain circulation in severe arterial hypertension. Br Med J 1973;3:507–10.

[7] Miller JD, Becker DP, Ward JD, et al. Significance of intracranial hypertension in severe head injury. J Neurosurg 1977;47:503–16.

[8] Lundberg N, Troupp H, Lorin H. Continuous recording of ventricular fluid pressure in patients with severe acute traumatic brain injury. A preliminary report. J Neurosurg 1965;22: 581–90.

[9] Giulioni M, Ursino M, Alvis iC. Correlations among intracranial pulsatility, intracranial hemodynamics, and transcranial doppler wave form: literature review and hypothesis for future studies. Neurosurgery 1988;22:807–12.

[10] Hassler W, Steinmetz H, Gawlowski J. Transcranial Doppler ultrasonography in raised intracranial pressure and in intracranial circulatory arrest. J Neurosurg 1988; 68:745–51.

[11] Greitz T, Gordon E, Kolmodin G, et al. Aortocranial and carotid angiography in determination of brain death. Neuroradiology 1973;5:13–9.

[12] Jalan R, Olde Damink SW, Deutz NE, et al. Moderate hypothermia prevents cerebral hyperemia and increase in intracranial pressure in patients undergoing liver transplantation for acute liver failure. Transplantation 2003;75(12):2034–9.

[13] Kerr ME, Weber BB, Sereika SM, et al. Effect of endotracheal suctioning on cerebral oxygenation in traumatic brain-injured patients. Crit Care Med 1999;27(12):2776–81.

[14] Kofke WA, Dong ML, Bloom M, et al. Transcranial Doppler ultrasonography with induction of anesthesia for neurosurgery. J Neurosurg Anesthesiol 1994;6:89–97.

[15] Aggarwal S, Kramer D, Yonas H, et al. Cerebral hemodynamic and metabolic changes in fulminant hepatic failure: a retrospective study. Hepatology 1994;19:80–7.

[16] Michenfelder J. The 27th Rovenstine lecture: neuroanesthesia and the achievement of professional respect. Anesthesiology 1989;70(4):695–701.

[17] Wilkins R. Cerebral vasospasm. Crit Rev Neurobiol 1990;6:51–77.

[18] Jaggi JL, Obrist WD, Gennarelli TA, et al. Relationship of early cerebral blood flow and metabolism to outcome in acute head injury. J Neurosurg 1990;72(2):176–82.

[19] Stocchetti N, Zanier ER, Nicolini R, et al. Oxygen and carbon dioxide in the cerebral circulation during progression to brain death. Anesthesiology. 103: p. 957–61.

[20] Stocchetti N, Zanier ER, Nicolini R, et al. Continuous recording and control of ventricular fluid pressure in neurosurgical practice. Acta Psychiatr Scand Suppl 1960;36(149): 1–193.

[21] Rosner M, Becker D. The etiology of plateau waves: a theoretical model and experimental observations. In: IS, Nagai H, Brock M, editors. Intracranial pressure. New York: Springer-Verlag; 1983. p. 301–6.

[22] Beaumont A, Hayaski K, Marmarou A, et al. Contrasting effects of dopamine therapy in experimental brain injury. J Neurotrauma 2001;18(12):1359–72.

[23] Matakas F, Von Waechter R, Knupling R, et al. Increase in cerebral perfusion pressure by arterial hypertension in brain swelling. A mathematical model of the volume-pressure relationship. J Neurosurg 1975;42(3):282–9.

[24] Raichle M, Posner J, Plum F. Cerebral blood flow during and after hyperventilation. Arch Neurol 1970;23:394–403.

[25] Lassen N. Control of cerebral circulation in health and disease. Circ Res 1974;34:749–60.

[26] Shapiro H. Intracranial hypertension: therapeutic and anesthetic considerations. Anesthesiology 1975;43:445–71.

[27] Shenkin H, Bouzarth W. Clinical methods of reducing intracranial pressure. N Engl J Med 1970;282:1465–71.

[28] Raichle M, Plum F. Hyperventilation and cerebral blood flow. Stroke 1972;3(5):566–75.

[29] Stringer W, et al. Hyperventilation-induced cerebral ischemia in patients with acute brain lesions: demonstration by xenon-enhanced CT. AJNR Am J Neuroradiol 1993;14(2): 475–84.

[30] Coles JP, Minhas PS, Fryer TD, et al. Effect of hyperventilation on cerebral blood flow in traumatic head injury: clinical relevance and monitoring correlates. Crit Care Med 2002; 30(9):1950–9.

[31] Muizelaar JP, Marmarou A, Ward JD, et al. Adverse effects of prolonged hyperventilation in patients with severe head injury: a randomized clinical trial. J Neurosurg 1991;75:731–9.

[32] Cruz J, Miner ME, Allen SJ, et al. Continuous monitoring of cerebral oxygenation in acute brain injury: injection of mannitol during hyperventilation. J Neurosurg 1990;73:725–30.

[33] Pierce E, Lambertsen C, Deutsch S. Cerebral circulation and metabolism during thiopental anesthesia and hyperventilation in man. J Clin Invest 1962;41:1664–71.

[34] Marshall LF, Shapiro HM, Rauscher A, et al. Pentobarbital therapy for intracranial hypertension in metabolic coma. Reye's syndrome. Crit Care Med 1978;6:1–5.

[35] Hartung H. Intracranial pressure after propofol and thiopental administration in patients with severe head trauma. Anaesthesist 1987;36:285–7.

[36] Larsen R, Hilfiker O, Radke J, et al. The effects of midazolam on the general circulation, the CBF and cerebral oxygen consumption in man. Anaesthesist 1981;30:18–21.

[37] Renou AM, Vernhiet J, Macrez P, et al. CBF and metabolism during etomidate anaesthesia in man. Br J Anaesth 1978;50:1047–51.
[38] Prior JG, Hinds CJ, Williams J, et al. The use of etomidate in the management of severe head injury. Intensive Care Med 1983;9:313–20.
[39] Vandesteene A, Trempont V, Engelman E, et al. Effect of propofol on CBF and metabolism in man. Anaesthesia 1988;45(Suppl):42–3.
[40] Sakabe T, Maekawa T, Ishikawa T, et al. The effects of lidocaine on canine metabolism and circulation related to the electroencephalogram. Anesthesiology 1974;40:433–41.
[41] Yano M, Nishiyama H, Yokota H, et al. Effect of lidocaine on ICP response to endotracheal suctioning. Anesthesiology 1986;64(5):651–3.
[42] Muizelaar J, Lutz Hd, Becker D. Effect of mannitol on ICP and CBF and correlation with pressure autoregulation in severely head-injured patients. J Neurosurg 1984;61: 700–6.
[43] Reichenthal E, Kaspi T, Cohen ML, et al. The ambivalent effects of early and late administration of mannitol in cold-induced brain oedema. Acta Neurochir Suppl (Wein) 1990;51: 110–2.
[44] Rosenberg GA, Barrett J, Estrada E, et al. Selective effect of mannitol-induced hyperosmolality on brain interstitial fluid and water content in white matter. Metab Brain Dis 1988;3: 217–27.
[45] Bell BA, Smith MA, Kean DM, et al. Brain water measured by magnetic resonance imaging. Correlation with direct estimation and changes after mannitol and dexamethasone. Lancet 1987;1:66–9.
[46] Chan P, Fishman R. Elevation of rat brain amino acids, ammonia and idiogenic osmoles induced by hyperosmolality. Brain Res 1979;161:293–301.
[47] Pollock A, Arieff A. Abnormalities of cell volume regulation and their functional consequences. Am J Physiol 1980;239:F195–205.
[48] McManus M, Strange K. Acute volume regulation of brain cells in response to hypertonic challenge. Anesthesiology 1993;78(6):1132–7.
[49] Kofke W. Mannitol: potential for rebound intracranial hypertension? J Neurosurg Anesthesiol 1993;5(1):1–3, [editorial; comment].
[50] Rudehill A, Gordon E, Ohman G, et al. Pharmacokinetics and effects of mannitol on hemodynamics, blood and cerebrospinal fluid electrolytes, and osmolality during intracranial surgery. J Neurosurg Anesthesiol 1993;5(1):4–12.
[51] Zornow M. Hypertonic saline as a safe and efficacious treatment of intracranial hypertension. J Neurosurg Anesthesiol 1996;8:175–7.
[52] Weed L, McKibben P. Pressure changes in the cerebro-spinal fluid following intravenous injection of solutions of various concentrations. Am J Physiol 1919;48:512–30.
[53] Worthley L, Cooper D, Jones N. Treatment of resistant intracranial hypertension with hypertonic saline. Report of two cases. J Neurosurg 1988;68(3):478–81.
[54] Qureshi AI, Suarez JI, Bhardwaj A, et al. Use of hypertonic (3%) saline/acetate infusion in the treatment of cerebral edema: effect on intracranial pressure and lateral displacement of the brain. Crit Care Med 1998;26(3):440–6.
[55] Schatzmann C, Heissler HE, Konig K, et al. Treatment of elevated intracranial pressure by infusions of 10% saline in severely head injured patients. Acta Neurochir Suppl 1998;71: 31–3.
[56] Vialet R, Albanèse J, Thomachot L, et al. Isovolume hypertonic solutes (sodium chloride or mannitol) in the treatment of refractory posttraumatic intracranial hypertension: 2 mL/kg 7.5% saline is more effective than 2 mL/kg 20% mannitol. Crit Care Med 2003;31:1683–7.
[57] Shackford SR, Bourguignon PR, Wald SL, et al. Hypertonic saline resuscitation of patients with head injury: a prospective, randomized clinical trial. J Trauma 1998;44(1):50–8.
[58] Simma B, Burger R, Falk M, et al. A prospective, randomized, and controlled study of fluid management in children with severe head injury: lactated Ringer's solution versus hypertonic saline. Crit Care Med 1998;26(7):1265–70.

[59] Khanna S, Daniel D, Bradley P, et al. Use of hypertonic saline in the treatment of severe refractory posttraumatic intracranial hypertension in pediatric traumatic brain injury. Crit Care Med 2000;28(4):1144–51.

[60] Peterson B, Khanna S, Fisher B, et al. Prolonged hypernatremia controls elevated intracranial pressure in head-injured pediatric patients. Crit Care Med 2000;28(4):1136–43.

[61] Tseng MY, Al-Rawi PG, Pickard JD, et al. Effect of hypertonic saline on cerebral blood flow in poor-grade patients with subarachnoid hemorrhage stroke 2003;34; 1389–96.

[62] Schwarz S, Schwab S, Bertram M, et al. Effects of hypertonic saline hydroxyethyl starch solution and mannitol in patients with increased intracranial pressure after stroke. Stroke 1998;29:1550–5.

[63] Suarez JI, Qureshi AI, Bhardwaj A, et al. Treatment of refractory intracranial hypertension with 23.4% saline. Crit Care Med 1998;26(6):1118–22.

[64] Horn P, Munch E, Vajkoczy P, et al. Hypertonic saline solution for control of elevated intracranial pressure in patients with exhausted response to mannitol and barbiturates. Neurol Res 1999;21(8):758–64.

[65] Suarez JI. Hypertonic saline for cerebral edema and elevated intracranial pressure. Cleve Clin J Med 2004;71(Suppl 1):S9–13.

[66] Brown M, Wade J, Marshall J. Fundamental importance of arterial oxygen content in the regulation of cerebral blood flow in man. Brain 1985;108(Pt 1):81–93.

[67] Floyd TF, Clark JM, Gelfand R, et al. Independent cerebral vasoconstrictive effects of hyperoxia and accompanying arterial hypocapnia at 1 ATA. [Clinical Trial. Journal Article]. J Appl Physiol 2003;95(6):2453–61.

[68] Nakajima S, Meyer JS, Amano T, et al. Cerebral vasomotor responsiveness during 100% oxygen inhalation in cerebral ischemia. Arch Neurol 1983;40(5):271–6.

[69] Fiskum G, Rosenthal RE, Vereczki V, et al. Protection against ischemic brain injury by inhibition of mitochondrial oxidative stress. J Bioenergetics and Biomembranes 2004;36(4): 347–52.

[70] Halsey JH Jr, Conger KA, Garcia JH, et al. The contribution of reoxygenation to ischemic brain damage. Journal of Cerebral Blood Flow & Metabolism 1991;11(6):994–1000.

[71] Mickel HS, Kempski O, Feuerstein G, et al. Prominent white matter lesions develop in Mongolian gerbils treated with 100% normobaric oxygen after global brain ischemia. Acta Neuropathologica 1990;79(5):465–72.

[72] Marsala J, Marsala M, Vanicky I, et al. Post cardiac arrest hyperoxic resuscitation enhances neuronal vulnerability of the respiratory rhythm generator and some brainstem and spinal cord neuronal pools in the dog. Neuroscience Letters 1992;146(2):121–4.

[73] Dings J, Meixensberger J, Jager A, et al. Clinical experience with 118 brain tissue oxygen partial pressure catheter probes. Neurosurgery 1998;43(5):1982–95.

[74] van den Brink WA, van Santbrink H, Steyerberg EW, et al. Brain oxygen tension in severe head injury. Neurosurgery 2000;46(4):876–8.

[75] Valadka AB, Gopinath SP, Contant CF, et al. Relationship of brain tissue PO2 to outcome after severe head injury. Crit Care Clin 1998;26(9):1576–81.

[76] van Santbrink H, van den Brink WA, Steyerberg EW, et al. Brain tissue oxygen response in severe traumatic brain injury. Acta Neruochir (Wein) 2003;145(6):429–38.

[77] Stiefel MF, Spiotta A, Gracias VH, et al. Reduced mortality rate in patients with severe traumatic brain injury treated with brain tissue oxygen monitoring. J Neurosurg 2005; 103(5):805–11.

[78] Meixensberger J, Vath A, Jaeger M, et al. Monitoring of brain tissue oxygenation following severe subarachnoid hemorrhage. Neurol Res 2003;25(5):445–50.

[79] Klein J. Normobaric pulmonary oxygen toxicity. Anesth Analg 1990;70(2):195–207.

[80] Gudeman SJ, Young HF, Miller JD, et al. Indications for operative treatment and operative technique in closed head injury. In: Becker D, Gudeman S, editors. Textbook of head injury. WB Saunders; 1989. p. 138–81.

[81] Kalia K, Yonas H. An aggressive approach to massive middle cerebral artery infarction. Arch Neurol 1993;50:1293–7.

[82] Manno EM, Atkinson JL, Fulgham JR, et al. Emerging medical and surgical management strategies in the evaluation and treatment of intracerebral hemorrhage. Mayo Clin Proc 2005;80(3):420–33.

[83] Cooper PR, Rovit RL, Ransohoff J. Hemicraniectomy in the treatment of acute subdural hematoma: a re-appraisal. Surg Neurol 1976;5:25–8.

[84] Delashaw JB, Broaddus WC, Kassell NF. Treatment of right hemispheric cerebral infarction by hemicraniectomy. Stroke 1990;21:874–81.

[85] Polin RS, Shaffrey ME, Bogaev CA. Decompressive bifrontal craniectomy in the treatment of severe refractory posttraumatic cerebral edema. Neurosurgery 1997;41:84–92.

[86] Schwab S, Steiner T, Aschoff A. Early hemicraniectomy in patients with complete middle cerebral artery infarction. Stroke 1998;29:1888–93.

[87] Doerfler A, Engelhorn T, Forsting M. Decompressive creniectomy for early therapy and secondary prevention of cerebral infarction. Stroke 2001;32:813–5.

[88] Forsting M, Reith W, Schabitz WR, et al. Decompressive creniectomy for cerebral infarction. An experimental study in rats. Stroke 1995;26:259–64.

[89] Kocher T. Die therapie des hirndruckes. In: Holder A, editor. Himerschutterung, hirndruck und chirurgische eingriffe bei hirnkrankheitten. Vienna: Alfred Holder; 1901. p. 262–6.

[90] Cushing H. The establishment of cerebral hernia as a decompressive measure for inaccessible brain tumor: With the description of intramuscular methods of making the bone defect in temporal and occipital regions. Surg Gynecol Obstet 1905;1:297–314.

[91] Cushing H. Subtemporal decompressive operations for the intracranial complications associated with bursting fractures of the skull. Ann Surg 1908;47:641–4.

[92] Carter BS, Ogilvy CS, Candia GJ. One-year outcome after decompressive surgery for massive nondominant hemispheric infarction. Neurosurgery 1997;40:1168–75.

[93] Kondziolka D, Fazl M. Functional recovery after decompressive craniectomy for cerebral infarction. Neurosurgery 1988;23:143–7.

[94] Munch E, Horn P, Schurer L. Management of severe traumatic brain injury by decompressive craniectomy. Neurosurgery 2000;47:315–23.

[95] Sahuquillo J, Arikan F. Decompressive craniectomy for the treatment of refractory high intracranial pressure in traumatic brain injury. Cochrane Database Syst Rev 2006;(1): CD003983.

[96] Kilincer C, Asil T, Utku U, et al. Factors affecting the outcome of decompressive craniectomy for large hemispheric infarctions: a prospective cohort study. Acta Neruochir (Wein) 2005;147(6):587–94.

[97] Albanese J, Leone M, Alliez JR, et al. Decompressive craniectomy for severe traumatic brain injury: evaluation of the effects at one year. Crit Care Clin 2003;31(10):2535–8, [see comment].

[98] Matta B, Lam A. Nitrous oxide increases cerebral blood flow velocity during pharmacologically induced EEG silence in humans. J Neurosurg Anesthesiol 1995;7(2):89–93.

[99] Reinstrup P, Ryding E, Algotsson L, et al. Distribution of cerebral blood flow during anesthesia with isoflurane or halothane in humans. Anesthesiology 1995;82(2):359–66.

[100] Mönkhoff M, Schwarz U, Gerber A, et al. The effects of sevoflurane and halothane anesthesia on cerebral blood flow velocity in children. Anesth Analg 2001;92(4):891–6.

[101] Matta BF, Heath KJ, Tipping K, et al. Direct cerebral vasodilatory effects of sevoflurane and isoflurane. Anesthesiology 1999;91(3):677–80.

[102] Kaisti KK, Långsjö JW, Aalto S, et al. Effects of sevoflurane, propofol, and adjunct nitrous oxide on regional cerebral blood flow, oxygen consumption, and blood volume in humans. Anesthesiology 2003;99(3):603–13.

[103] Kolbitsch C, Lorenz IH, Hörmann C, et al. Sevoflurane and nitrous oxide increase regional cerebral blood flow (rCBF) and regional cerebral blood volume (rCBV) in a drug-specific manner in human volunteers. Magn Reson Imaging 2001;19(10):1253–60.

[104] Mielck F, Stephan H, Buhre W, et al. Effects of 1 MAC desflurane on cerebral metabolism, blood flow and carbon dioxide reactivity in humans. Br J Anaesth 1998;81(2):155–60.

[105] Mielck F, Stephan H, Weyland A, et al. Effects of one minimum alveolar anesthetic concentration sevoflurane on cerebral metabolism, blood flow, and CO2 reactivity in cardiac patients. Anesth Analg 1999;89(2):364–9.

[106] Fraga M, Rama-Maceiras P, Rodiño S, et al. The effects of isoflurane and desflurane on intracranial pressure, cerebral perfusion pressure, and cerebral arteriovenous oxygen content difference in normocapnic patients with supratentorial brain tumors. Anesthesiology 2003;98(5):1085–90.

[107] Ornstein E, Matteo RS, Weinstein JA, et al. Accelerated recovery from doxacurium-induced neuromuscular blockade in patients receiving chronic anticonvulsant therapy. J Clin Anesth 1991;3:108–11.

[108] Nishiyama T, Matsukawa T, Yokoyama T, et al. Cerebrovascular carbon dioxide reactivity during general anesthesia: a comparison between sevoflurane and isoflurane. Anesth Analg 1999;89(6):1437–41.

[109] Statler KD, Alexander H, Vagni V, et al. Comparison of seven anesthetic agents on outcome after experimental traumatic brain injury in adult, male rats. J Neurotrauma 2006; 23(1):97–108.

[110] Warner DS. Isoflurane neuroprotection: a passing fantasy, again? Anesthesiology 2000; 92(5):1226–8.

[111] Wise-Faberowski L, Pearlstein RD, Warner DS. NMDA-induced apoptosis in mixed neuronal/glial cortical cell cultures: the effects of isoflurane and dizocilpine. J Neurosurg Anesthesiol 2006;18(4):240–6.

[112] Wei H, Kang B, Wei W, et al. Isoflurane and sevoflurane affect cell survival and BCL-2/ BAX ratio differently. Brain Res 2005;1037(1-2):139–47.

[113] Hoffman WE, Charbel FT, Edelman G, et al. Comparison of the effect of etomidate and desflurane on brain tissue gases and pH during prolonged middle cerebral artery occlusion. Anesthesiology 1998;88(5):1188–94.

[114] Hoffman WE, Charbel FL, Edelman G, et al. Thiopental and desflurane treatment for brain protection. Neurosurgery 1998;43(5):1050–3.

[115] Lorenz IH, Kolbitsch C, Hörmann C, et al. Influence of equianaesthetic concentrations of nitrous oxide and isoflurane on regional cerebral blood flow, regional cerebral blood volume, and regional mean transit time in human volunteers. Br J Anaesth 2001;87(5):691–8.

[116] Lorenz IH, Kolbitsch C, Hörmann C, et al. The influence of nitrous oxide and remifentanil on cerebral hemodynamics in conscious human volunteers. Neuroimage 2002;17(2): 1056–64.

[117] Aono M, Sato J, Nishino T. Nitrous oxide increases normocapnic cerebral blood flow velocity but does not affect the dynamic cerebrovascular response to step changes in end-tidal P(CO2) in humans. Anesth Analg 1999;89(3):684–9.

[118] Phirman JR, Shapiro HM. Modification of nitrous oxide-induced intracranial hypertension by prior induction of anesthesia. Anesthesiology 1977;46(2):150–1.

[119] Russell GB, Snider MT, Richard RB, et al. Hyperbaric nitrous oxide as a sole anesthetic agent in humans. Anesth Analg 1990;70:289–95.

[120] Kofke WA, Stiller RL, Rose ME. Comparison of extracellular dopamine concentration in awake unstressed and postsurgical nitrous oxide sedated rats. J Neurosurg Anesthesiol 1995;7(4):280–3.

[121] Dziewit JA, Guo J, Kofke WA. No neuroexcitation by nitrous oxide in unstressed young and old mice. J Neurosurg Anesthesiol 2006;18(4):292–3.

[122] Jevtovic-Todorovic V, Todorovic SM, Mennerick S, et al. Nitrous oxide (laughing gas) is an NMDA antagonist, neuroprotectant and neurotoxin. Nat Med 1998;4(4):460–3.

[123] Eisenberg HM, Frankowski RF, Contant CF, et al. High-dose barbiturate control of elevated intracranial pressure in patients with severe head injury J Neurosurg. J Neurosurg 1988;69:15–23.

[124] Schulte am Esch J, Pfeifer G, Thiemig I. [Effects of etomidate and thiopentone on the primarily elevated intracranial pressure (ICP) (author's transl)]. Anaesthesist 1978;27(2):71–5, [in German].

[125] Preziosi P, Vacca M. Adrenocortical suppression and other endocrine effects of etomidate. Life Sci 1988;42:477–89, [review].

[126] McConnel JR, Ong CS, McAllister JL, et al. Propylene glycol toxicity following continuous etomidate infusion for the control of refractory cerebral edema. Neurosurgery 1996;38(1): 232–3.

[127] Gemma M, Tommasino C, Cerri M, et al. Intracranial effects of endotracheal suctioning in the acute phase of head injury. J Neurosurg Anesthesiol 2002;14(1):50–4.

[128] Jamali S, Archer D, Ravussin P, et al. The effect of skull-pin insertion on cerebrospinal fluid pressure and cerebral perfusion pressure: influence of sufentanil and fentanyl. Anesth Analg 1997;84(6):1292–6.

[129] Kofke WA, Attaallah AF, Kuwabara H, et al. Neuropathologic effects in rats and neurometabolic effects in humans of high-dose remifentanil. Anesth Analg 2002;94:1229–36.

[130] Kofke WA, Garman RH, Rose ME, et al. Opioid neurotoxicity: fentanyl-induced exacerbation of forebrain ischemia in rats. Brain Research 1999;818:326–34.

[131] Kofke WA, Garman RH, Janosky J, et al. Opioid neurotoxicity: neuropathologic effects of different fentanyl congeners and effects of hexamethonium-induced normotension. Anesth Analg 1996;83:141–6.

[132] Kofke WA, Garman RH, Stiller RL, et al. Opioid neurotoxicity: fentanyl dose response effects in rats. Anesth Analg 1996;83:1298–306.

[133] Kofke WA, Garman RH, Tom WC, et al. Alfentanil-induced hypermetabolism, seizure, and neuropathology in rats. Anesth Analg 1992;75:953–64.

[134] Kofke WA, Garman RH, Rose ME, et al. Opioid neurotoxicity: fentanyl-induced exacerbation of cerebral ischemia in rats. Brain Res 1999;818:326–34.

[135] Statler KD, Kochanek PM, Dixon CE, et al. Isoflurane improves long-term neurologic outcome versus fentanyl after traumatic brain injury in rats. J Neurotrauma 2000;17(12): 1179–89.

[136] Sullivan PM, Sinz EH, Gunel E, et al. A retrospective comparison of remifentanil versus methohexital for anesthesia in electroconvulsive therapy. J ECT 2004;20(4):219–24.

[137] Sinz EH, Kofke WA, Garman RH. Phenytoin, midazolam, and naloxone protect against fentanyl-induced brain damage in rats. Anesth Analg 2000;91(6):1443–9.

ELSEVIER
SAUNDERS

ANESTHESIOLOGY
CLINICS

Anesthesiology Clin
25 (2007) 605–630

Electrophysiologic Monitoring in Neurosurgery

Leslie C. Jameson, MD*, Daniel J. Janik, MD,
Tod B. Sloan, MD, MBA, PhD

*University of Colorado at Denver and Health Sciences Center,
4200 East 9th Ave, Denver, CO 80262, USA*

Electrophysiologic monitoring is a commonly used tool in the operating room to improve surgical decision making and patient outcome. Recent articles have extensively reviewed the methodology, the anatomy, the effects of anesthesia drugs, and patient physiologies' impact on electrophysiologic monitoring [1–19]. Thus, the purpose of this article is to review the application of these tools during neurosurgical procedures.

Electrophysiologic mapping techniques allow for the identification of specific neurological structures, so the surgical approach to pathology can avoid key structures or identify specific target regions for lesioning or stimulation. Similarly, monitoring techniques allow for operations on neural structures by preventing surgical incursions into adjacent functional structures. In general, monitoring and mapping techniques depend on the unique characteristics of the tissues that allow electrophysiologic stimulation or recording. These techniques are useful for procedures on the brain, brainstem, spinal cord, and peripheral nervous system.

Mapping techniques of the cerebral cortex

Direct cortical recordings of electroencephalography or electrocorticography (ECoG) is commonly used to identify or map seizure foci. ECoG recordings are often made during awake craniotomies or postoperatively from specialized grids placed during general anesthesia; recording electrodes are placed over brain areas suggested by magnetic resonance imaging (MRI), functional MRI, or positron emission tomography imaging, to be

---

* Corresponding author.
E-mail address: leslie.jameson@uchsc.edu (L.C. Jameson).

1932-2275/07/$ - see front matter © 2007 Elsevier Inc. All rights reserved.
doi:10.1016/j.anclin.2007.05.004   *anesthesiology.theclinics.com*

the locus of the seizure activity (Fig. 1) [20]. Continuous ECoG recordings from the cortical grids over the next 3 to 5 days allow the neurosurgeon to locate the area involved in the seizure activity. A craniotomy is again performed and the grids and seizure foci removed. The anesthetic management for the removal of the seizure foci can either be a general anesthetic or regional anesthesia with mild sedation. In both situations, stimulation of the brain can be performed to either induce electroencephalography (EEG) defined seizure-like activity or classic spike and dome waveform. In conscious patients, stimulation can be used to identify symptoms similar to the seizure prodrome or to disrupt brain function in the areas at risk, such as speech, language, sensation, or motor function. Identification of the functional brain improves the likelihood of a complete resection of the seizure focus or tumor, while avoiding damage to functional areas [21].

The identification of the speech area is usually done awake. When awake testing cannot be used, functional MRI can be done preoperatively to suggest functional areas. Recent studies suggest that identification of Broca's or Wernicke's area may be possible through the use of cortical-cortical evoked

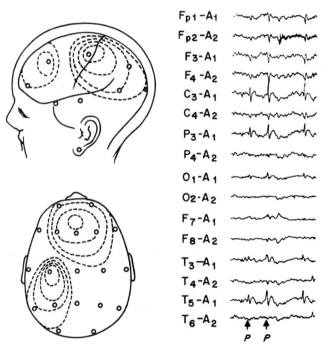

Fig. 1. Cortical Mapping of a seizure focus. Dipole mapping on the scalp (left) shows upward deflection in locations C3, P3 and T5, downward deflection in locations Fp1, Fp2, F3 and F4, consistent with a seizure generator deep in the parasaggital region. (*Modified from* Daly DD. Epilepsy and syncope. Daly D, Pedley T, editors. Current practice of clinical electroencephaloigraphy. New York: Raven Press; 1990. p. 277; with permission.)

potentials [22,23]. Here, stimulation of these areas produces an evoked response in the oro-facial area of the motor cortex or vocalis muscles of the larynx, indicating a functional connection [24]. In the future these functional connections may provide similar information as that obtained during an awake craniotomy, when performing an awake craniotomy is not possible or undesirable.

For removal of seizure foci or tumors near the sensory or motor strip, the location of these regions can be mapped in an awake patient who provides feedback on their perception, movement, or sensation in response to stimulation. Similar results are obtained in an anesthetized patient using electrophysiologic recordings or electromyography (EMG). The sensory cortex can be identified by locating the primary cortical peak of the somatosensory evoked potential (SSEP), which is generated in the sensory strip (Fig. 2) [25]. Both monopolar recording and bipolar recording will show a typical response when located over the surface of that region. Bipolar recording produces a reversal of polarity across the gyrus between the sensory and motor regions. This reversal occurs because the generator of the response is located deep in the sulcus [26–28]. This technique identifies the sensory-motor

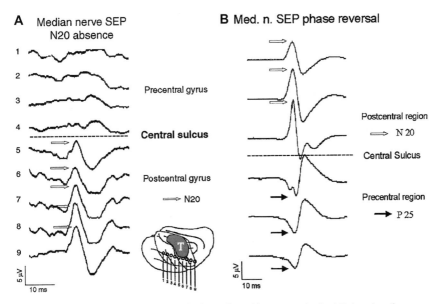

Fig. 2. SSEP mapping of the sensory strip is conducted by two methods. (*A*) A series of monopolar recordings moving anterior to the sulcus progressively posteriorly (note locations on brain figure); note the absence of a traditional N20 and SSEP recording when the electrode is anterior to the sensory strip. (*B*) Bipolar recordings in similar pairs of electrode positions; note the phase reversal when the electrode pair crosses the central sulcus between the sensory and motor areas. (*Reproduced from* Neuloh G, Schramm J. Intraoperative neurophysiological mapping and monitoring for supratentorial procedures. In: Deletis V, Shils JL, editors. Neurophysiology and neurosurgery. New York: Academic Press; 2002. p. 355, 357; with permission.)

cortex in 100% [25,28] of patients and is quite useful because MRI localization of the central sulcus is often inaccurate [28]. Identification of the sensory-motor strip can help the surgeon map a safe approach for the removal of more deeply seated tumors that affect the motor cortex.

Monitoring is becoming routine in stereotactic neurosurgery for movement disorders. Here, lesions in relevant deep brain structures or deep brain stimulators are placed for treatment of Parkinson's disease, essential tremor, and dystonia [17]. The monitoring becomes useful because the targets for effective surgery are deep, difficult to approach surgically, and not always effectively visualized or located by image guided neuronavigation systems. Here electrophysiologic recording of the target tissue is used to improve accuracy without reducing safety [29]. High resolution MRI is used to estimate the major coordinates using imaging target boundaries. However, since variations in human anatomy and imaging errors provide a resolution of between 1.5 mm and 5 mm, when compared with anatomic reference atlases [2], microelectrode EEG recordings are used to improve localization. These EEG recordings are used to find specific neuronal firing signatures as well as changes in movement induced activity (especially with procedures for movement disorders) (Fig. 3) [17]. Finally, electrical stimulation of the electrode can test the clinical effectiveness and side effects of an implanted stimulation electrode at that location.

Monitoring techniques for use during surgery on the cerebral cortex

Electrophysiologic monitoring of the brain has frequently been done to look for the occurrence of cerebral ischemia, such as during intracranial and extracranial vascular surgery. Although a variety of techniques have been used, the classic method is the EEG. The EEG allows monitoring a large surface area of the cerebral cortex by using multiple scalp electrodes. Each EEG electrode provides a continuous view of a spherical region about 2 cm to 3 cm in diameter; this area consists of superficial pyramidal cells, primarily in cortical layers 3, 5, and 6 [30]. These pyramidal layers are extremely sensitive to both hypoxia and ischemia, with detectable change occurring within 30 seconds to 5 minutes [31]. Characteristic changes in EEG occur with decreases in cerebral blood flow (Table 1) [32]. Regions that have the highest metabolic rate or are furthest from the major supply arteries (ie, boundary regions) are most sensitive to hypoperfusion, making the best electrode locations dependent on the specific area at risk for ischemia.

EEG monitoring during carotid endarterectomy (CEA) can be incorporated into a decision algorithm as the primary method to determine if cerebral ischemia is present. This is an effective monitor primarily because the area at risk is the watershed area perfused by the middle cerebral artery. EEG electrode placements vary from few parietal-temporal leads, with its

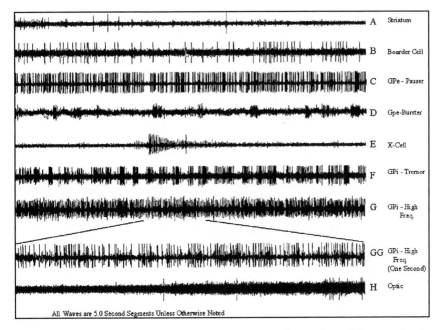

Fig. 3. Representative tracings from a microelectrode-recording probe used for targeting the globus pallidus interna (GPi) for deep brain stimulator placement. Note the different electronic signature of each region assist in the optimal electrode location. (*Reprinted from* Shils JL, Tagliati M, Alterman RL. Neurophysiological monitoring during neurosurgery for movement disorders. In: Deletis V, Shils JL, editors. Neurophysiology in neurosurgery. Boston: Academic Press; 2002. p. 428; with permission.)

emphasis on the perfusion area of the middle cerebral, to a full 32-lead montage. Many patients with carotid artery disease have other cerebrovascular diseases, making full EEG monitoring desirable because it allows assessment of more generalized hypoperfusion related to blood pressure and cardiac output.

The rapid response to changes in perfusion with the flattening of the hemisphere is a major advantage of EEG monitoring recording (Fig. 4) [33]. Ischemic changes (see Table 1) that do not rapidly respond to increases in blood pressure may be an indication for carotid bypass shunt placement. Since routine shunt use increases the risk of embolic stroke, methods such as the EEG can help the clinician limit shunt placement to only those patients who have clear ischemic changes after clamping the carotid artery during endarterectomy. The changes in the EEG have also been used to estimate the ischemic time that causes irreversible neuronal injury resulting in a clinical stroke [34]. Ischemic stroke has become an infrequent cause of postoperative neurologic injury, possibly reflecting the effectiveness of the monitoring modality and the anesthetic and surgical response to the information. In one study with 658 subjects, all monitored with EEG, only 34 developed

Table 1
Effect of decreasing cerebral blood flow on normal electroencephalographic activity in patients
during a general anesthetic

Estimated CBF (ml/100gm/min)	Expected EEG effect	Severity of injury
35–70	Normal	None
25–35	Loss of fast beta frequencies; often not seen during general anesthesia	Mild reversible
18–25	Increase in theta to <25% or decrease in amplitude >50%	Mild reversible
12–18	Increase in theta >25% or delta <25% and amplitude >50%	Moderate reversible
8–10	Suppression of all frequencies	Severe cell death
Below 8	No activity or isoelectric ECG may be present	Loss of neurons

Effect of decreasing cerebral blood flow (CBF) on normal EEG activity in patients during a general anesthetic. Depth of anesthetic will influence the EEG response caused by the change normally seen with the administration of hypnotic drugs.
Data from Refs. [31,32,42].

a postoperative neurological deficit and only 7, or 20% of this group, had computed tomographic (CT) findings that supported hypoperfusion as the cause [35].

As with any other monitor, EEG monitoring for CEA is not perfect and may be associated with either false positives or negatives [36]. One study

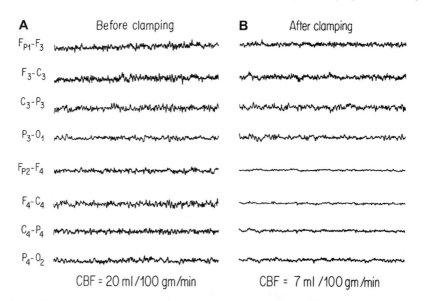

Fig. 4. EEG recording during carotid endarterectomy. Note flattening in the hemisphere where the cerebral blood flow was reduced after carotid cross clamping (7 cc/min/100gm). (*Reproduced from* Daube J, Harper CM, Litchy W. Intraoperative monitoring. In: Daly D, Pedley T, editors. Current practice of clinical electroencephaloigraphy. New York: Raven Press; 1990. p. 743; with permission.)

compared EEG changes with functional changes seen in patients who underwent CEA with a cervical block, and with the number of patients having EEG during general anesthesia. Approximately 7% of the cervical block patients were true positives (both neurological and EEG change indicating ischemia); 15% of the general anesthesia patients had EEG changes supporting ischemia, suggesting a possible 8% false positive rate. The general anesthesia group also often had bilateral changes, suggesting the cardiovascular effects of the anesthetic put the patient at risk. Thus, the EEG may be detecting real events that do not occur during regional anesthesia [37]. Another shortcoming of EEG monitoring is that after a recent stroke (less than 6 weeks), identification of ischemic change is often not possible [38].

The cost of EEG monitoring and the expertise needed for interpretation has led to research into the use of commercial processed EEG monitors. Pattern changes in the alpha, beta, and delta frequencies suggest algorithms could be developed to allow effective processed-EEG analysis that would be indicative of major and minor ischemia [39]. None of the currently available single channel monitors have been found to be reliable at detecting ischemia, even in awake patients [40]. No data is available to evaluate the possibility that processed EEG monitors that monitor right and left frontal areas provide an accurate indication of ischemic change. Unfortunately, two thirds of the postoperative strokes are focal embolic events and would not be detected by EEG monitoring of any variety. Thus, more ideal intraoperative monitoring may include transcranial doppler, for detection of emboli that may most benefit from a change in surgical technique, in combination with monitoring of EEG, for detection of situations that would most benefit from manipulation of oxygenation and blood pressure [31,38,41].

The SSEP has also been used for the detection of cerebral ischemia. Because of signal averaging, the SSEP changes more slowly than the EEG and studies suggest the SSEP is less sensitive to ischemia than the EEG. When the neural tissue at risk includes SSEP monitored regions, the SSEP appears more specific than the EEG. This is particularly true when the ischemia includes the subcortical areas [42]. A variety of primate studies suggest that the loss of 50% of the cortical SSEP amplitude corresponds to a regional cerebral blood flow of 14 mL/100 g/min to 16 mL/100 g/min. This is above the regional cerebral blood flow associated with infarction, suggesting that dysfunction should be reversible [11]. Meta-analysis of EEG and SSEP monitoring suggest that used together, EEG and SSEP are useful in identifying ischemia with CEA, and improve neurologic outcome [11].

Other combined uses of EEG and SSEP include testing the effects of vessel occlusion during interventional radiology for carotid artery angioplasty and deliberate occlusion of various arterial vessels, including aneurysms and arterio-venous malformations (AVM) [43,44]. Because it can require up to 15 minutes for an ischemic effect to be detected using SSEP, the effectiveness is limited. In some of these cases the intravascular injection of barbiturates causing the reversible loss of the evoked response suggests that the vessel injected may be a critical vessel.

The ability of electrophysiology to detect ischemia during intracerebral surgery has also made it useful for the detection of a variety of situations where there is a risk of reduced blood flow in supratentorial regions. These include inadvertent vessel occlusion, vasospasm, ischemia from retractor pressure, suboptimal vessel clip application, and relative hypotension, and has prompted surgical changes, including stopping coagulation or dissection, applying papaverine, and changing the area and style of dissection [25]. In particular, SSEP and motor evoked potentials (MEP) are useful monitors in surgery of AVMs and cavernous malformations in the pericentral region of the brain. The MEP is also a valuable monitor during vascular surgery involving deep brain and brainstem structures near the motor pathways [45].

In supratentorial surgery, the main use for SSEP monitoring is in aneurysm surgery of the anterior circulation. For anterior cerebral artery aneurysms, the lower extremity SSEP is most useful because of the vascular territory involved. Upper extremity SSEP is useful for surgery on the middle cerebral artery and for aneurysms of the internal carotid artery unless the aneurysm is at the bifurcation. In vascular cases, the use of both lower and upper extremity responses may be important if perforating arteries are involved. With aneurysms, one study stated that changes in the SSEP monitoring caused the surgeon to change the procedure in 11.3% of the surgeries, presumably resulting in better patient outcome [46]. The SSEP is not useful in surgery of the posterior circulation.

Motor evoked potential monitoring is useful in intracranial aneurysm surgery when perforating arteries may be at risk to deep structures, including the motor pathways in the corona radiata, internal capsule, cerebral peduncle, basis pontis, and pyramids [12]. For cortical surgery, MEP can be produced by direct cortical stimulation rather than transcranial stimulation. This has the advantage of an unambiguous stimulation location [12]. As with direct cortical stimulation for mapping of the motor cortex, seizure activity may be induced in susceptible patients. All patients will have a stimulation threshold for seizure activity, a condition easily treated by irrigation with iced saline. EEG monitoring is essential to detecting the after discharges that signal such activation, and can signal a spread of the stimulation to adjacent areas that could produce misleading motor activity.

Since multiple vascular territories can be affected with procedures, such as aneurysm and AVM, both SSEP and MEP monitoring are useful for the detection of ischemia. This is particularly true with resection or embolization with AVMs located near the central region or close to the sensory-motor pathways. Here, test occlusion of AVM feeders can be assessed for the compromising of nearby normal tissue before permanent manipulation.

Using both MEP and SSEPs for monitoring has been suggested for tumors near the motor cortex, motor tracts (including in the brainstem), and insula, and include cavernous angiomas [25]. In these cases the monitoring strategy is to continue resection until the MEP or SSEP is altered. Although not all motor deficits are avoided, the combined MEP-SSEP monitoring is considered essential by some to limit unnecessary morbidity [25].

Monitoring anesthetic drug effect

The EEG detects ischemia by loss of synaptic activity when the energy supply to neurons is compromised. Many other factors can cause loss of synaptic function and changes in the EEG. Anesthetic agents depress synaptic function; this drug effect produces a reduction in metabolism that may enhance the ability of the neurons to tolerate mild ischemia [47]. An EEG-determined burst suppression is the typical desired endpoint. The change in pattern of synaptic activity is also used to characterize the global effect of anesthetic agents during anesthetic drug administration [19].

The majority of anesthetic drugs alter the EEG by producing an initial excitatory stage, characterized by desynchronization and with increased relative power (proportional amount of a frequency present) of faster alpha and beta frequencies [48]. This fast beta activity is most prominent in the frontal regions and moves posterior as the anesthetic drug effect increases. Concomitantly, a prominent area of EEG synchronization in the alpha range (8 Hz–13 Hz) develops over the more posterior regions and moves to the frontal regions, an action referred to as the "anterior shift" or "frontal dominance." The general synchrony of the EEG appears to be related to a pacemaker-like influence from the thalamus or brainstem [49]. With a loss of consciousness from anesthetic and sedative agents, there is a common set of observations which include: a marked drop in gamma-band activity (25 Hz–50 Hz), an increase in slower frequency patterns (theta, delta), a great increase in power in the frontal electrodes, a marked increase in synchrony of the EEG, and an uncoupling of interaction between frontal and parietal regions and across the midline [50].

In general, most anesthetics reduce EEG amplitude and frequency by reducing the amount of synaptic activity. Increasing anesthetic drug dose causes progressive slowing until the EEG achieves burst suppression (where periods of EEG activity are interspersed with periods of a flat EEG) and, finally, electrical silence or a flat EEG [51]. Further, the EEG pattern is not uniform, with some anesthetic drugs increasing activity and others depressing activity. Most anesthetics in current clinical use, such as isoflurane, sevoflurane, desflurane, and propofol, follow a depressive pattern; previously used volatile agents produced EEG excitation or seizure-like motor activity under some physiologic conditions (eg, enflurane with hyperventilation). Modern volatile anesthetics produce burst suppression, usually at minimum alveolar concentrations (MAC) of 1.5.

Based on the observations of a gradual shift of EEG power to slower frequencies, and then loss of activity, attempts have been made to develop a depth of anesthesia monitor. Reliably assessing anesthetic depth requires complex analysis of the combination of amplitude, frequency, variability, topography, and frontal EMG. The easiest anesthetic states to detect are the awake state and that of intense synaptic depression (isoelectricity). Each anesthetic agent (based on the receptor involved in their action) has a characteristic EEG profile for the transition from the awake to unconscious state. Thus, no single EEG signature or pattern is common among all anesthetic agents because they produce their myriad of effects in different ways. Processed EEG devices vary in how they mathematically transform the EEG to determine the transition from awake to unconscious, and what their dimensionless numeric index (ranging from 0–100, where 0 is deeply asleep and 100 is awake) represents on the continuum from deeply anesthetized to awake. This value does not reflect drug-specific differences; for example, ketamine and nitrous oxide produce increased EEG activity that increases the reported dimensionless number, despite increased hypnosis [52].

Aspect Medical's bispectral index (BIS) has the longest clinical experience and the largest number of peer reviewed publications. It uses an unknown combination of power spectrum and bispectrum from a single frontal EEG channel to calculate the BIS value. Bispectral analysis, also referred to as the bispectrum, is a mathematical technique that incorporates the phase relationships between waves by determining the phase coupling between different frequencies. The degree of EEG phase relationship is thought to be inversely related to the number of independent EEG pacemakers. Increasing synchrony occurs within the brain with deepening anesthesia. The mathematical weight of each analysis changes with level of consciousness as defined by the selected EEG parameters, with all calculations being reported as a BIS number.

The Danmeter cerebral state monitor (Danmeter A/S) calculates a cerebral state index using analysis of four calculated parameters derived from the single EEG channel. EMG is not used. The difference between the parameter ratios is used to indicate the shift in EEG energy from higher to lower frequencies. It also uses the amount of burst suppression in each 30-second period. The four parameters are analyzed using fuzzy logic to create the index.

Entropy (GE Healthcare) describes the degree of asynchrony or variability of the EEG. The algorithm for calculation of entropy in the EEG signal has been published [53], but the monitor determines two separate entropy values. State entropy is an index ranging from 0 to 91 (awake), using EEG frequencies from 0.8 Hz to 32 Hz, and is thought to reflect the cortical state of the patient. Response entropy ranges from 0 to 100 (awake), and is calculated using a frequency range from 0.8 Hz to 47 Hz so that it includes EMG-dominated frequencies. Thus the response entropy will also respond to the increased EMG activity possibly resulting from inadequate analgesia. Little is published on the mathematical algorithm used to produce the index numbers.

The Narcotrend (Monitor-Technik) uses the discontinuous nature of the EEG analysis, and defined EEG "stages" are calculated using an unspecified multivariate statistical algorithm derived from multiple mathematical transformations. The defined EEG stage is calculated based on a single EEG channel. The SEDLine (Hospira) algorithm is based on a four-lead EEG recorded from a five-forehead-electrode array. The SEDLine analysis depends on the well recognized shift in power, between the frontal and occipital areas, that occurs during loss of consciousness and increasing hypnotic drug effect. The proprietary mathematical analysis includes EEG power, frequency, and coherence between bilateral brain regions [54]. The SNAPII (Everest Biomedical) calculation is based on a spectral mathematical analysis of EEG activity in the 0-Hz to18-Hz and 80-Hz to 420-Hz frequency ranges, and a burst suppression algorithm.

The literature is silent in defining the efficacy of these processed EEG monitors over a broad range of clinical uses. Practitioners use them to guide anesthetic dosing for management of cardiovascular perturbation and reduction of intraoperative awareness. Their value as a monitor of anesthetic effect is still evolving; at present they appear more an index of sedation and hypnosis than analgesia. However, they may have a particular application in neurosurgery to gauge anesthetic management during the total intravenous anesthesia needed for some of the electrophysiological monitoring techniques (eg, MEPs).

Mapping of the brainstem

Similar to supratentorial mapping, electrophysiologic techniques have been used in the brainstem for localization of structures during surgery and identification of surgical pathways to deeper regions. Once considered untouchable, tumors in the brainstem are now routinely approached surgically [55]. Mapping and monitoring of the brainstem allows meticulous surgical techniques, avoiding unplanned injury to neural structures [55]. A variety of "safe" entry zones have been identified in relation to normal brainstem structures; however, because these are based on anatomical landmarks which may become distorted by the growth of lesions, mapping techniques are critical (Fig. 5). These techniques are based on recording muscle activity following stimulation of motor nuclei VII, IX to X, and XII on the floor of the fourth ventricle [16,56–58].

Other mapping techniques include: localizing structures which may be in the operative field; identifying the facial nerve, which may be intertwined or obscured by an acoustic neuroma; finding structures for surgical resection (ie, the use of the auditory nerve can help find the cleavage plane with the vestibular nerve for sectioning of the latter); or recording from the trigeminal nerve after facial stimulation, for sectioning for trigeminal neuralgia [59].

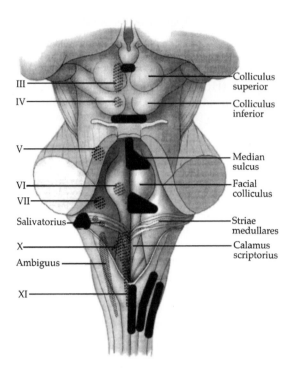

Fig. 5. Positions of the cranial nerve-motor nuclei in the brainstem and relatively safe entry zones (black regions) for surgical access to deep structures. (*Modified from* Bricolo A, Sala F. Surgery of brainstem lesions. In: Deletis V, Shils JL, editors. Neurophysiology in neurosurgery. Boston: Academic Press; 2002. p. 271; with permission.)

Brainstem motor mapping of the corticospinal tract is done using a hand-held stimulator and then recording compound muscle action potentials (CMAP) [16]. This technique has been found helpful in midbrain tumors where the corticospinal tract is difficult to identify or in surgery near the cerebral peduncle and ventral medulla [16,55].

Monitoring techniques during surgery on the brainstem

Monitoring during brainstem surgery is useful to reduce the risk of unintended neural morbidity. Cranial nerves are susceptible to damage because of their small size, limited epineurium, and complicated course. The damage occurs from surgical disruption, manipulation, or ischemia, resulting in paresis, paralysis, and possibly chronic pain. EMG provides continuous and immediate feedback to the surgeon, which allows the surgeon to change the approach to avoid permanent damage. EMG is more resistant to the depressant effects of anesthetics and other physiologic variables, such as temperature and blood pressure [6]. EMG monitoring records motor unit potentials (MUP). Neurotonic discharges are high-frequency intermittent or continuous bursts of MUPs, usually caused by mechanical (compression, contusion, rubbing, manipulation, irrigation, stretching) or metabolic (ischemia) stimuli to the nerve in question (Fig. 6) [60]. Bursts may last less than 200 ms, with single or multiple MUPs firing at 30 Hz to 100 Hz, or they can be long trains of continuous discharges lasting 1 to 30 seconds [6]. The best recording conditions are with the use of pairs of small needle electrodes placed deep within the belly of a muscle innervated by the nerve at risk. Bipolar nerve root stimulation minimizes current spread to adjacent nerves, but monopolar probes minimize the chance of subthreshold stimulation. Nerves or cranial nerve nuclei are stimulated proximal to the site of potential operative injury, allowing assessment of nerve integrity and function. Amplitude reduction in a facial nerve (CN VII) CMAP correlates with

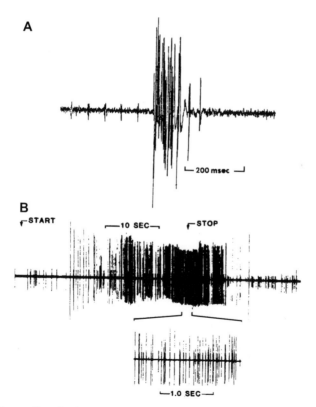

Fig. 6. EMG recordings from muscle during monitoring during surgery near motor nerves. The upper trace (*A*) shows a single, brief burst of muscle activity from nerve irritation. The lower trace (*B*) shows sustained "neurotonic" activity from injurious nerve irritation. Note the difference in time scales. (*From* Prass RL, Luders H. Acoustic (loudspeaker) facial electromyographic monitoring: part 1. Evoked electromyographic activity during acoustic neuroma resection. Neurosurgery 1986;19:395, 397; with permission.)

immediate and long-term paralysis [61]. After sharp transection of a nerve, stimulation of the distal segment may still evoke a CMAP response, which could be interpreted inaccurately to indicate an intact neural pathway.

As described in Table 2, monitoring can be accomplished from all cranial nerves with motor components. Damage to lower cranial nerve nuclei (IX–XII) can lead to dyspnea, severe dysphagia, and aspiration requiring tracheostomy, even when the injury is unilateral. Oculomotor nerves (III, IV, andVI) are not commonly monitored, but may be of value during tumor removal in the region of the cavernous sinus or intraventricular tumors [62]. EMG monitoring is useful in surgery with hyperactive cranial nerves and cranial nerve compression syndromes, including trigeminal neuralgia (V), hemifacial spasm (VII), and vago-glossal-pharyngeal neuralgia (IX, X) [14]. EMG monitoring of the facial nerve during surgery in the cerebello-pontine angle has become a standard of care because of the frequent risk of facial nerve injury [63,64]. In addition to neurotonic discharges, monitoring the latency, from intentional stimulation to the muscle response, can help differentiate between the different cranial nerves. The close proximity of nerve fibers and cranial nerve nuclei can lead to accidental stimulation, causing a motor response in several muscle groups. This is particularly

Table 2
Nerve roots and muscles commonly monitored

Nerve		Muscle
Spinal cord		
Cervical	C 2–4	Trapezoids, sternocleidomastoid
	C 5, 6	Biceps, deltoid
	C 6, 7	Flexor carpi radialis
Thoracic	C 8–T 1	Adductor pollicis
	T 2–6	Specific intercostals
	T 5–12	Specific area of rectus abdominus
Lumbar	L 2	Adductor longus
	L 2–4	Vastus medialis
Sacral	L 4–S 1	Tibialis anterior
	L 5–S 1	Peroneus longus
	S 1, 2	Gastrocnemius
	S 2–4	Anal sphincter
Cranial nerves		
Oculomotor	III	Superior, medial, inferior rectus
Trochlear	IV	Superior oblique
Trigeminal	V	Masseter
Abducens	VI	Lateral rectus
Facial	VII	Obicularis oculi, oris; mentalis, temporalis
Glossopharyngeal	IX	Pharyngeal muscles
Vagus	X	Vocal cords
Spinal accessory	XI	Trapezius, sternocleidomastoid
Hypoglossal	XII	Tongue

notable for temporalis (CN VII) and masseter (CN V) muscle stimulation when EMG is recorded in the orbicularis oculi and oris (CN VII) [64].

Auditory brainstem response (ABR), also referred to as brainstem auditory evoked response or BAER, monitoring in acoustic neuroma surgery may help reduce risk of surgical damage to the acoustic nerve [65]. The traditional ABR recordings require a relatively long averaging period (1000 repetitions at 11.7 Hz), allowing surgical difficulties to go undetected for a period of time. Traditional ABR predict intact hearing if they are present at the end of the procedure, but do not guarantee the quality of residual hearing. In addition, loss of ABR during the procedure does not predict hearing loss [66]. Recording directly from the auditory nerve or from the surface of the cochlear nucleus is effective when the extracranial portion of the nerve, the cochlea, and the labyrinthine artery are at risk. Direct nerve recordings provide a rapid response and the loss of signal reliably predicts hearing loss. Cerebello-pontine angle recordings are also rapid and can monitor the distal and proximal portions of the nerve.

In surgery on tumors of the posterior fossa, monitoring of cranial nerve EMG has been shown to correlate with postoperative neurologic status. In a study of pediatric patients undergoing surgery for removal of tumors in the brainstem, where the lower cranial nerves (IX, X, XII) were monitored, a positive EMG event in one nerve was associated with a postoperative deficit in 73% of the subjects, and temporary increases in EMG activity in all three nerves was always associated with a deficit. Postoperative aspiration pneumonia or need for tracheotomy was always associated with intraoperative EMG activity in at least one of these nerves [67].

Monitoring cranial nerve function outside the brainstem is also useful. Monitoring recurrent laryngeal and superior laryngeal branches as a surrogate for the vagus nerve (CN X) is often used in neck dissections, thyroid removal, and anterior cervical spine fusions. EMG monitoring is performed by placing needle electrodes in the cricothyroid or vocalis muscles, or using contact electrodes on an endotracheal tube. With a reported incidence of recurrent laryngeal nerve injury following surgery of the thyroid at 2.3% to 5.2%, investigators have found laryngeal EMG useful [68]. Unfortunately, EMG is only a reliable diagnostic tool if prior test stimulation results in a positive response; negative responses may be due to altered nerve function, stimulation of nonnerve tissue, or equipment malfunction [69]. Nonetheless, EMG monitoring has been found to reduce the risk of damage to the vagus nerve [68,70].

ABR, SSEP and EMG monitoring is used to assess the general integrity of the brainstem structures near the surgical site or under retractors. Spontaneous EMG activity may be helpful but an absolute correlation with outcome has not been established [71,72]. In addition, SSEP and ABR can only monitor the functional integrity of about 20% of the brainstem [73]. Changes in ABR are more sensitive than vital signs in detecting brainstem injury [74]. With surgery close to the cerebral peduncles or the ventral medulla, injury to the corticospinal tracts is a concern and monitoring with MEP is important [75–77]. Monitoring MEPs of the face and hand muscu-lature can assess the corticospinal and cortico-bulbar tracts, particularly for tumors in the posterior fossa [16].

Mapping of the spinal cord

For surgery within the spinal cord, the identification of the midline for an entrance myelotomy is usually key to minimizing damage to the cord. Because the SSEP tracts follow the dorsal columns which lie adjacent to the midline, stimulation of the lower extremity and recording from a series of contacts across the posterior aspect of the cord allow for the identification of the dorsal median sulcus when distorted anatomy (eg, from a tumor) would otherwise make this difficult (Fig. 7) [78]. Unfortunately, because of the loss of the SSEP tracts by the myelotomy, monitoring of the SSEP may not be possible in up to 30% of the cases [79]. This problem is less fre-quent in children below the age of 9 or 10 because the pathways are more laterally located [15].

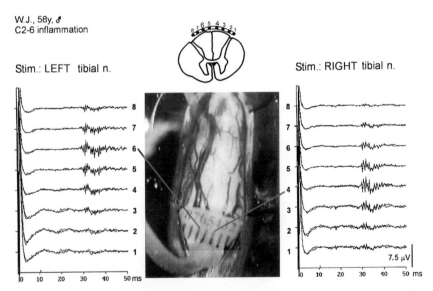

Fig. 7. Spinal cord mapping using Surface electrodes and the SSEP. Note the epidural SSEP recording shows a maximal amplitude from the left- and right-sided stimulation at electrodes 6 and 4, respectively, suggesting the midline for myelotomy is under electrode 5. (*Reproduced from* Krzan MJ. Intraoperative neurophysiological mapping of the spinal cord's dorsal col-umns. In: Deletis V, Shils JL, editors. Neurophysiology in neurosurgery. New York: Academic Press; 2002. p. 158; with permission.)

Alternatively, some investigators use posterior spinal cord contacts to stimulate the cord electrically and record descending responses (antidromically conducted sensory responses) in peripheral nerves [80]. Similar stimulation and recording techniques have been used to stimulate within the spinal cord to identify the descending motor tracts. For identification of the motor tracts, stimulation within the spinal cord shortly after transcranial stimulation produces a collision which blocks the D-wave or the muscle response, identifying the location of the tract [3,79–81].

Monitoring techniques for spinal cord surgery

Monitoring has been used during neurosurgical procedures that revolve around external spinal cord compression or spinal column bony abnormalities. In general, when the entire spinal cord is affected by the surgical maneuvers or pathology, SSEP monitoring is highly predictive of neurological outcome. This has been documented by the Scoliosis Research Society and the European Spinal Deformities Society [82]. SSEP monitoring during scoliosis correction is now a standard in many high volume centers.

MEP monitoring has also become common during spinal column surgery because the SSEP may miss a motor injury. Two recent studies examined outcome and reported a high correlation of MEP changes with outcome [83]. In the largest study, 11.3% of the subjects had MEP change; in the five subjects with permanent MEP change, all had partial or permanent neurologic injury [84]. In cervical spine surgery, monitoring of MEP is believed to decrease morbidity, in part because it may allow differentiation between cervical cord myelopathy and peripheral neuropathy [85,86].

For monitoring of spinal cord surgery, MEPs can be monitored using two methodologies. First is the traditional recording of muscle action potentials after multipulse transcranial stimulation; second is the spinal cord monitoring of the D-wave in the corticospinal tract. The amplitude of the D-wave is considered a semiquantitative assessment of the number of preserved fibers in the fast conducting fibers of the corticospinal tract [16], and correlates better with long-term functional motor outcome than does the muscle response or EMG [15]. The CMAP response also monitors the supportive systems of the spinal cord (non-corticospinal tracts) and proprio-spinal system [16]. When the D-wave amplitude is unchanged or reduced less than 50%, the patient will have postoperative motor function, even if a temporary loss of a muscle response is seen. Transient postoperative paralysis, lasting several hours to days, is thought to be due to a loss of accessory motor pathways (eg, propriospinal systems that facilitate the corticospinal pathway) [4]. Because as little as 10% of the CT fibers may be necessary for motor function, the warning criteria for D-wave change is often a 30% to 50% loss before surgery is halted or abandoned [16]. Using combined D-wave and CMAP monitoring, the outcome from intramedullary spinal cord surgery is 100% sensitive and 91% specific [16]. Other techniques, such as descending neurogenic evoked potentials, neurogenic MEPs, and spinal to spinal evoked responses, used to monitor the spinal cord during spine reconstruction are less useful during intramedullary spinal cord surgery.

The use of both SSEP and MEP is recommended when surgery involves risks to specific vascular structures or specific regions within the spinal cord. Hence, combined monitoring has been conducted during the removal of spinal cord tumors or arteriovenous malformations [15]. Studies report an excellent correlation with monitoring and clinical outcome [87,88]. With AVMs, the monitoring has allowed provocative testing of the vascular supply to determine the safety of vessel sacrifice. In this case, test clamping or the injection of sodium amytal, which blocks gray matter neural activity of MEP, and lidocaine, which blocks white matter conduction of SSEP or MEP, helps identify when vascular supply to lesions involves critical pathways [89].

Because of the risk for damage to the spinal cord, both SSEP and MEP are usually monitored with spine surgery cephalad to the termination of the cord (L1–L2). Below this level the MEP is often omitted and monitoring of reflex nerve pathways, such as the H-reflex, is used. These reflex monitoring techniques have become popular for monitoring in regions of the spinal cord where traditional evoked responses are not useful, such as cauda equina, or when motor evoked potentials are not recordable or contraindicated.

The H-reflex is the result of electrical stimulation of the peripheral nerve, which activates the lowest threshold Ia fibers. The ascending volley activates the motoneurons via synaptic reflex pathways in the spinal cord, producing a muscle response (Fig. 8) [13]. The H-reflex is thus a reflection of these reflex pathways and the excitability of the motoneurons. This is useful to monitor the gray matter at the level of the reflex, as well as more cephalad influences. Hence, changes in the descending pathways of the corticospinal, rubrospinal, vestibulospinal, and reticulospinal systems can alter the response [90].

The H-reflex is best monitored in the flexors of the upper extremity and the extensors of the lower extremity (eg, gastrocnemius from posterior tibial nerve stimulation), although it has been recorded in over 20 muscles throughout the hand, arm, leg, foot, and jaw [13]. A sustained, significant loss of the response strongly correlates with a new onset motor deficit [9].

EMG monitoring is more sensitive than SSEP during spinal column surgery for detecting radiculopathy [7]. SSEP may fail to alert the surgeon to individual nerve root damage because multiple nerve roots contribute to the cortical response [10]. Radiculopathy may be caused by improper placement of instrumentation, such as pedicle screws, which violate the bony wall of the pedicle and exert pressure on adjacent nerve roots. Placement of pedicle screws is done under direct vision and with the aid of intraoperative radiographs, but these are unreliable. Holes and screws can be

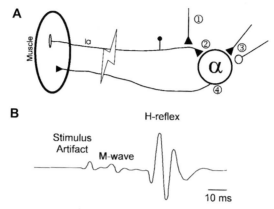

Fig. 8. H-reflex pathway and typical muscle response. The reflex arc is initiated by stimulation of the peripheral nerve (which produces the M wave) and activates the alpha motor neuron in the spinal gray matter, producing the second muscle activity (the H-reflex). Modulation of the response includes (1) presynaptic inhibition, (2) homosynaptic depression, (3) descending spinal tract influences, and (4) intrinsic alpha motor neuron membrane excitability. (*Reproduced from* Misiaszek JE. The H-reflex as a tool in neurophysiology: its limitations and uses in understanding nervous system function. Muscle Nerve 2003;28:145; with permission.)

stimulated with a monopolar probe, and recordings are made from needle electrodes in appropriate muscles. Both constant current and constant voltage can be effectively used. The bone cortex has a higher resistance to current flow than soft tissue; therefore, low stimulus thresholds will indicate a breach in the posterior bony wall holding the screw and should prompt either exploration of the screw placement or removal and repositioning. Stimulus thresholds for various situations are presented in Table 3 [7]. It is important to note that chronically compressed nerves, through mechanisms of axonotmesis, have a much higher threshold for stimulation than normal nerves. Direct nerve root stimulation distal to the pedicle should be employed when the patient presents with a radicular motor deficit, to

Table 3

Stimulus thresholds for normal healthy nerve roots, chronically compressed nerve roots, and normal and misplaced pedicle hole and screws

Structure	Stimulus threshold, (in milliamperes)
Normal nerve root	2.2 (0.2–5.7)
Chronically compressed nerve root	6.3–20
Normal hole	30.4 (16.5–44.3)
Normal screw	24 (12.1–35.9)
Misplaced hole	3.4 (1–6)
Misplaced screw	3.5 (1–6)

Data from Holland NR. Intraoperative electromyography. J Clin Neurophysiol 2002;19:444–53.

establish a control threshold necessary for the pedicle screw to stimulate the nerve [91]. With regards to anesthetic technique during spinal column surgery, Holland [92] has found it to be possible to effectively monitor EMG with up to 75% neuromuscular blockade, but requires careful titration of neuromuscular blocking agents. Data derived from multiple prospective studies and case series performed during cervical, thoracic, and lumbosacral procedures of the spinal column support the sensitivity of EMG monitoring in detecting malpositioned hardware, as well as the usefulness of multimodality monitoring (EMG, SSEP) in preventing nerve root injury [93–99].

EMG monitoring has also proven useful in monitoring the nerve roots that collectively form the cauda equina. Procedures, such as release of tethered cord and tumor excision, carry the risk of damage to nerve roots innervating the muscles of the leg, anal, and urethral sphincters. Damage to these roots is extremely debilitating, and every effort is sought to avoid this complication. It may be difficult, even with microscope assistance, to separate nervous from nonfunctional tissue. Spontaneous and evoked EMG recordings aid in identification of nerves. There will be a difference in the stimulation threshold of filum terminale fibers, compared with motor nerve fibers of up to 100 to 1 [100]. As with other spinal surgery, a multimodality approach is used. Suggested techniques include spontaneous and evoked EMG, including anal sphincter, urethral sphincter, bladder pressure, tibial nerve SSEP, and MEP. Urethral sphincter EMG may be recorded using a bladder catheter with electrodes attached two centimeters from the inflating balloon [101]. Although bladder pressure is simple to measure, it measures primarily stimulated responses, and therefore does not provide the immediate and continuous feedback desired. It can be argued that anal sphincter EMG will provide the needed information about the bladder because the innervation of both arises from the second through fourth sacral segments [102]. The cauda equina can be mapped during surgery using evoked EMG, peripheral sensory stimulation with surgical field recording, motor evoked potentials, cortical sensory evoked potentials, and the bulbocavernosus reflex [8].

Mapping of the peripheral nervous system

Operations for repair of nerves damaged by trauma can benefit from neurophysiologic monitoring, by guiding the surgeon's decision to graft, reapproximate the nerve, or do nothing. Blunt trauma typically leaves nerves in continuity with varying degrees of internal disruption. If the damage is neuropraxic or axonotmetic, then the nerve can be expected to recover over time by remyelination or axon growth. The presence of a nerve action potential recording over the injured segment of such a nerve that has been surgically exposed will indicate the presence of regeneration, making a grafting procedure unnecessary. Absence of recordable action potentials will indicate more severe disruption and neurotmetic injury and will require grafting for satisfactory outcome. In the case of a nerve root avulsion, action potentials can still be recorded because the injury is proximal to the dorsal root ganglion. Recording of cortical SSEP responses after stimulation of the proximal segment will indicate that the injury is distal to the ganglion [7]. For these reasons, electrophysiologic mapping has been used in evaluation of neuroma-in-situ and in brachial plexus lesions to identify neural sections, which maintain some motor or sensory continuity (where time will improve function), or where no continuity exists (where surgical reanastimosis or neural graft will improve outcome).

Dorsal rhizotomy, for reduction of severe incapacitating spasticity (often the result of cerebral palsy), is facilitated by electrophysiologic mapping. In these patients the spasticity is thought to result from hyperactivity of sensory rootlets devoid of adequate supraspinal control. This hyperactivity spreads to adjacent myotomes, resulting in excessive leg and foot tone and reflex muscle activity. Thus, intraoperative stimulation and recording of adjacent myotomes identifies the rootlets to be sectioned [16,103]. Usually these rootlets are between L2 and S2; because rootlets at S2 may be involved, pudendal mapping of rootlets to the anal sphincter and urogential system is useful to minimize bowel and bladder complications.

Monitoring techniques during peripheral nerve surgery

Monitoring the peripheral nervous system includes spinal nerve roots as well as the plexus and individual nerves of the limbs, and is typically performed to prevent surgical injury or guide surgical repair. Injury may occur during procedures on the spinal column, with or without in situ instrumentation, and during removal of tumors from or untethering of the cauda equina. EMG monitoring follows the principles outlined for cranial nerve monitoring, namely that either spontaneous or evoked activity is correlated to surgical events; the activity is either neurotonic discharges or CMAP. Neurotonic discharges will alert the neurophysiologist, and hence the surgeon, to irritation of neural tissue, and the CMAP will allow identification of individual nerve roots and bony pedicles. When monitoring the EMG of the spinal nerve roots, it is important to select muscles which allow identification of discrete myotomes covering the area of potential surgical insult.

Summary

Electrophysiologic mapping and monitoring has become commonplace in neurosurgery to improve surgical decision making and refine procedures, while reducing undesired neural morbidity. Similar to how the introduction of the operating microscope and stereotactic imaging procedures have allowed the neurosurgeon to better see the structural aspects of their procedures, electrophysiologic testing and monitoring have allowed a functional assessment of these structures. As such, these procedures enhance the operating techniques and decision-making capabilities of the surgeon, so as to improve the effectiveness of the surgery and reduce the risk of undesired morbidity. Like the other techniques, this has allowed the development of neurosurgical procedures in ways not visualized before their introduction.

References

[1] Barkley GL, Baumgartner C. MEG and EEG in epilepsy. J Clin Neurophysiol 2003;20: 163–78.

[2] Bootin M. Deep brain stimulation: overview and update. J Clin Monit Comput 2006;20: 341–6.

[3] Cioni B, Meglio M, Rossi GF. Intraoperative motor evoked potentials monitoring in spinal neurosurgery. Arch Ital Biol 1999;137:115–26.

[4] Deletis V. Intraoperative neurophysiology and methodologies used to monitor the functional integrity of the motor system. In: Deletis V, Shils JL, editors. Neurophysiology in neurosurgery. Boston: Academic Press; 2002. p. 25–51.

[5] Harper CM, Daube JR. Facial nerve electromyography and other cranial nerve monitoring [see comment]. J Clin Neurophysiol 1998;15:206–16.

[6] Harper CM. Intraoperative cranial nerve monitoring. Muscle Nerve 2004;29:339–51.

[7] Holland NR. Intraoperative electromyography. J Clin Neurophysiol 2002;19:444–53.

[8] Kothbauer KF, Novak K. Intraoperative monitoring for tethered cord surgery: an update. Neurosurg Focus 2004;16:1–5.

[9] Leppanen RE. Intraoperative applications of the H-reflex and F-response: a tutorial. J Clin Monit Comput 2006;20:267–304.

[10] Leppanen RE, Abnm D, American Society of Neurophysiological M. Intraoperative monitoring of segmental spinal nerve root function with free-run and electrically-triggered electromyography and spinal cord function with H-reflexes and F-responses. A position statement by the American Society of Neurophysiological Monitoring. J Clin Monit Comput 2005;19:437–61.

[11] Lopez JR. The use of evoked potentials in intraoperative neurophysiologic monitoring. Phys Med Rehabil Clin N Am 2004;15:63–84.

[12] MacDonald D. Intraoperative motor evoked potential monitoring: overview and update. J Clin Monit Comput 2006;20:347–77.

[13] Misiaszek JE. The H-reflex as a tool in neurophysiology: its limitations and uses in understanding nervous system function. Muscle Nerve 2003;28:144–60.

[14] Moller AR. Intraoperative neurophysiologic monitoring. 2nd edition. Totowa (NJ): Humana Press; 2006.

[15] Sala F, Krzan MJ, Deletis V. Intraoperative neurophysiological monitoring in pediatric neurosurgery: why, when, how? Childs Nerv Syst 2002;18:264–87.

[16] Sala F, Lanteri P, Bricolo A. Motor evoked potential monitoring for spinal cord and brain stem surgery. Adv Tech Stand Neurosurg 2004;29:133–69.

[17] Shils JL, Tagliati M, Alterman RL. Neurophysiological monitoring during neurosurgery for movement disorders. In: Deletis V, Shils JL, editors. Neurophysiology in neurosurgery. Boston: Academic Press; 2002. p. 405–48.

[18] Jameson LC, Sloan TB. Monitoring of the brain and spinal cord. Anesthesiol Clin North America 2006;24:777–91.

[19] Jameson LC, Sloan TB. Using EEG to monitor anesthesia drug effects during surgery. J Clin Monit Comput 2006;20:445–72.

[20] Daly DD. Epilepsy and syncope. In: Daly D, Pedley T, editors. Current practice of clinical electroencephaloigraphy. New York: Raven Press; 1990. p. 269–332.

[21] MacDonald DB, Pillay N. Intraoperative electrocorticography in temporal lobe epilepsy surgery. Can J Neurol Sci 2000;27(Suppl 1):S85–91 [discussion: S92–6].

[22] Greenlee JD, Oya H, Kawasaki H, et al. A functional connection between inferior frontal gyrus and orofacial motor cortex in human. J Neurophysiol 2004;92:1153–64.

[23] Matsumoto R, Nair DR, LaPresto E, et al. Functional connectivity in the human language system: a cortico-cortical evoked potential study. Brain 2004;127:2316–30.

[24] Rodel RM, Olthoff A, Tergau F, et al. Human cortical motor representation of the larynx as assessed by transcranial magnetic stimulation (TMS). Laryngoscope 2004;114: 918–22.

[25] Neuloh G, Schramm J. Intraoperative neurophysiological mapping and monitoring for supratentorial procedures. In: Deletis V, Shils JL, editors. Neurophysiology and neuro-surgery. New York: Academic Press; 2002. p. 339–401.

[26] Wood CC, Spencer DD, Allison T, et al. Localization of human sensorimotor cortex during surgery by cortical surface recording of somatosensory evoked potentials. J Neurosurg 1988;68:99–111.

[27] Berger MS, Kincaid J, Ojemann GA, et al. Brain mapping techniques to maximize resection, safety, and seizure control in children with brain tumors. Neurosurgery 1989;25:786–92.

[28] Cedzich C, Taniguchi M, Schafer S, et al. Somatosensory evoked potential phase reversal and direct motor cortex stimulation during surgery in and around the central region. Neurosurgery 1996;38:962–70.

[29] Maciunas RJ, Galloway RL Jr, Latimer JW. The application accuracy of stereotactic frames. Neurosurgery 1994;35:682–94 [discussion: 694–5].

[30] Ebersole JS. EEG source modeling. The last word. J Clin Neurophysiol 1999;16:297–302.

[31] Jordan KG. Emergency EEG and continuous EEG monitoring in acute ischemic stroke. J Clin Neurophysiol 2004;21:341–52.

[32] Arnold M, Sturzenegger M, Schaffler L, et al. Continuous intraoperative monitoring of middle cerebral artery blood flow velocities and electroencephalography during carotid endarterectomy. A comparison of the two methods to detect cerebral ischemia. Stroke 1997;28:1345–50.

[33] Daube J, Harper CM, Litchy W. Intraoperative monitoring. In: Daly D, Pedley T, editors. Current practice of clinical electroencephaloigraphy. New York: Raven Press; 1990. p. 739–79.

[34] Deriu GP, Milite D, Mellone G, et al. Clamping ischemia, threshold ischemia and delayed insertion of the shunt during carotid endarterectomy with patch. J Cardiovasc Surg (Torino) 1999;40:249–55.

[35] Krul JM, van Gijn J, Ackerstaff RG, et al. Site and pathogenesis of infarcts associated with carotid endarterectomy. Stroke 1989;20:324–8.

[36] Findlay JM, Marchak BE, Pelz DM, et al. Carotid endarterectomy: a review. Can J Neurol Sci 2004;31:22–36.

[37] Illig KA, Sternbach Y, Zhang R, et al. EEG changes during awake carotid endarterectomy. Ann Vasc Surg 2002;16:6–11.

[38] Allain R, Marone LK, Meltzer J, et al. Carotid endarterectomy. Int Anesthesiol Clin 2005; 43:15–38.

[39] Visser GH, Wieneke GH, van Huffelen AC. Carotid endarterectomy monitoring: patterns of spectral EEG changes due to carotid artery clamping. Clin Neurophysiol 1999;110: 286–94.

[40] Deogaonkar A, Vivar R, Bullock RE, et al. Bispectral index monitoring may not reliably indicate cerebral ischaemia during awake carotid endarterectomy [see comment]. Br J Anaesth 2005;94:800–4.

[41] Sloan MA. Prevention of ischemic neurologic injury with intraoperative monitoring of selected cardiovascular and cerebrovascular procedures: roles of electroencephalography, somatosensory evoked potentials, transcranial doppler, and near-infrared spectroscopy. Neurol Clin 2006;24:631–45.

[42] Ragazzoni A, Chiaramonit R, Zaccara G, et al. Simultaneous monitoring of multichannel somatosensory evoked potentials and electroencephalogrm during carotid endarterectomy: a comparison of the two methods to detect cerbral ischemia. Clin Neurophysiol 2000;111: S138.

[43] Dietz A, von Kummer R, Adams HP, et al. [Balloon occlusion test of the internal carotid artery for evaluating resectability of blood vessel filtrating cervical metastasis of advanced head and neck cancers—Heidelberg experience]. Laryngorhinootologie 1993;72:558–67 [in German].

[44] Cloughesy TF, Nuwer MR, Hoch D, et al. Monitoring carotid test occlusions with continuous EEG and clinical examination. J Clin Neurophysiol 1993;10:363–9.

[45] Neuloh G, Schramm J. Motor evoked potential monitoring for the surgery of brain tumours and vascular malformations. Adv Tech Stand Neurosurg 2004;29:171–228.

[46] Schramm J, Zentner J, Pechstein U. Intraoperative sep monitoring in aneurysm surgery. Neurol Res 1994;16:20–2.

[47] Sakai H, Sheng H, Yates RB. Isoflurane provides long-term protection against focal cerebral ischemia in the rat. Anesthesiology 2007;106:92–9.

[48] Stockard J, Bickford R. The neurophysiology of anesthesia. In: Gordon E, editor. A basis and practice of neuroanesthesia. New York: Excerpta Medica; 1981. p. 3–50.

[49] Newman J. Thalamic contributions to attention and consciousness [comment]. Conscious Cogn 1995;4:172–93.

[50] John ER, Prichep LS, Kox W, et al. Invariant reversible QEEG effects of anesthetics [see comment][Erratum appears in Conscious Cogn 2002 Mar;11(1):138. Note: diMichele F [corrected to diMichele F]]. Conscious Cogn 2001;10:165–83.

[51] Rampil IJ. A primer for EEG signal processing in anesthesia [see comment]. Anesthesiology 1998;89:980–1002.

[52] Hirota K. Special cases: ketamine, nitrous oxide and xenon. Best Pract Res Clin Anaesthesiol 2006;20:69–79.

[53] Chen X, Tang J, White PF, et al. A comparison of patient state index and bispectral index values during the perioperative period. Anesth Analg 2002;95:1669–74.

[54] Drover DR, Lemmens HJ, Pierce ET, et al. Patient State Index: titration of delivery and recovery from propofol, alfentanil, and nitrous oxide anesthesia. Anesthesiology 2002; 97:82–9.

[55] Bricolo A, Sala F. Surgery of brainstem lesions. In: Deletis V, Shils JL, editors. Neurophysiology in neurosurgery. Boston: Academic Press; 2002. p. 267–89.

[56] Strauss C, Lutjen-Drecoll E, Fahlbusch R. Pericollicular surgical approaches to the rhomboid fossa. Part I. Anatomical basis [see comment]. J Neurosurg 1997;87:893–9.

[57] Strauss C, Romstock J, Nimsky C, et al. Intraoperative identification of motor areas of the rhomboid fossa using direct stimulation [see comment]. J Neurosurg 1993;79:393–9.

[58] Morota N, Deletis V, Epstein FJ. Brainstem mapping. In: Deletis V, Shils JL, editors. Neurophysiology in neurosurgery. Boston: Academic Press; 2002. p. 319–35.

[59] Stechison MT, Moller A, Lovely TJ. Intraoperative mapping of the trigeminal nerve root: technique and application in the surgical management of facial pain. Neurosurgery 1996; 38:76–81 [discussion: 81–2].

[60] Prass RL, Luders H. Acoustic (loudspeaker) facial electromyographic monitoring: part 1. Evoked electromyographic activity during acoustic neuroma resection. Neurosurgery 1986; 19:392–400.

[61] Harner SG, Daube JR, Ebersold MJ, et al. Improved preservation of facial nerve function with use of electrical monitoring during removal of acoustic neuromas. Mayo Clin Proc 1987;62:92–102.

[62] Jannetta PJ. Cranial rhizopathies. In: Youmans JR, editor. Neurosurgical surgery. Philadelphia: W.B. Saunders; 1990. p. 4169–82.

[63] Consensus statement 9. National Institutes of Health (NIH). Consensus Development Conference. Washington, DC, December 11–13, 1991.

[64] Daube JR. Intraoperative monitoring of cranial motor nerves. In: Schramm J, Moller A, editors. Intraoperative neurophysiologic monitoring in neurosurgery. New York: Springer-Verlag; 1991. p. 246–67.

[65] Fischer C. Intraoperative brainstem auditory evoked potential (BAEP) monitoring in acoustic neuroma surgery. In: Schramm J, Moller A, editors. Intraoperative neurophysiologic monitoring in neurosurgery. New York: Springer-Verlag; 1991. p. 187–92.

[66] Levine RA. Monitoring auditory evoked potentials during cerebellopontine angle tumor surgery: relative value of electrocochleogtraphy, brainstem auditry evoked potentials, and cerebellopontine angle recordings. In: Schramm J, Moller A, editors. Intraoperative neurophysiologic monitoring in neurosurgery. New York: Springer-Verlag; 1991. p. 193–213.

[67] Glasker S, Pechstein U, Vougioukas VI. Monitoring motor function during resection of tumours in the lower brain stem and fourth ventricle. Childs Nerv Syst 2006;22:1288–95.

[68] Petro ML, Schweinfurth JM. Transcricothyroid, intraoperative monitoring of the vagus nerve. Arch Otolaryngol Head Neck Surg 2006;132:624–8.

[69] Snyder SK, Hendricks JC. Intraoperative neurophysiology testing of the recurrent laryngeal nerve: plaudits and pitfalls. Surgery 2005;138:1183–91 [discussion: 1191–2].

[70] Pearlman RC, Isley MR, Ruben GD, et al. Intraoperative monitoring of the recurrent laryngeal nerve using acoustic, free-run, and evoked electromyography. J Clin Neurophysiol 2005;22:148–52.

[71] Grabb PA, Albright AL, Sclabassi RJ, et al. Continuous intraoperative electromyographic monitoring of cranial nerves during resection of fourth ventricular tumors in children. J Neurosurg 1997;86:1–4.

[72] Schlake HP, Goldbrunner R, Siebert M, et al. Intra-operative electromyographic monitoring of extra-ocular motor nerves (Nn. III, VI) in skull base surgery. Acta Neurochir (Wien) 2001;143:251–61.

[73] Fahlbusch R, Strauss C. [Surgical significance of cavernous hemangioma of the brain stem]. Zentralbl Neurochir 1991;52:25–32 [in German].

[74] Angelo R, Moller AR. Contralateral evoked brainstem auditory potentials as an indicator of intraoperative brainstem manipulation in cerebellopontine angle tumors. Neurol Res 1996;18:528–40.

[75] Pechstein U, Cedzich C, Nadstawek J, et al. Transcranial high-frequency repetitive electrical stimulation for recording myogenic motor evoked potentials with the patient under general anesthesia. Neurosurgery 1996;39:335–43 [discussion: 343–4].

[76] Deletis V, Sala F, Morota N. Intraoperative neurophysiological monitoring and mapping during brainstem surgery: a modern approach. Operative Techniques in Neurosurgery 2000;3:109–13.

[77] Deletis V, Kothbauer KF. Intraoperative neurophysiology of the corticospinal tract. In: Stalberg E, Sharma HS, Olsson Y, editors. Spinal cord monitoring. New York: Springer; 1998. p. 421–44.

[78] Krzan MJ. Intraoperative neurophysiological mapping of the spinal cord's dorsal columns. In: Deletis V, Shils JL, editors. Neurophysiology in neurosurgery. New York: Academic Press; 2002. p. 153–68.

[79] Deletis V, Bueno De Camargo A. Interventional neurophysiological mapping during spinal cord procedures. Stereotact Funct Neurosurg 2001;77:25–8.

[80] Quinones-Hinojosa A, Gulati M, Lyon R, et al. Spinal cord mapping as an adjunct for resection of intramedullary tumors: surgical technique with case illustrations. Neurosurgery 2002;51:1199–206 [discussion: 1206–97].

[81] Deletis V. Intraoperative neurophysiology of the corticospinal tract of the spinal cord. Suppl Clin Neurophysiol 2006;59:107–12.

[82] Nuwer MR, Dawson EG, Carlson LG, et al. Somatosensory evoked potential spinal cord monitoring reduces neurologic deficits after scoliosis surgery: results of a large multicenter survey. Electroencephalogr Clin Neurophysiol 1995;96:6–11.

[83] MacDonald DB, Al Zayed Z, Khoudeir I, et al. Monitoring scoliosis surgery with combined multiple pulse transcranial electric motor and cortical somatosensory-evoked potentials from the lower and upper extremities. Spine 2003;28:194–203.

[84] Langeloo DD, Lelivelt A, Louis Journee H, et al. Transcranial electrical motor-evoked potential monitoring during surgery for spinal deformity: a study of 145 patients. Spine 2003;28:1043–50.

[85] Freedman B, Potter B. Managing neurologic complications in cervical spine surgery. Curr Opin Orthop 2005;16:169–77.

[86] Christakos A. The value of motor and somatosensory evoked potentials in evaluation of cervical myelopathy in the presence of peripheral neuropathy. Spine J 2004;29:e239–47.

[87] Lorenzini NA, Schneider JH. Temporary loss of intraoperative motor-evoked potential and permanent loss of somatosensory-evoked potentials associated with a postoperative sensory deficit. J Neurosurg Anesthesiol 1996;8:142–7.

[88] Herdmann J, Lumenta CB, Huse KO. Magnetic stimulation for monitoring of motor pathways in spinal procedures. Spine 1993;18:551–9.

[89] Guerit JM. Neuromonitoring in the operating room: why, when, and how to monitor? Electroencephalogr Clin Neurophysiol 1998;106:1–21.

[90] Leis AA, Zhou HH, Mehta M, et al. Behavior of the H-reflex in humans following mechanical perturbation or injury to rostral spinal cord. Muscle Nerve 1996;19:1373–82.

[91] Holland NR, Lukaczyk TA, Riley LH 3rd, et al. Higher electrical stimulus intensities are required to activate chronically compressed nerve roots. Implications for intraoperative electromyographic pedicle screw testing. Spine 1998;23:224–7.

[92] Holland NR. Intraoperative electromyography during thoracolumbar spinal surgery. Spine 1998;23:1915–22.

[93] Reidy DP, Houlden D, Nolan PC, et al. Evaluation of electromyographic monitoring during insertion of thoracic pedicle screws. J Bone Joint Surg Br 2001;83:1009–14.

[94] Bose B, Wierzbowski LR, Sestokas AK. Neurophysiologic monitoring of spinal nerve root function during instrumented posterior lumbar spine surgery. Spine 2002;27:1444–50.

[95] Raynor BL, Lenke LG, Kim Y, et al. Can triggered electromyograph thresholds predict safe thoracic pedicle screw placement? [see comment] Spine 2002;27:2030–5.

[96] Shi YB, Binette M, Martin WH, et al. Electrical stimulation for intraoperative evaluation of thoracic pedicle screw placement. Spine 2003;28:595–601.

[97] Gunnarsson T, Krassioukov AV, Sarjeant R, et al. Real-time continuous intraoperative electromyographic and somatosensory evoked potential recordings in spinal surgery: correlation of clinical and electrophysiologic findings in a prospective, consecutive series of 213 cases. Spine 2004;29:677–84.

[98] Krassioukov AV, Sarjeant R, Arkia H, et al. Multimodality intraoperative monitoring during complex lumbosacral procedures: indications, techniques, and long-term follow-up review of 61 consecutive cases [see comment]. J Neurosurg Spine 2004;1:243–53.

[99] Djurasovic M, Dimar JR 2nd, Glassman SD, et al. A prospective analysis of intraoperative electromyographic monitoring of posterior cervical screw fixation [see comment]. J Spinal Disord Tech 2005;18:515–8.

[100] Quinones-Hinojosa A, Gadkary CA, Gulati M, et al. Neurophysiological monitoring for safe surgical tethered cord syndrome release in adults. Surg Neurol 2004;62:127–33, [discussion: 133–5].

[101] Paradiso G, Lee GY, Sarjeant R, et al. Multi-modality neurophysiological monitoring during surgery for adult tethered cord syndrome. J Clin Neurosci 2005;12:934–6.

[102] Kothbauer K, Schmid UD, Seiler RW, et al. Intraoperative motor and sensory monitoring of the cauda equina. Neurosurgery 1994;34:702–7 [discussion: 707].

[103] Abbott R. Sensory rhizotomy for the treatment of childhood spasticity. In: Deletis V, Shils JL, editors. Neurophysiology in neurosurgery. Boston: Academic Press; 2002. p. 219–30.

ELSEVIER
SAUNDERS

Anesthesiology Clin
25 (2007) 631–653

ANESTHESIOLOGY
CLINICS

Risks and Benefits of Patient Positioning During Neurosurgical Care

Irene Rozet, MD[a], Monica S. Vavilala, MD[a,b,c],*

[a]Department of Anesthesiology, University of Washington,
325 Ninth Avenue, Seattle, WA 98134, USA
[b]Department of Pediatrics, University of Washington, 325 Ninth Avenue,
Seattle, WA 98134, USA
[c]Department of Neurological Surgery, University of Washington,
325 Ninth Avenue, Seattle, WA 98134, USA

Positioning of the surgical patient is an important part of anesthesia care and attention to the physical and physiologic consequences of positioning can help prevent serious adverse events and complications. The general principles of patient positioning of the anesthetized and awake neurosurgical patient are discussed in this article.

General principles

Ideal patient positioning involves balancing surgical comfort against the risks related to the patient position. Therefore, patient positioning during surgery should be considered during the preoperative evaluation [1].

Patient positioning is typically attended to after induction of general anesthesia and placement of arterial and venous lines. Positioning is the joint responsibility of the surgeon and anesthesiologist. Positioning of the neurosurgical patient is challenging and requires adequate anesthetic depth, maintenance of hemodynamic stability, evidence of appropriate oxygenation, and preservation of invasive monitors. Disconnection of intravenous or arterial catheters and tracheal tube during body positioning and during rotation or movement of the operating table is often required, sometimes creating a complete "blackout" state, when the patient may not be monitored or oxygenated [2]. This is especially dangerous in trauma patients,

* Corresponding author. Harborview Medical Center, Box 359724, 325 Ninth Avenue, Seattle, WA 98104-2499.
E-mail address: vavilala@u.washington.edu (M.S. Vavilala).

1932-2275/07/$ - see front matter © 2007 Elsevier Inc. All rights reserved.
doi:10.1016/j.anclin.2007.05.009
anesthesiology.theclinics.com

who are at risk of thromboembolism, and in patients with hemo- or pneumothoraces who are dependent on functioning chest tubes. Therefore, pulse oximetry and blood pressure should be monitored throughout positioning, whenever possible, and chest tubes should not be clamped. Specifically, positioning of the head and neck requires special attention. Positioning of the body should be based on general guidelines according to the Practice Advisory of American Society of Anesthesiologists (ASA) (Table 1) [1].

Head positioning

Patient positioning for craniotomies and the majority of spine procedures begins with positioning of the head. Knowledge of the neurosurgical approach to head positioning is important for anesthesiologists because evaluation of whether the patient can tolerate the desired intraoperative positioning, particularly during long procedures, is essential.

The ideal position of the head is the position that provides optimal surgical approach to the target brain area and is based on the two principles: (1) an imaginary trajectory from the highest point at the skull surface to the area of interest in the brain should be the shortest distance between the two points, and (2) whenever possible, the exposed surface of the skull and an imaginary perimeter of craniotomy should be parallel to the floor [3].

Types of craniotomies

There are five classic surgical approaches for craniotomies: frontal, temporal, occipital, parietal, and posterior fossa. These approaches provide extensive "regional" exposure of the entire lobes and are currently used, occasionally, when exposure of large areas is required (eg, decompressive craniectomy). In modern neurosurgery, six standard types of craniotomies, derived from the regional craniotomies by miniaturization of the area of exposure or combination of their different parts, are used: (1) anterior parasagittal, (2) frontosphenotemporal (pterional), (3) subtemporal, (4) posterior parasagittal, (5) midline suboccipital, and (6) lateral suboccipital (Fig. 1) [3].

Fixation of the head

For craniotomies or burr holes, the head can be positioned on the horseshoe headrest (or doughnut), or skeletally fixed with the three- or four-pins fixation device. The Mayfield frame is a three-pin device that is used for fixation during craniotomies; a four-pin rigid frame is usually used for burr holes and functional neurosurgical procedures (eg, implantation of deep brain stimulators). For prone positioning, the head may be positioned on a foam pillow, headrest, or fixed with the Mayfield frame.

Application of a skeletal fixation device and tightening of pins on the scalp has a profound stimulating effect, leading to tachycardia and hypertension. Since severe hypertension during pin fixation may cause rupture of untreated cerebral aneurysms, pins may be placed only after the anesthesia team has preempted the hemodynamic effects of fixation. Local infiltration of the skin should be used whenever possible in every awake, as well as anesthetized patient, and the dose of local anesthetic should be recorded. In patients under general anesthesia, anesthesia should be deepened with either a bolus of intravenous anesthetic agent (eg, propofol 0.5–1 mg/kg) or with deepening of the inhalational anesthetic. The dose of the anesthetic given should be titrated to the estimated depth of anesthesia and arterial blood pressure. Therefore, standard monitoring and invasive blood pressure monitoring should commence before application of pins. In cases when invasive blood pressure monitoring is unavailable (eg, during an emergency, such as head trauma), a bolus of an anesthetic agent should be given before the application of pins, titrated to the noninvasive blood pressure value.

Benefits of the skeletal head holder consist of immobility of the head and surgical comfort. Risks of the head holder include bleeding from the pins sites, air embolism (especially in the sitting position, where placement of antibiotic ointment on pins is advocated for prevention of air embolism), and scalp and eye laceration. Pressure alopecia has been described after using a horseshoe headrest [4].

Head and neck positioning: head rotation, hyperflexion, hyperextension, and lateral flexion

Manipulation of the head and neck during positioning may have serious consequences, including quadriplegia and cerebral infarction. Even in healthy individuals, slight movement of the head and neck may lead to mechanical stress of arteries and veins supplying the brain and cervical spinal cord [5]. Blood flow in the vertebral arteries, which are located in the narrow foramina in the transverse processes along the cervical spine, decreases on the side ipsilateral to the direction of head turning. Hyperflexion of the head and neck may decrease blood flow in vertebral and carotid arteries, leading to brain stem and cervical spine ischemia, resulting in quadriparesis and quadriplegia. Patients with osteophytes, arthritis or vascular atherosclerosis are also at risk for cerebral ischemia, secondary to inappropriate head and neck movement [6]. During positioning, the head can typically be safely rotated between 0 degrees and 45 degrees away from the body. If more rotation is needed, a roll or pillow placement under the opposite shoulder is recommended [4]. Maintaining two to three finger-breadths thyromental distance is recommended during neck flexion. The patient's preoperative ability to move the neck without neurological consequences, such as paresthesias, pain, or dizziness may limit or dictate the extent of intraoperative head and neck positioning. Hyperflexion, hyperextension, lateral flexion or rotation should be avoided.

Table 1
Summary of specific physiological changes and risks and benefits with positioning for neurosurgical procedures

Position	Cardiovascular	Respiratory	Central nervous	Benefits	Risks
Supine	Compared to upright, awake and anesthetized: VR ↑, SV ↑, CO ↑ HR ↓ SVR ↔ SBP ↔, MAP↓ ↔	Compared to upright: FRC ↓, TLC ↓ atelectasis of the dependent lung zones; Qs/Qt ↔ V/Q mismatch ↑	Compared to upright: JVF ↔ JVR ↓ → CPP ↔ → CSF drainage may be impaired	The easiest position	Often needs head flexion/extention/rotation Ulnar and peroneal nerve injury
Modifications: *a) lawn-chair* *b) reverse Trendelenburg*	*Improvement of the VR from the lower extremities*	*Improvement of ventilation of the dependent lung zones*	*Improvement of the cerebral venous, lymphaticand CSF drainage*		
Lateral	Compared to supine, anesthetized: VR ↓, SV ↓, CO↓ HR↑ SVR↑, PVR ↑ SBP ↓, MAP↓	Compared to supine: FRC ↓, TLC ↓ Qs/Qt ↑↑ V/Q mismatch ↑↑ atelectasis of the dependent lung	Compared to supine: JVF ↑ ↔ JVR ↓ ↔ with neck flexion: JVF↓, JVR↑, ICP↑	Optimal approach to the temporal lobe	Brachial plexus injury Ear and eye injury Suprascapular nerve injury (of the dependent shoulder)
Modification: *park-bench*					*Stretch injuries (axillary trauma)* *Decreased perfusion to the dependent arm*

	Cardiovascular	Respiratory	ICP / Venous	Benefits	Risks
Prone	Compared to supine, awake: VR↓, SV↓; HR↑↔; SVR↑, PVR↑; SBP↑↔, MAP↑↔. In anesthetized patient: VR↓, SV↓, CO↓↔; HR↑, SVR↑, PVR↑; SBP↓↔, MAP↓↔	Compared to supine: increase in upper airway resistance (Wilson frame and chest rolls); FRC↑↔, TLC↑; V/Q mismatch↓ less atelectasis in lungs	Compared to supine: a) neutral to the heart JVF↑↔; JVR↓↔; b) lower than heart JVF↑, JVR↓, venous congestion; ICP↑	Optimal posterior approach to spine; Less risk for VAE (compared to sitting)	The most difficult position; Difficult access to airway; Pressure sores of soft tissues; Eye injury; Blindness; Bleeding (compared with sitting)
Modification: Concorde					*Neck and head hyperflexion: venous congestion of the face, nose, and tongue, epystarchis, chin necrosis, cerebral venous obstruction, increase of ICP, quadriplegia*
Sitting	Compared to supine, awake: VR↓, SV↓, CO↓; HR↑, SVR↑, PVR↑	Compared to supine: TLC↑, FRC↑; Qs/Qt↓	Compared to supine: JVF↓, JVR↑; ICP↓↓	Optimal approach to posterior fossa; Low ICP	Venous air embolism (VAE); Paradoxical air embolism; Arterial Hypotension

(continued on next page)

Table 1 (*continued*)

Position	Cardiovascular	Respiratory	Central nervous	Benefits	Risks
	SBP ↑↔↓, MAP↓ ↔↑ In anesthetized patient: VR↓↓, SV ↓, CO↓ HR↑, SVR↑, PVR ↑ SBP ↓, MAP ↓	V/Q mismatch ↓ less atelectasis in lungs	CPP ↔ Good cerebral venous and CSF drainage	Minimal bleeding (compared with prone) Access to airway	Pneumocephalus Paraplegia, Quadriplegia Macroglossia
Three - quarters	different changes, resemble lateral or prone	changes, resemble lateral or prone	different changes, resemble lateral or prone	Less risk for VAE (compared with sitting) Better access to airway (compared with prone)	Difficult position Brachial plexus injury Pressure sores Compartment syndrome of the dependent upper extremity Pudendal nerve injury

Changes of physiologic parameters in cardiovascular, respiratory, and central nervous system are presented as observed in anesthetized subjects. Changes in cardiovascular system are presented in awake and anesthetized subjects, where **HR** is heart rate, **SV** is stroke volume, **VR** is venous return, **CO** is cardiac output, **SBP** is systolic blood pressure, **TLC** is total lung capacity, **FRC** is functional residual capacity, **Qs/Qt** is intrapulmonary shunt, **V/Q** mismatch is ventilation/perfusion mismatch, **ICP** is intracranial pressure, **JVF** is jugular venous flow, **JVR** is jugular venous resistance, **CPP** is cerebral perfusion pressure, ↑ is to increase, ↓ is to decrease, and ↔ is no change.

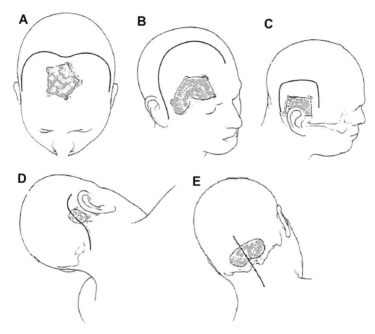

Fig. 1. Types of Standard Craniotomies: (*A*) Anterior parasagittal craniotomy is a miniaturization of the frontal regional craniotomy along the midline. (*B*) Frontosphenotemporal craniotomy is a combination of two regional craniotomies: anterior-inferior portion of the frontal regional craniotomy with the anterior portion of the temporal regional craniotomy. (*C*) Subtemporal craniotomy is a miniaturization of the temporal regional craniotomy along with the middle fossa floor. (*D*) Lateral suboccipital craniotomy is a miniaturization of the posterior fossa regional craniotomy along with the midportion of cerebellum. (*E*) Midline suboccipital craniotomy is a miniaturization of the frontal regional craniotomy along the midline. (*Adapted from* Clatterbuck RE, Tamargo RJ. Surgical positioning and exposures for cranial procedures. In: Winn RH, editor. Youmans Neurological Surgery. 5th edition. Philadelphia: Saunders; 2004; with permission.)

Benefits include surgical comfort and optimal access to the target area. Risks and complications of head positioning include: cervical strain, leading to postoperative discomfort and pain; necrosis of the chin; brachial plexus injury; obstruction of the cerebral lymphatic and venous outflow, leading to face, neck, and airway swelling; macroglossia, leading to the airway obstruction; obstruction of cerebro-spinal fluid flow; and obstruction of vertebral or carotid arteries, leading to the brain stem ischemia and quadriplegia. Impairment of cerebral venous outflow, especially during prolonged surgery, can potentially cause intraoperative brain swelling, increased intracranial pressure (ICP), ischemia and cerebral infarction [7]. Jugular veins and vertebral venous plexuses are the major venous pathways from the brain. Because jugular veins tend to collapse with change of the body position (eg, in a sitting position) [8], vertebral venous drainage may predominate [9]. Collapse or obstruction of jugular veins and stretching or obstruction of the vertebral venous plexus should be avoided during head and neck positioning.

Monitoring during head positioning

First, since increase in ICP can reflect impaired venous drainage, measuring ICP can be helpful during head positioning. In patients with in situ ICP monitoring, we recommend monitoring ICP, with the goal of maintaining normal ICP at less than 20 mm Hg. Repositioning to achieve a normal ICP may be needed. Second, jugular bulb pressure (JBP) monitoring is an alternative to direct ICP monitoring. Jugular bulb pressure and jugular venous saturations can both be measured using a retrograde jugular bulb catheter. Monitoring JBP allows the anesthesiologist to continuously measure and record intracranial venous pressure and compare it to central venous pressure (CVP). When CVP and JBP are measured and monitored continuously, obstruction of the jugular vein can be quickly recognized (JBP exceeds CVP). If the patient is supine, and pressure transducers are placed at the level of the heart, JBP and CVP are usually equal, or JBP may be higher by 1 to 2 cm H_2O. During head-up tilt, placement of the pressure transducers should be considered. If both transducers are placed at the same level (usually at the ear tragus to reflect middle cerebral artery pressure), JBP will be higher than CVP; with head-down tilt, JBP is lower than CVP. If each transducer is placed near its reference level (CVP at the level of the right atrium and JBP at the level of tragus), there should be no change in pressures compared with the baseline. The most important sign of proper head positioning is that JBP remains the same. Any elevation of JBP requires evaluation. Once technical errors are excluded (check for kinking of the catheter, flush the catheter), partial obstruction of venous outflow and repositioning of the head should be considered.

Body positioning

There are six basic body positions used in neurological surgery: supine, lateral, prone, concorde, sitting, and three-quarters. Additionally, there are significant circulatory and respiratory changes, with changes in body position, in both awake and anesthetized patients. These changes may affect blood-gas exchange and cerebral hemodynamics. The most significant physiologic changes and benefits and risks with different body positions used in neurosurgery are summarized in Box 1.

Supine position

The supine or dorsal decubitus position, is the most frequently used position in neurosurgery and is used for cranial procedures, carotid endarterectomies, and for anterior approaches to the cervical and lumbar spine (Fig. 2). Benefits of this position are that it is the simplest position because it does not require special instrumentation, it is easily achievable, and it usually does not require disconnection of the tracheal tube and invasive

Box 1. Summary of task force consensus on the prevention of perioperative peripheral neuropathies relevant to positioning for neurosurgery

Preoperative assessment
- Ascertain that patients can comfortably tolerate the anticipated operative position.

Upper extremity positioning
- Arm abduction should be limited to 90° in supine patients; patients who are positioned prone may comfortably tolerate arm abduction greater than 90°.
- Position arms to decrease pressure on ulnar groove (humerus). When arms are tucked at the side, neutral forearm position is recommended. When arms are abducted on armboards, either supination or a neutral forearm position is acceptable.
- Prolonged pressure on the radial nerve in the spiral groove of the humerus should be avoided.
- Extension of the elbow beyond a comfortable range may stretch the median nerve.

Lower extremity positioning
- Prolonged pressure on the peroneal nerve at the fibular head should be avoided.
- Neither extension nor flexion of the hip increase the risk of femoral neuropathy.

Protective padding
- Padded armboards may decrease the risk of upper extremity neuropathy.
- The use of chest rolls in laterally positioned patients may decrease the risk of upper extremity neuropathies.
- Padding at the elbow and at the fibular head may decrease the risk of upper and lower extremity neuropathies, respectively.

Equipment
- Properly functioning automated blood pressure cuffs on the upper arms do not affect the risk of upper extremity neuropathies.
- Shoulder braces in steep head-down positions may increase the risk of brachial plexus neuropathies.

Postoperative assessment
- A simple postoperative assessment of extremity nerve function may lead to early recognition of peripheral neuropathies.

- Charting specific position actions during the care of patients may result in improvements of care by: (1) helping practitioners focus attention on relevant aspect of patient positioning, and (2) providing information that continuous improvement processes can use to lead to refinement in patient care.

  (Adapted from American Society of Anesthesiologists Task Force on the Prevention of Perioperative Peripheral Neuropathies: Practice Advisory for the Prevention of Perioperative Peripheral Neuropathies. Anesthesiology 2000;92: 1168–82).

monitors. The risk of this position is that head rotation or flexion is often required to create optimal surgical conditions.

There are three types of supine positioning used in neurosurgery. The horizontal position is achieved when the patient is lying on his or her back on a straight table (see Fig. 2A). This position does not provide optimal positioning of the hip and knee joint and is poorly tolerated, even for a short time, by conscious patients. Skin to metal contact should be prevented, and arms must be padded or restrained along the body or positioned on arm boards. Bony contact points at elbows and heels should be padded. The lawn-chair (contoured) position is a modification of the horizontal position, with 15-degree angulation and flexion at the trunk-thigh-knee, and provides more physiological positioning of the lumbar spine, hips and knees (see Fig. 2B). A blanket, soft (gel) cushion, or pillow can be placed under the knees to keep them flexed. The other advantage of the lawn-chair position is that it includes a slight head elevation, with improvement of venous drainage from the brain, and a slight leg elevation, which can improve venous return to the heart. The head-up tilt or reverse Trendelenbourg position usually involves a 10 degree to 15 degree repositioning from the horizontal axis to provide optimal venous drainage from the brain (see Fig. 2C).

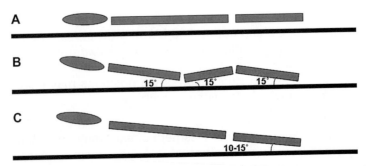

Fig. 2. Types of supine positioning: (*A*) horizontal position, (*B*) lawn-chair (contoured) position and, (*C*) reverse Trendelenbourg position.

Hemodynamics and ventilation

Because each 2.5-cm change of vertical height from the reference point at the level of the heart leads to a change of mean arterial pressure by 2 mm Hg in the opposite direction [10], and because the venous compartment is a low pressure compartment, venous return to the heart depends on body position. Head-down tilt increases venous return from the lower extremities, but increases venous congestion in the upper part of the body. If the head is tilted below the level of the heart, venous pressure in the cerebral veins increases in proportion to the hydrostatic pressure gradient. Even after short procedures, postoperative headache, congestion of the conjunctivae, and nasal mucosa may be observed. Therefore, to improve venous drainage from the brain, the head should be positioned above the level of the heart using reverse Trendelenbourg positioning or with flexion of the table. The head can typically be safely rotated to 45 degrees relative to the body, but if more rotation is needed, a roll or pillow should be placed under the contralateral shoulder.

In conscious subjects, change in body position does not usually cause profound changes in blood pressure because of the baroreceptor (from aortic arch and carotid sinus) reflexes and renin-angiotensin-aldosterone system. During anesthesia, hemodynamic instability may develop due to impaired compensatory mechanisms and the effect of anesthetic agents [11]. Adverse hemodynamic changes are not common in supine positioning.

Pulmonary blood flow may change profoundly with changes in patient position [12]. Perfusion and ventilation are best in the dependent parts of the lungs (Fig. 3). In anesthetized patients, positive-pressure ventilation provides the best ventilation to the nondependent lung zones. During head-up tilt, ventilation of the dependent lung is improved by displacement of the abdominal viscera downward from the diaphragm.

Lateral position

The lateral position is used as a surgical approach for patients requiring temporal lobe craniotomy, skull base, and posterior fossa procedures, as well as for the retroperitoneal approach to thoracolumbar spine (Figs. 4A, B). The benefits of this position are that it provides the best surgical approach to the temporal lobe. The risks include brachial plexus injuries, stretch injuries, pressure palsies, and possible occurrence of ventilation-perfusion mismatch.

Hemodynamics and ventilation

Lateral positioning leads to gravitational changes of the ventilation-perfusion relationship in the lung. The best perfusion occurs in the dependent lung zones. In a conscious patient in the lateral position, Zone 3 West is occupying the dependent 18 cm of lung tissue. Lung tissue above 18 cm from bed level is not perfused (see Fig. 3) [13]. During general

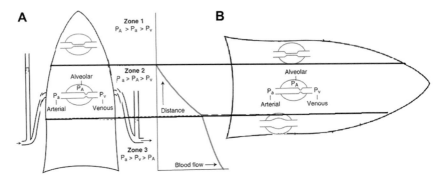

Fig. 3. West zones of the Lungs. This is a schematic presentation of the ventilation-perfusion relationships in the lungs, which shows dependency of the venous pressure on gravity, where (*A*) is the upright position, (*B*) is the supine position, P_a is arterial pressure, P_A is alveolar pressure, and P_V is venous pressure. Perfusion in the lungs is established in Zone 3, at the point when venous pressure overcomes alveolar pressure. (*From* West JB, Dollery CB, Naimark A. Distribution of blood flow in isolated lung; relation to vascular and alveolar pressures. J Appl Physiol 1964;19:713–24; with permission.)

anesthesia and positive pressure ventilation, the nondependent lung zones are ventilated better relative to the dependent zones, worsening ventilation-perfusion mismatch.

Special attention is required for positioning of the patient's dependent (lower) arm because of the potential danger of axillary artery compression and brachial plexus injury. The dependent arm can be positioned in a hanging or ventral position and may be rested on a low padded arm board, inserted between the table and head fixator (See Fig. 4A). Alternatively, the forearm can be hung on a pillow and towels wrapped over the arm and forearm. The shoulder should be abducted, and the elbow flexed (See Fig. 4B). An axillary roll, inflatable pillow or a gel pad should be placed under the upper chest (not directly in the axilla) to take pressure off of the dependent shoulder and prevent arm ischemia, brachial plexus injury, and compartment syndrome. It is also critical to support the patient's head with a pillow or gel pad to minimize angulation of the cervical spine, which may be achieved with the simultaneous inflation of the both inflatable pillows under the chest and the head [14]. If there is no arterial line, palpation of the radial pulse of the dependent forearm can be helpful in verifying optimal positioning. The nondependent (upper) arm may be positioned on the "airplane" armrest or on a pillow placed anterior to the patient's body.

The park-bench position is a modification of lateral position and provides the surgeon with better access to the posterior fossa, as compared with the lateral position. The upper arm is positioned along the lateral trunk and the upper shoulder is taped toward the table. The lower extremities should be slightly flexed, and a pillow should be placed between the legs (particularly the knees). Reverse Trendelenbourg and marked flexion of

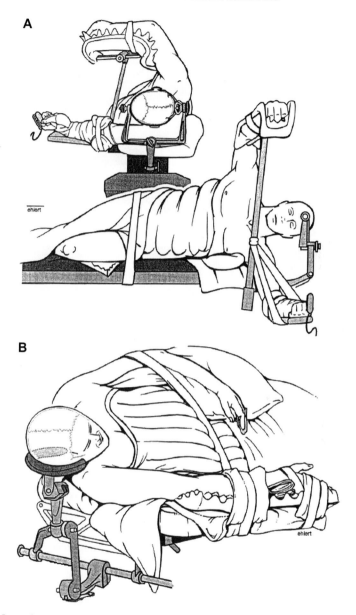

Fig. 4. Lateral positioning. (*A*) Dependent arm is hung under the operating table, an upper arm is placed on the arm board. (*B*) Dependent arm is positioned on the operating table and an arm board, an upper arm is placed over the trunk on the pillow. (*Adapted from* Goodkin R, Mesiwala A. General principles of operative positioning. In: Winn RH, editor. Youmans Neurological Surgery. 5th edition. Philadelphia: Saunders; 2004; with permission.)

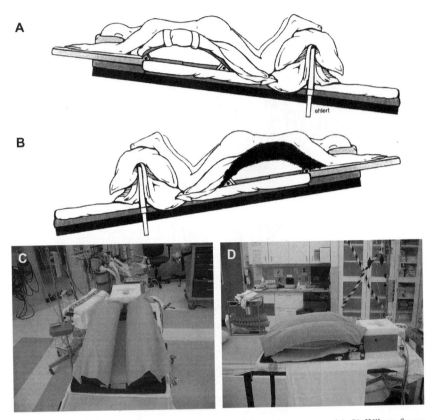

Fig. 5. Prone positioning and the main frames used for spine surgery. (*A–D*) Wilson frame.
Positioning on the Wilson frame: abdomen is partially compressed, pelvis is partially supported,
legs are positioned below the trunk, head is positioned on the pillow (*Adapted from* Goodkin R,
Mesiwala A. General principles of operative positioning. In: Winn RH, editor. Youmans Neurological Surgery. 5th edition. Philadelphia: Saunders; 2004; with permission.); (*E–H*) Andrews
frame. Positioning on the Andrews frame: abdomen hangs free, pelvis is partially supported,
legs are positioned below the heart, head is positioned on the foam pillow, or headrest. Andrews
frame (OSI ANDREWS SST 3000 model 5820 Spine Surgery Table, Ideal Medical, Monroe,
GA, www.idealmedicalequipment.com). Relton Hall frame. Positioning on the Relton Hall
frame: abdomen hangs free, pelvis is supported, legs are positioned below the heart, head is
positioned on the foam pillow or headrest; Relton Hall frame. (*Adapted from* Relton JE,
Hall JE. An operation frame for spinal fusion. A new apparatus designed to reduce hemorrhage
during operation. J Bone Joint Surg Br 1967;49(2):327–32; with permission.) (*I–M*) Jackson table. Positioning on the Jackson table. Step I: the patient is lying on the Jackson table. Step II:
Jackson frame is put over the patient, the thoracic pad is adjusted to support shoulders and thoracic cage, two side pelvic pads are adjusted to the pelvis, and two other side pads are adjusted
to support the thighs. The patient is compressed between the table and the frame. Step III: after
the flipping into prone position has been completed and the Jackson table has been removed
from the patient's back, the patient is lying on the Jackson frame. The patient's abdomen hangs
free, pelvis is supported, legs are supported and are positioned at the heart level, and the head
may be positioned on a foam pillow or headrest, or may be fixed with the Mayfield frame.
Jackson table, Jackson frame.

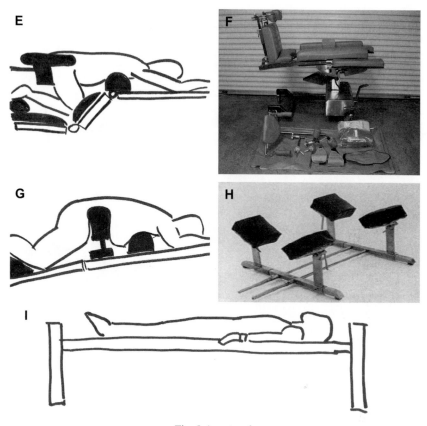

Fig. 5 (*continued*)

the legs at hips and knees should be avoided, as it can lead to the lower extremity venous stasis and decrease of venous return to the heart. Leg wrapping with compression bandages can be used to prevent venous pooling.

Prone position

The prone position is commonly used for approaches to the posterior fossa, suboccipital region, and posterior approaches to spine (Fig. 5A–M). The benefits of this position are that it is a good position for posterior approaches, and there is a lower incidence of venous air embolism compared with the sitting position. The risks are that logistically, this is the most difficult positioning because of challenges associated with providing adequate oxygenation, ensuring adequate ventilation, maintaining hemodynamics, and securing intravenous lines and the tracheal tube. Access to the patients'

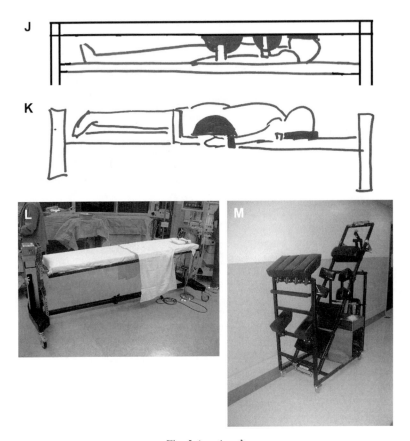

Fig. 5 (*continued*)

airway is poor. Pressure sores, vascular compression, brachial plexus in-juries, air embolism, blindness, and quadriplegia can occur.

Hemodynamics and ventilation

Turning the patient prone from the supine position increases intra-abdominal pressure, decreases venous return to the heart, and increases systemic and pulmonary vascular resistance [15]. With the head-up tilt or in kneeling position with flexed lower extremities, pooling of venous blood in the lower part of the body occurs, decreasing venous return and causing hypotension [16]. Although the cardiovascular responses to turning prone have not been fully characterized, data suggest that left-ventricular ejection fraction and cardiac index may decrease, potentially causing hemodynamic instability [15,17,18].

Oxygenation and oxygen delivery, however, may improve with prone positioning because of improved matching of ventilation and perfusion.

The relationship between ventilation and perfusion may be improved for three reasons: (1) perfusion of the entire lungs improves [12], (2) increase in intra-abdominal pressure decreases chest wall compliance, which under positive-pressure ventilation, improves ventilation of the dependent zones of the lung, and (3) previously atelectatic dorsal zones of the lungs may open.

Characteristic challenges with prone positioning include disconnection of pulse oximetry, arterial line, and tracheal tube, leading to hypoventilation, desaturation, hemodynamic instability, and altered anesthetic depth. To prevent anesthesia disasters, pulse oximetry and the arterial line should be left connected during the turn whenever possible. Monitoring of invasive blood pressure is especially important in patients with heart or lung disease and trauma patients. For uncomplicated elective surgeries, when invasive blood pressure monitoring is not used, standard ASA monitoring should be applied.

The patient is usually anesthetized in the supine position, and is then turned prone on chest rolls or on a special frame. The head should be kept in the neutral position. All catheters, invasive monitors, and the tracheal tube should be carefully secured before turning the patient prone. Pressure sores (of breasts, penis, soft tissue at the bone points, ears, eyes) are the most frequent complications of prone positioning [4]. Therefore, special frames, such as the Wilson, Relton-Hall frame, Andrews frame, and Jackson table and frame (see Figs. 5A–M), which provide support to the chest but leave the abdominal wall and pelvis free, are often used. Chest rolls may be used to support the chest wall, and allow free movement of the chest and abdominal wall. Free movement of the abdominal region is desirable for 3 reasons: (1) improved excursion of the diaphragm, and improved oxygenation ventilation, (2) a decrease in intra-abdominal pressure and decreased surgical bleeding, and (3) improvement of venous return from lower extremities and pelvis. The breast should not be exposed to pressure.

The effects of the prone position on hemodynamic stability and respiratory mechanics are frame dependent [16,19–21]. Positioning on the Jackson table provides the most stable hemodynamics and does not increase dynamic lung compliance (See Figs. 5I–M) [19–21].

Eyes, nose, and ears should be protected against pressure and eyelids should be closed. If the head is positioned on a specially designed pillow (with holes for the eyes and nose), the eyes and nose should be periodically checked for lack of pressure (no less than once every 30 minutes) and the head should be repositioned if needed. Blindness is a rare occurrence (in about 0.2% of cases), but it is a devastating complication of spine surgery during prone position, where prolonged surgery and the magnitude of the blood loss may be risk factors [22]. Positioning of the head at the body level, or higher, avoiding the head-down position and associated venous congestion are essential. On the other hand, elevation of the head for posterior fossa surgery or cervical spine surgery may increase the risk for air embolism.

The upper extremities may be positioned along the body or abducted on to padded armboards. If abduction is used, great care must be exercised to avoid hyperextension of the arms to prevent brachial plexus injury.

The Concorde position is a modification of the prone position (Fig. 6). This is the best positioning for surgical approach to occipital transtentorial and supracerebellar infratentorial area. The head is typically skeletally fixed and flexed, but may be laterally flexed if needed. The body is positioned in reverse Trendelenburg and chest rolls are placed under the trunk. The arms are tucked alongside to the trunk, and the knees are flexed. Specific complications include necrosis of the chin and an obstruction of cerebral venous outflow.

Sitting position

This position is most commonly used for posterior fossa surgery and cervical laminectomy (Fig. 7). The benefit of this position is that it provides optimal surgical exposure for posterior fossa surgery because tissue retraction and risks of cranial nerve damage are reduced, cerebral venous drainage is improved and bleeding is less. The patient's airway is accessible to the anesthesiologist.

Risks include venous air embolism (VAE), paradoxical air embolism, bradycardia, or cardiac arrest because of brain stem manipulations. Macroglossia, upper airway obstruction [23], pneumocephalus [24], subdural hematoma, and quadriplegia [25] have also been reported. Despite well-described risks involved with the sitting position, there is no evidence of increased mortality rate [26–28]. A recent national survey has demonstrated that the sitting position is still used for posterior fossa surgery in about half of the practices in the USA [2]. Relative contraindications to the sitting position include open ventriculoatrial shunt, signs of cerebral ischemia when upright and awake, right-to-left shunt, as with patent foramen ovale, and cardiac instability.

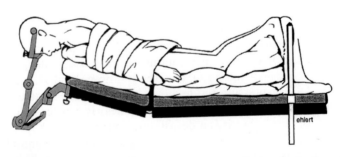

Fig. 6. Concorde positioning. The head is flexed, arms are tucked to the trunk, and legs are flexed at the knees. (*Adapted from* Goodkin R, Mesiwala A. General principles of operative positioning. In: Winn RH, editor. Youmans Neurological Surgery. 5th edition. Philadelphia: Saunders; 2004; with permission.)

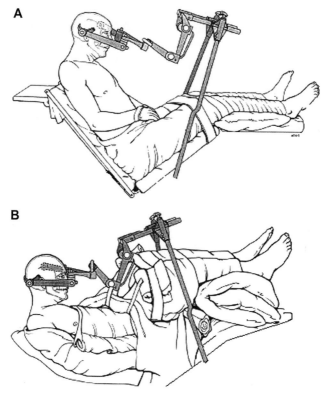

Fig. 7. Sitting positioning: (*A*) classical sitting position, (*B*) modified (semirecumbent) position. (*Adapted from* Goodkin R, Mesiwala A. General principles of operative positioning. In: Winn RH, editor. Youmans Neurological Surgery. 5th edition. Philadelphia: Saunders; 2004; with permission.)

Hemodynamics and ventilation

The classic sitting position causes postural hypotension in about one third of patients, and 2% to 5% of patients suffer severe hypotension (decrease in blood pressure more than by half from baseline) [29]. The major hemodynamic consequence is a decrease in venous return, leading to a decrease in cardiac output and hypotension. Therefore, hemodynamic instability and cardiac disease are relative contraindications for prone positioning. Wrapping of the legs with elastic bandages (eg, ACE bandage) prevents pooling of blood in the lower extremities and should be applied in every case. The modified sitting (semirecumbent) position provides better venous return and less hemodynamic instability (see Fig. 7B). With head-up tilt, venous drainage via internal jugular veins is improved, which results in decreased intracranial pressure. However, jugular veins may also collapse in the sitting position [8], and careful head positioning to avoid hyperflexion and hyperextension is required to prevent stretching or obstruction of the vertebral venous outflow.

Ventilation in the sitting position is improved, when compared with the supine position, because of a downward shift of the diaphragm, which decreases intra-abdominal pressure, improves ventilation of the dependent zones, and decreases ventilation-perfusion mismatch. However, low perfusion pressure secondary to decreased venous return may affect oxygenation. Therefore, preventing hypovolemia and maintaining normal pulmonary perfusion pressure are crucial for maintaining an adequate oxygen delivery in the sitting position.

Venous air embolism

The mechanisms of VAE include negative venous pressure and exposure of veins and boney venous sinuses to air. When the site of surgery is exposed to air and located above the level of the heart, air may be entrained in the veins and boney venous sinuses, and air may enter the pulmonary circulation. A large VAE may decrease cardiac output by creating an airlock and decreasing left ventricular output. The incidence of VAE in the sitting position may approximate 20% to 50% when precordial Doppler monitoring is used for detection [30], and 76% with transesophageal echocardiography (TEE) used for detection [31]. Patent foramen ovale should be excluded before every case, as it is a source of paradoxical air embolism. Therefore, a preoperative "bubble test" in conscious patients using TEE or transthoracic echocardiography is advocated by some investigators if the sitting position is considered [32].

In addition to standard monitoring, precordial transthoracic Doppler is recommended for early detection of VAE [25]. Although TEE is more sensitive in detecting VAE, precordial Doppler is inexpensive, readily available, easy to use, and noninvasive. Optimal placement of the precordial probe should be guided by the recognizing the highest pitch over the right upper sternal border with the intravenous injection of agitated saline. When precordial Doppler or TEE are unavailable, VAE should be considered when end-tidal CO_2 suddenly decreases in the presence of hypotension, not explained by other causes. An atrial catheter (multiorifice or single orifice) placed at the high level of the right atrium may be helpful for air aspiration. Correct positioning may be verified using intravenous electrocardiography, chest radiography, or TEE. However, the therapeutic value of the right atrial catheter may be limited. The most important treatments for VAE include irrigation of the surgical site with saline, rescue head-down tilt or left lateral positioning, and cardiovascular support with administration of inotropes.

Other complications

The incidence of postoperative pneumocephalus in the sitting position may reach 100% [20], and may be due to negative cerebral spinal fluid pressure or residual air during closure of the dura. Therefore, nitrous oxide should be discontinued 20 to 30 minutes before completion of the procedure. However, pneumocephalus can develop even without the use of nitrous oxide and may persist for weeks after surgery. Life-threatening tension pneumocephalus is rare (3%) [28].

Quadriplegia is a rare but devastating complication and results from cervical spine ischemia with neck and head hyperflexion. Elderly patients with cervical spine deformities and vascular pathologies have higher risk [6]. During positioning, sufficient distance between the chin and neck (at least two finger-breadth) is recommended to avoid neck hyperflexion.

Three-quarter prone position (lateral oblique, or semiprone)

The three-quarter prone position is used for posterior fossa and parieto-occipital surgery (Fig. 8). The benefit of this position is that the risk of VAE is lower when compared with the sitting position. Risks include bleeding, brachial plexus injury, pressure sores, and macroglossia. The issues with hemodynamics and ventilation in this position are similar to those with lateral and prone positioning.

The principles of three-quarter positioning resemble those for the lateral position, but the head may be placed on the table and the dependent (lower) arm may be placed behind the body (coma or sleeping position). If a suboccipital approach is required, the nondependent (upper) shoulder should be taped down toward the foot. However, this can cause additional stretching of the brachial plexus (maneuvers to prevent brachial plexus injury are discussed in "Lateral Position" section).

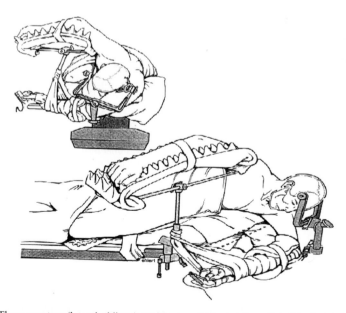

Fig. 8. Three-quarters (lateral oblique) positioning. (*Adapted from* Goodkin R, Mesiwala A. General principles of operative positioning. In: Winn RH, editor. Youmans Neurological Surgery. 5th edition. Philadelphia: Saunders; 2004; with permission.)

Summary

Positioning of the patient for neurological surgery is an important part of anesthesia care and poses many technical and physiological challenges. As discussed, recognition of the physiological changes with positioning and careful and meticulous positioning may decrease unwanted complications.

References

[1] American Society of Anesthesiologists Task Force on the prevention of perioperative peripheral neuropathies: practice advisory for the prevention of perioperative peripheral neuropathies. Anesthesiology 2000;92:1168–82.

[2] Shapiro H, Drummond J. Neurosurgical anesthesia. In: Miller RD, editor. Anesthesia. 4th edition. New York: Churchill Livingstone Inc.; 1994. p. 1897–946.

[3] Clatterbuck R, Tamargo R. Surgical positioning and exposures for cranial procedures. In: Winn H, editor. Youmans neurological surgery. 5th edition. Philadelphia: Sounders, Elsevier Inc.; 2004. p. 623–45.

[4] Goodkin R, Mesiwala A. General principles of operative positioning. In: Winn HR, editor. Youmans neurological surgery. 5th edition. Sounders, Elsevier Inc.; 2004. p. 595–621.

[5] Toole JF. Effects of change of head, limb and body position on cephalic circulation. N Engl J Med 1968;279:307–11.

[6] Vandam L. Positioning of patients for operation. In: Rogers M, Tinker J, Covino B, et al, editors. Principles and practice of anesthesiology. St. Louis: Mosby-Year Book, Inc.; 1993. p. 703–18.

[7] Todd M, Warner D. Neuroanesthesia: a critical review. In: Rogers MC, Tinker J, Covino B, et al, editors. Principles and practice of anesthesiology. St Luis (MO): Mosby-Year Book, Inc.; 1993. p. 1599–648.

[8] Cirovic S, Walsh C, Fraser WD, et al. The effect of posture and positive pressure breathing on the hemodynamics of the internal jugular vein. Aviat Space Environ Med 2003;74:125–31.

[9] Epstein HM, Linde HW, Crampton AR, et al. The vertebral venous plexus as a major cerebral venous outflow tract. Anesthesiology 1970;32:332–7.

[10] Enderby GE. Postural ischaemia and blood-pressure. Lancet 1954;266:185–7.

[11] Cucchiara R, Faust R. Patient positioning. In: Miller RD, editor. Miller's anesthesia. 4th edition. New York: Churchill Livingstone Inc.; 1994. p. 1057–74.

[12] West JB, Dollery CT, Naimark A. Distribution of blood flow in isolated lung. Relation to vascular and alveolar pressures. J Appl Physiol 1964;19:713–24.

[13] Kaneko K, Milic-Emili J, Dolovich MB, et al. Regional distribution of ventilation and perfusion as a function of body position. J Appl Physiol 1966;21:767–77.

[14] Della Valle AG, Salonia-Ruzo P, Peterson MGE, et al. Inflatable pillows as axillary support devices during surgery performed in the lateral decubitus position under epidural anesthesia. Anesth Analg 2001;93:1338–43.

[15] Toyota S, Amaki Y. Hemodynamic evaluation of the prone position by transesophageal echocardiography. J Clin Anesth 1998;10:32–5.

[16] Yokoyama M, Ueda W, Hirakawa M, et al. Hemodynamic effect of the prone position during anesthesia. Acta Anaesthesiol Scand 1991;35:741–4.

[17] Hering R, Wrigge H, Vorwerk R, et al. The effects of prone positioning on intraabdominal pressure and cardiovascular and renal function in patients with acute lung injury. Anesth Analg 2001;92:1226–31.

[18] Sudheer PS, Logan SW, Ateleanu B, et al. Haemodynamic effects of the prone position: a comparison of propofol total intravenous and inhalation anaesthesia. Anaesthesia 2006; 61:138–41.

[19] Wadsworth R, Anderton JM, Vohra A. The effect of four different surgical prone positions on cardiovascular parameters in healthy volunteers. Anaesthesia 1996;51:819–22.

[20] Palmon SC, Kirsch JR, Depper JA, et al. The effect of the prone position on pulmonary mechanics is frame dependent. Anesth Analg 1998;87:1175–80.

[21] Dharmavaram S, Jellish WS, Nockels RP, et al. Effect of prone positioning systems on hemodynamic and cardiac function during lumbar spine surgery: an echocardiographic study. Spine 2006;31:1388–93.

[22] Practice advisory for perioperative visual loss associated with spine surgery: a report by the American Society of Anesthesiologists task force on perioperative blindness. Anesthesiology 2006;104:1319–28.

[23] Ellis SC, Bryan-Brown CW, Hyderally H. Massive swelling of the head and neck. Anesthesiology 1975;42:102–3.

[24] Di Lorenzo N, Caruso R, Floris R, et al. Pneumocephalus and tension pneumocephalus after posterior fossa surgery in the sitting position: a prospective study. Acta Neurochir (Wien) 1986;83:112–5.

[25] Hitselberger WE, House WF. A warning regarding the sitting position for acoustic tumor surgery. Arch Otolaryngol 1980;106:69.

[26] Matjasko J, Petrozza P, Cohen M, et al. Anesthesia and surgery in the seated position: analysis of 554 cases. Neurosurgery 1985;17:695–702.

[27] Young ML, Smith DS, Murtagh F, et al. Comparison of surgical and anesthetic complications in neurosurgical patients experiencing venous air embolism in the sitting position. Neurosurgery 1986;18:157–61.

[28] Duke DA, Lynch JJ, Harner SG, et al. Venous air embolism in sitting and supine patients undergoing vestibular schwannoma resection. Neurosurgery 1998;42:1282–6 [discussion: 6–7].

[29] Black S, Cucchiara R. Tumor surgery. In: Cucchiara RF, Michenfelder SBJD, editors. Clinical neuroanesthesia. 2nd edition. New York 10011, 1998:334–66.

[30] Porter JM, Pidgeon C, Cunningham AJ. The sitting position in neurosurgery: a critical appraisal. Br J Anaesth 1999;82:117–28.

[31] Papadopoulos G, Kuhly P, Brock M, et al. Venous and paradoxical air embolism in the sitting position. A prospective study with transoesophageal echocardiography. Acta Neurochir (Wien) 1994;126:140–3.

[32] Standefer M, Bay JW, Trusso R. The sitting position in neurosurgery: a retrospective analysis of 488 cases. Neurosurgery 1984;14:649–58.

ELSEVIER
SAUNDERS

Anesthesiology Clin
25 (2007) 655–674

ANESTHESIOLOGY
CLINICS

Perioperative Pain Management in the Neurosurgical Patient

Jose Ortiz-Cardona, MD, Audrée A. Bendo, MD*

Department of Anesthesiology, SUNY Downstate Medical Center, 450 Clarkson Avenue, Box 6, Brooklyn, NY 11203–2098, USA

The perioperative management of pain in neurosurgical patients is a controversial topic with management decisions based mainly on reports of anecdotal experiences. There is no consensus regarding the standardization of pain control in this patient population. The small number of evidence-based reports and conflicting conclusions found in the literature has resulted in inconsistent practice, and in most cases suboptimal care.

In the last decade, improved awareness and advances in the practice of pain management have resulted in the implementation of diverse techniques to achieve adequate analgesia in this undertreated group of patients. This has led to an increased number and quality of studies and clinical trials to this effect.

This article provides information about the various techniques and approaches, based on the latest research and clinical trials conducted in this patient population. Specifically, the physiology of pain in patients undergoing brain or spine surgery, the different modalities for pain control, and the diverse choice of drugs, with their associated risks and benefits, are reviewed.

Undertreatment of pain in neurosurgical patients: causes and consequences

Pain is a complex syndrome causing emotional and physical distress, which results in adverse physiologic impact to several organ systems (Table 1), ultimately affecting patient recovery and general well-being. There is evidence that pain after neurosurgical procedures is more severe than expected [1,2], which may result in undertreatment by the perioperative

---

* Corresponding author.
E-mail address: jose.ortiz@downstate.edu (J. Ortiz-Cardona).

1932-2275/07/$ - see front matter. Published by Elsevier Inc.
doi:10.1016/j.anclin.2007.05.003

anesthesiology.theclinics.com

Table 1
Physiologic sequelae of pain

Organ system response to pain	
Respiratory	Increased skeletal muscle tension
	Decreased total lung compliance
Endocrine	Increased adrenocorticotropic hormone, cortisol, glucagon, epinephrine, aldosterone, antidiuretic hormone, catecholamines, and angiotensin II
	Decreased insulin and testosterone
Cardiovascular	Increased myocardial work (mediated by catecholamines, angiotensin II)
Immunologic	Lymphopenia
	Depression of reticuloendothelial system
	Leukocytosis
	Reduced killer T-cell cytotoxicity
Coagulation effects	Increased platelet adhesiveness
	Diminished fibrinolysis
	Activation of coagulation cascade
Gastrointestinal	Increased sphincter tone
	Decreased smooth muscle tone
Genitourinary	Increased sphincter tone
	Decreased smooth muscle tone

Data from Lubenow TR, Ivankovich AD, Barkin RL. Management of acute postoperative pain. In: Barash PG, et al, editors. Clinical anesthesia. 5th edition. Philadelphia: Lippincott Williams & Wilkins; 2006. p. 1411.

team. Recent studies describe pain after craniotomy as moderate to severe and inadequately treated in approximately 50% of patients [3–7]. Postoperative pain management in craniotomy patients is a challenge to the acute pain service provider. Because neurosurgical patients require frequent neurologic examinations, typical postoperative opioid therapy for analgesia is often inappropriate. Aggressive postoperative analgesia management may result in an unintended risk of producing an overly sedated patient, which could mask new neurologic deficits. The need to detect any change in mental status in a timely fashion may overshadow the timely treatment of pain. In addition, some neurosurgical patients may not be able effectively to communicate their need for analgesics because of altered mental status or neurologic deficits. The dilemma for the acute pain service providers is that inadequate analgesia may lead to agitation, hypertension, shivering, and vomiting, which may increase the risk of intracranial bleeding or other neurologic complications [3].

In patients undergoing spine procedures, pain is often a source of significant preoperative distress. Most of these patients have become "chronic pain patients," requiring high, sometimes massive doses of narcotics to achieve satisfactory analgesia. Postoperative pain management for these patients can be problematic if a one-dimensional approach for pain control is used. For example, if opioids are the sole agent administered, caregivers may be reluctant to order the high doses needed to achieve analgesia because of a fear of respiratory depression or other side effects. The implementation of a multimodal approach to manage pain is more often required in this patient population than in non–opioid dependent patients.

Physiology of pain

Pain, as defined by the International Association for the Study of Pain, is an unpleasant sensory and emotional experience associated with actual or potential tissue damage, or described in terms of such damage or both. It is an individual experience, with unique properties varying from patient to patient. The best way to assess whether a patient has pain and to what degree is simple: ask them. Because it is a subjective perception, the reliance on more physiologic objective measures, like changes in heart rate and blood pressure, or the absence of such, does not necessarily translate into adequate treatment.

Pain is sensed by nociceptors, free nerve endings located in the skin, muscles, joints, and mucosa, and in visceral organs. Mechanical nociceptors respond to stimuli, such as sharp, pricking pain, and are supplied by myelinated A delta afferent nerve fibers. These are fast conducting, and posses a low threshold for activation. Polymodal nociceptors respond to high-intensity mechanical or chemical stimuli, and cold-hot stimuli, and are supplied by unmyelinated, slow C fibers.

Tissue injury triggers the release of inflammatory mediators, substance P and calcitonin-gene related peptides, inducing vasodilatation, plasma extravasation at the site of injury, and activation of nociceptors [8]. Impulses generated at these peripheral receptors travel by the primary afferent neurons to the dorsal horn of the spinal cord. At this site, integration of peripheral nociceptive and descending modulatory input occurs, and synapsis with wide dynamic range second-order neurons occurs. First-order neurons also communicate with the cell bodies of the sympathetic nervous system and ventral motor nuclei, either directly or through internuncial neurons [9]. The second-order neuron transmits pain, temperature, and light touch to the central nervous system. They synapse at the thalamus, where third-order neurons relay information to the somatosensory cortex. Along the way to the thalamus, they also send axonal branches in the regions of the reticular formation, nucleus raphe magnus, periaqueductal gray, and other areas in the brainstem. Substance P, γ-aminobutyric acid, glycine, dopamine, serotonin, somatostatin, norepinephrine, enkephalin, bradykinin, histamine, prostaglandins, L-glutamate, aspartate, corticotrophin-inhibiting peptide, and neuropeptide Y are among the numerous mediators that play a role in the complex modulation of nociceptive stimuli occurring peripherally and centrally, and as such, provide potential targets for pharmacologic intervention.

Pain experienced by patients after craniotomy seems to be of somatic origin, most likely involving the scalp, pericranial muscles, and soft tissue, and from manipulation of the dura mater [4,10]. There is a strong correlation between the site of the surgical wound and the source of pain experienced by patients, with the subtemporal and suboccipital surgical routes yielding the highest incidence of postoperative pain [4].

The scalp receives its innervations from branches originating at the cervical plexus and the trigeminal nerve. The anterior scalp is innervated by the supraorbital and supratrochlear nerves, divisions of the frontal nerve (ophthalmic division of trigeminal nerve). The temporal scalp region is supplied by the zygomaticotemporal (maxillary division of trigeminal nerve), temporomandibular, and auriculotemporal nerves (mandibular division of trigeminal nerve). The occipital scalp region receives its sensory innervations from nerves originating in the cervical plexus: greater auricular, and the greater, lesser, and least occipital nerves. The dura mater is innervated by nerves that accompany the meningeal arteries.

Methods of analgesic delivery for postoperative pain after craniotomy

Regional analgesia

Scalp block

The scalp block, often performed before the insertion of cranial pins into the periosteum in patients undergoing awake craniotomy procedures, has also been studied as an adjunct for treating pain after craniotomies (Fig. 1). It has been shown to be effective in providing transitional analgesia, similar to that of intravenous morphine, in the immediate postoperative period following a remifentanil-based anesthetic [11]. Scalp blocks decrease the amount of rescue pain medication requests, increase the time between the end of surgery and the first request for postoperative analgesics, and lower pain score values in the early postoperative period [12]. Lower pain scores lasting up to 48 hours have been described, and a preemptive analgesic

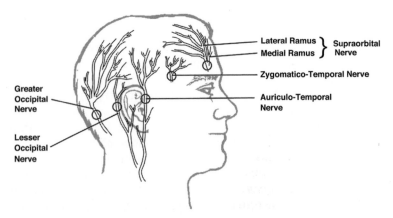

Fig. 1. Cutaneous nerves providing sensory innervation to the scalp. Open circles designate the points at which the nerves can be blocked most easily with local anesthetic injections.

mechanism has been hypothesized [10]. The technique, as described and modified by Pinosky and colleagues [13], involves the injection of local anesthetic through the whole thickness of the scalp, onto the outer margin of the skull, in an area from the postauricular region, through the operative preauricular temporal site, and then crossing the glabella up to the preauricular and postauricular regions of the contralateral sites. Great care must be exercised at the preauricular site to avoid injection into the temporalis artery and to stay above the zygomatic arch, avoiding undesired anesthesia of the facial nerve. The choice of local anesthetic can be made by individual preference or availability. In general, bupivacaine 0.5% with epinephrine 1:200,000 is recommended because it is long-acting. As always indicated, the total dose administered must be less than the recommended maximum dose for patient weight, and intravascular injection must be avoided. Because of the vascular nature of the scalp, it is common to observe cardiovascular evidence of epinephrine absorption following this block. The major advantage of using this technique is that it provides transitional analgesia without compromising neurologic examination. It does not affect the patient's mental status or motor or sensory function, and provides ideal conditions for postoperative neurologic assessment. The scalp block can be performed after skin closure, using the technique described previously, in patients undergoing supratentorial craniotomies with minimal side effects and a good safety profile [10–13].

Wound infiltration

Preincision local anesthetic scalp infiltration is often used in neurosurgical practice to blunt the systemic responses to craniotomy and to minimize bleeding with skin incision (because of the epinephrine used with the local anesthetic). There is insufficient evidence either supporting or discouraging the use of local anesthetic wound infiltration after craniotomy as a means to improve postoperative analgesia, reduce opioid requirements, or reduce time to first pain medication request. Law-Koune and colleagues [14] studied wound infiltration with either 0.375% bupivacaine with epinephrine or 0.75% ropivacaine after skin closure, and found that both can decrease the morphine requirements during the first 2 postoperative hours, but with no significant effect on visual analog scale (VAS) scores when compared with placebo. A study using preincision wound infiltration of bupivacaine 0.25% showed no benefit in postoperative pain relief or decrease in postoperative analgesic requirements [15].

Although more research is warranted, wound incision site infiltration does not seem to be as effective as the scalp block in improving postcraniotomy pain scores. In general, one should not expect preincisional scalp infiltration to provide postoperative analgesia in craniotomy patients. Local anesthetic wound infiltration after skin closure, however, may prove beneficial in providing some transitional pain control in the immediate postoperative period.

Parenteral opioids

Parenteral opioids remain the cornerstone for managing moderate to severe pain, especially in the postoperative period after major surgery. The mechanism of action of opioids involve the stimulation of μ and κ receptors located centrally (brainstem, hypothalamus, limbic system, substantia gelatinosa of the spinal cord) and peripherally (gastrointestinal tract, peripheral histamine receptors). Activation of opioid receptors leads to inhibition of voltage-gated calcium channels and an increase in potassium influx, causing a reduction in neuronal excitability. In a broader picture, opioids inhibit the transmission of painful stimuli from the afferent first neuron to the second neuron at the dorsal horn of the spinal cord, both by presynaptic and postsynaptic mechanisms. They also activate the descending inhibitory pathways that go from the midbrain, rostral ventromedial medulla, ending in the dorsal horn of the spinal cord. There has also been evidence suggesting a peripheral action of opioids involving immune cells located at the inflammation site [16].

Although intermittent systemic administration of opioids was a standard method for postoperative analgesia in the past, this strategy may result in periods of oversedation (peak opiate effect) followed by periods of inadequate analgesia (through opiate effect). Other methods, like patient-controlled analgesia (PCA) with morphine or oxycodone, have also been used effectively in postcraniotomy patients [17,18]. Although sufficient to achieve adequate analgesia, opioids have side effects that can adversely affect patients' recovery from surgery. For example, nausea, vomiting, decreased gastrointestinal motility leading to constipation, pruritus, respiratory depression, and oversedation can all result in the need for additional pharmacologic intervention, and eventually an increased length of inpatient hospital stay. The occurrence of postoperative sedation is especially troubling because of the need for frequent postoperative neurologic examinations. Concern over producing excessive postoperative sedation may lead to the clinician providing high-risk patients with inadequate analgesia. Some side effects caused by opioids are mediated primarily by receptors located in the periphery (nausea, vomiting, pruritus). These dose-dependent side effects, although not as problematic as respiratory depression and sedation, can limit the use of high-dose opioids. Peripheral opioid antagonists, such as nalmefene, have been shown to decrease significantly the need for antiemetics and antipruritic medications in patients receiving intravenous morphine PCA.

Nalbuphine, an opioid agonist-antagonist, has been studied for postoperative pain control after supratentorial craniotomy by Verchere and colleagues [3]. They found 0.15 mg/kg to be effective in maintaining VAS score below 30 mm when used in combination with paracetamol.

Nonsteroidal anti-inflammatory drugs

These drugs can be divided into arylpropionic acids (ibuprofen, naproxen, flurbiprofen, ketoprofen); indole acetic acids (indomethacin, etodolac);

heteroaryl acetic acids (diclofenac, ketorolac); enolic acids (piroxicam, phenylbutazone); and alkanones (nabumetone). Their mechanism of action involves the reversible, nonselective inhibition of the cyclooxygenase (COX) enzymes COX-1 and COX-2. COX acts on arachidonic acid to initiate a chain of reactions that result in the synthesis of prostaglandins (PGD_2, PGE_2, PGI_2 [prostacyclin], PGF_2) and thromboxane. COX-1 is expressed constitutively in the brain and spinal cord. Among its various physiologic functions, it protects the gastric mucosa and provides vascular hemostasis. COX-2, induced by growth factors, cytokines, and tumor promoters, seems to be the dominant source of prostaglandins during inflammation and chronic disease. COX-2 enzyme has also been shown to be constitutively expressed in the brain and spinal cord with further up-regulation after persistent noxious stimuli [19]. Analgesia is achieved by central and peripheral inhibition of prostaglandin-mediated amplification of chemical and mechanical irritants on the sensory pathways. There is also evidence supporting a spinal analgesic mechanism of nonsteroidal anti-inflammatory drugs (NSAIDs) [19].

Although NSAIDs are effective in providing analgesia, they can lead to platelet dysfunction and increased bleeding times, which may be devastating in neurosurgery patients [1]. They have limited use in the immediate postoperative period, especially in cases in which patients are at increased risk for bleeding, such as aneurysm repair, arteriovenous malformation resection, and hematoma evacuations.

COX-2 inhibitors (rofecoxib, celecoxib, meloxicam, nimesulide) selectively inhibit the COX-2 enzyme, effectively achieving anti-inflammatory and analgesic results, but sparing the side effects of nonselective COX inhibitors, such as prolonged postoperative bleeding, and gastrointestinal bleeding. They also spare the nausea, vomiting, respiratory depression, and sedation seen with opioid analgesics. Renal dysfunction characterized by sodium retention and decreased glomerular filtration rate warrants similar precautions as those followed with traditional NSAIDs [20].

There has been concern about the risk of cardiovascular disease among patients receiving chronic COX-2 inhibitor therapy. This was first noted after rofecoxib caused a fourfold increase in the incidence of myocardial infarction compared with naproxen in the Vioxx Gastrointestinal Outcomes Research trial. It seems that inhibition of prostacyclin synthesis, but not thromboxane synthesis, by these agents shifts the coagulation-anticoagulation balance toward the procoagulant effect of thromboxane. This study was performed on patients receiving the medication for a prolonged period of time (more than 18 months), leaving unanswered the question about COX-2 inhibitor safety for short-term use, as is the case in postoperative pain control. A review of randomized controlled trials available on rofecoxib [21] concluded that rofecoxib, 50 mg as a single dose, is effective as an oral analgesic for postoperative pain, with side effects reported to be less frequent than with placebo. Further studies exploring the safety of this drug and the incidence of thromboembolic events when they are used over a short period of time is warranted.

Paracetamol (acetaminophen): N-acetyl-p-aminophenol

Analgesic mechanism of N-acetyl-p-aminophenol (acetaminophen) involves the central inhibition of cyclooxygenases, with weak peripheral effects. It is nevertheless devoid of side effects commonly observed with the use of NSAIDs [22]. Verchere and colleagues [3] studied the use of acetaminophen for postoperative pain after supratentorial craniotomy and concluded that acetaminophen alone (30 mg/kg IV 1 hour before the end of surgery and every 6 hours thereafter) is not sufficient to provide adequate analgesia for this kind of surgery. Intravenous acetaminophen is not yet available in the United States for clinical use. When nalbuphine or tramadol were added to this regimen, VAS levels of less than 30 mm were achieved and maintained in the immediate postoperative period. Acetaminophen's opioid-sparring effect has not proved to be significant [22].

Alpha-2 adrenergic agonists

The use of alpha-2 adrenergic agonists for pain management has gained popularity in recent years. Dexmedetomidine, a potent and highly selective alpha-2 agonist in presynaptic neurons in the spinal cord dorsal horn, provides sedation and analgesia without respiratory depression [23]. Clinical applications of dexmedetomidine for several procedures, such as awake craniotomy, preoperative sedation of patients with aneurysmal subarachnoid hemorrhage, and fiberoptic tracheal intubation, have been described [24–26]. The administration of dexmedetomidine before the completion of major inpatient surgical procedures has been associated with opioid-sparing effects, reducing morphine requirements by as much as 60% [27]. Another study has demonstrated a potential preemptive analgesic effect [28].

Further research with this interesting class of drugs is needed to assess the adequacy of pain control versus side effects following craniotomy. The ability to bring a patient from sedation to arousal immediately for neurologic examinations in the postanesthesia care unit is invaluable. This class of drugs may prove very helpful in providing transitional analgesia from surgical anesthesia to the postanesthesia care unit.

N-methyl-D-aspartate receptor antagonists

N-methyl-D-aspartate antagonists are administered as adjuvant pain management drugs. N-methyl-D-aspartate receptors are ligand-gated ion channels that permit the passage of calcium, sodium, and potassium into the cell. These receptors are activated by glycine and glutamate and do not open at resting membrane potentials. Glutamate, a major excitatory neurotransmitter in the central nervous system, has a significant role in the modulation of pain at the level of the spinal cord, especially in the sensitization of nociceptors after exposure to noxious stimuli, increasing the magnitude and duration of neurogenic responses to pain, even after the initial peripheral input is stopped [29]. These agents do not possess intrinsic analgesic properties, but rather carry out their antinociceptive effects by inhibiting central sensitization to painful stimuli.

Low-dose ketamine (as an IV bolus, or infusion) and dextromethorphan by oral or intramuscular (IM) route have been studied as part of a multimodal pain management approach as adjuvants to opioid therapy and preemptive analgesics. The administration of dextromethorphan, 120 mg, IM 30 minutes before incision in patients undergoing abdominal surgery resulted in a longer time to the first request for analgesic medication in the immediate postoperative period, and a decrease in the amount of IV PCA opioid use with less incidence of hypoxemia [30]. In a systematic qualitative review of the literature by McCartney and colleagues [31], the effect of preoperative N-methyl-D-aspartate antagonists on reducing postoperative pain and analgesic consumption beyond the clinical duration of action of the target drug was reviewed. Dextromethorphan and ketamine were found to have significant immediate and preventive analgesic benefits in 67% and 58%, respectively, of studies reviewed. The use of ketamine in postcraniotomy patients may be precluded by the undesirable increase in intracranial pressure that can be seen after administration of this drug. Dextromethorphan when used as described by Helmy [30], however, may be a valuable adjuvant in the multimodal approach to pain management after craniotomy.

Postoperative pain management after spine surgery

Considerations for postoperative pain management after spine surgery

Hundreds of thousands of spine surgeries are performed in the United States each year, and it is well known that spine surgery patients report high-severity postoperative pain [32,33]. Several studies have investigated risk factors for postoperative pain after spine surgery. These include psychologic, social profile, and preoperative pain severity [34–37]. The use of minimally invasive neurosurgical techniques may decrease the occurrence of significant postoperative pain [38,39], but these techniques are not widely performed. The typical spine surgery patient has endured back pain chronically, with a good number of them on long-term pharmacologic analgesic therapy, sometimes requiring very large doses of analgesics and narcotics. Patients presenting to the operating room for surgical revision after the so-called "failed back syndrome" may be very challenging to provide adequate postoperative analgesia because of high baseline opiate requirements and significant anxiety for having to go through the perioperative experience once again. In addition, these patients require frequent neurologic examinations to assess for any possible postoperative deterioration that may require immediate intervention. Patient cooperation and awareness are vital to ensure a positive surgical outcome.

It is not sufficient to provide pain relief that is adequate for patients only at rest. The importance of early ambulation on surgical outcomes, nonsurgical complications, and hospital length of stay is well known. "Time to ambulation" is frequently used when evaluating the adequacy of analgesia and is an important milestone on the way to postsurgical recovery. To facilitate early ambulation, adequate analgesia and patient safety are essential. With these considerations in mind, the characteristics of pain after spine surgery and the various techniques available to provide postoperative analgesia are now discussed.

Characteristics of back pain

A detailed description of the etiology, diagnosis, and management of back pain, acute or chronic, in the perioperative setting may be obtained [40–42]. In brief, the sensation of back pain can originate in different structures, mediated by nociceptors and mechanoreceptors capable of eliciting a painful sensation. These include the vertebrae, intervertebral disk, dura and nerve root sleeves, facet joint capsules, muscles, ligaments, and fascia. Innervation is by the posterior rami of the spinal nerve roots, which are linked to the sympathetic and parasympathetic nerves, and to the major somatic and motor nerves innervating the upper extremities (cervical spine); the thorax (thoracic spine); abdomen; pelvis; and the lower extremities (lumbar spine). Inflammation in these structures or mechanical compression of the nerves in this area causes pain. Given this interconnectivity, the occurrence of referred pain is not uncommon in these patients. Klimek and colleagues [34] observed that referred pain far exceeded local and diffuse pain in the preoperative period in patients scheduled for spine surgery. After the surgery, pain was mostly local, and in those patients in whom referred pain persisted, VAS scores were higher. Referred pain is mostly neuropathic pain, which although does not respond well to conventional pain therapy, is often relieved by treatment with anticonvulsants and antidepressant medications [43–45].

There seems to be no significant difference in the severity of pain when comparing cervical, thoracic, and lumbar spine surgeries [34,46]. Postoperative pain after spinal surgeries is proportional to the number of vertebrae included in the operation and with regard to its invasiveness [47].

Methods of pain management after spine surgery

Parenteral administration

Opioids
Opioids have been used in combination with other analgesics or alone, sometimes with good results, sometimes with less than optimal results.

Opioids are excellent drugs for pain control, but the dose is often not optimized because of fear of sedation and respiratory depression, or because patients do not tolerate the doses required for adequate analgesia without experiencing unpleasant side effects. Although in the past opioids were often administered pro re nata, superior postoperative analgesia occurs in patients treated with IV opioid PCA than with intermittent IM opioid administration [48]. Those who had previously received IM injections also reported that PCA was easy to use and provided better analgesia [49]. Although PCA is the preferred method for postoperative opioid-based analgesia, an opioid-only regimen can have many side effects and should not be seen as the only choice to achieve an appropriate level of analgesia. A multidrug approach may lead to better patient satisfaction and decreased doses of opioids (opioid-sparing effect), which should result in a decreased risk of side effects.

Nonsteroidal anti-inflammatory drugs

Reports from several studies promote the use of NSAIDS in the perioperative period, but scarce information exists on their use for postoperative analgesia after spine surgery. Different routes of administration, different dosing regimens, and different drugs within this group have been studied. Some research has shown that the use of NSAIDS as the sole medication for pain control after spine surgery is not sufficient to provide adequate analgesia [50], but when combined with opioids, the combination results in much better results than with either one alone [51–54].

Ketorolac, given IM or IV, is the most investigated drug among the NSAIDS. It has good analgesic potency and its opioid-sparing capacity has been well documented [51–54]. Because its onset of action is not immediate (about 30–60 minutes after IM injection), its use in severe acute pain in the postoperative period is best as an adjuvant to opioids, rather than as a sole agent. There is also a concern regarding the deleterious effects of NSAIDS on bone healing, because of the importance of PGE_2 in the early stages of bone healing [55]. High-dose (120–240 mg/d), but not low-dose, ketorolac has been associated with nonunion following spine fusion surgery [56]. Low-dose ketorolac, in the absence of contraindications, may be a safe and effective adjuvant to an opioid-based regimen for acute postoperative pain management after spine surgery.

Steroids

A small number of studies have assessed the use of IV corticosteroids to reduce postoperative pain. Steroids are anti-inflammatory drugs that inhibit phospholipase A_2, but another mechanism of action involving a decrease in the expression of substance P at the dorsal root ganglion has been hypothesized [57]. The threshold of at least one type of peripheral nociceptors is lowered by certain endogenous chemicals liberated during the inflammatory process [58]. Some patients may still complain of radicular referred pain after the surgery, probably associated with nerve root inflammation. On that basis, the effect of IV dexamethasone after skin incision on postoperative pain has been studied. Intraoperative IV injection of 40-mg dexamethasone reduces postoperative radicular leg pain and narcotic use in patients after single-level herniated lumbar disk surgery [59,60]. Likewise, a lower dose of dexamethasone (10 mg IV intraoperatively) helped to reduce analgesic requirements in patients undergoing lumbar, but not cervical, diskectomy [60]. Larger trials are needed to confirm or refute these findings.

Acetaminophen

Propacetamol, an injectable prodrug of acetaminophen (not available in this form in the United States), has been studied to determine its analgesic efficacy and opioid-sparing effects in the postoperative period [61,62]. Its mechanism of action may involve centrally and peripherally located sites [63,64], possibly involving inhibition of prostaglandins [65] and activation of descending serotoninergic inhibitory pathways [66]. In patients in whom NSAIDS may be contraindicated or where there is concern about postoperative hemostasis, paracetamol may be a useful alternative as adjunct to opioid therapy.

Cyclooxygenase-2 inhibitors

Reports of adverse effects on bone healing by NSAIDS led to the investigation of the effects by COX-2 inhibitors on bone healing. COX-2–dependent PGE_2 produced at the early stage of bone healing is a prerequisite for efficient skeletal repair [55]. A study on healing bone fractures showed a decrease in osteogenesis potential after the cells were treated with celecoxib [67]. Reuben [56,68] studied the efficacy of the short-term use of COX-2 inhibitors for postoperative pain, opioid-sparing properties, and the effects on bone healing after spine fusion surgery. He concluded that the perioperative administration of celecoxib, given 1 hour before the induction of anesthesia and every 12 hours after surgery for the first 5 postoperative days, resulted in a significant reduction in postoperative pain and opioid use following spine fusion surgery. In addition, short-term administration had no apparent effect on the rate of nonunion. Similar to N-acetyl-p-aminophenol, COX-2 inhibitors do not affect platelets and bleeding time as do NSAIDS. These drugs can be used as alternative drugs for pain management in patients in whom hemostasis is an issue. Until more evidence is gathered, however, their use remains controversial in surgeries involving bone healing because of the potential for adverse effects.

Neuraxial administration: intrathecal

Opioids

Intrathecal (IT) opioids are extensively used for the management of acute pain in the perioperative period. The pharmacokinetics of different IT administered opioids has been extensively studied [69]. Lipophilic opioids, such as fentanyl, alfentanil, and sufentanil, have a faster onset of action but shorter duration of action (2–4 hours) compared with morphine (18–24 hours with a delayed onset of analgesia). Achieving adequate analgesia from IT opioids depends on the rate and extent to which opioids distribute from the cerebrospinal fluid to opioid receptors in the spinal cord dorsal horn as opposed to competing extraspinal sites. Because of its extended duration of action and its lower incidence of neurotoxicity, preservative-free morphine could be the drug of choice if the use of an IT opioid is intended for pain relief in the postoperative period. The same side effect profile that accompanies the IV injection of morphine applies to IT administration. Nausea, vomiting, pruritus, urinary retention (up to 35% incidence), and respiratory depression (early and delayed) can be seen in most patients who receive doses in excess of 0.3 mg. The need for monitoring for oversedation and respiratory depression assumes that the patient has a hospital stay of at least 24 hours after administration of IT morphine. Compared with the more lipophilic opioids, this drug is not recommended for ambulatory procedures. In addition, prolonged continuous infusion of drug through an IT catheter is not recommended because of the risk of cauda equina syndrome [70].

Studies evaluating the administration of IT morphine after spine surgery are limited. Urban and colleagues [71] studied the use of IT morphine (20 µg/kg) for postoperative analgesia after elective multilevel spine fusion surgery with good results. He reported that patients were comfortable immediately after surgery, remained pain free for a longer period, and required significantly less additional narcotic. Several studies also investigated the use of IT morphine as a single bolus, with doses ranging from 2 to 20 µg/kg, for pain relief after anterior or posterior spine fusion [72,73]. Postoperative analgesia was prolonged up to 36 hours after surgery, and there was a decrease in the need for supplemental analgesia. IT opiods can be easily administered by the surgeon when the thecal sac is exposed. Although this therapy provides effective analgesia, it is also associated with respiratory depression following spine surgery [74].

Local anesthetics

Experience with the IT administration of local anesthetics for postoperative pain management is mostly in combination with opioids or other adjuvants. Various studies have analyzed with favorable results the postoperative continuous IT administration of bupivacaine and morphine in the treatment of pain after selective dorsal rhizotomy [75,76]. Doses of up to 0.6 µg/kg/h of morphine with bupivacaine (40 µg/kg/h) have been associated with good analgesic effect, a decrease in the need for parenteral narcotics, and minimum side effects.

Other agents

Other adjuncts to IT-administrated local anesthetics have been studied mainly for orthopedic procedures. The addition of drugs like clonidine

[77] and neostigmine [78] to IT local anesthetics has been shown to prolong sensory and motor block. Prolonged block is not desirable in the early post-operative period after spine surgery, because of the need to assess neurologic function of the lower extremities. Clinical studies evaluating the use for these medications in conjunction with IT morphine are needed to determine whether their known analgesic effects result in a decrease in opioid require-ments and better pain scores after spine surgery. One study found that com-bining IT morphine (250 µg) with IT clonidine (25 or 75 µg) reduced the need for supplemental analgesics and improved pain control after total knee arthroplasty [79].

Studies in experimental animals suggest that spinally administered ketor-olac may be useful in treating postoperative pain caused by its inhibition of COX-1 enzyme [80,81]. The safety profile has been studied for up to 6 months after administration; no significant complications have been reported [82]. The study also reports, however, that the IT administration of selective COX-2 inhibitors has minimal analgesic effects. To date, there are no human studies assessing the efficacy of these drugs after IT administration.

Neuraxial administration: epidural

Opioids, local anesthetics, and the combination of both

There are several clinical trials studying the efficacy and safety of epidural administration of drugs for postoperative pain control following different procedures. When compared with IT administration, epidural opioids have a better safety margin and a lower incidence of dose-dependent respi-ratory depression and urinary retention. There is controversy as to whether this more invasive procedure is superior to the standard IV or IM route after spine surgery.

Opioids affect the modulation of nociceptive input mainly by acting on receptors in the dorsal horn without producing motor or sympathetic block-ade. Because of this, opioids are potentially very useful in the treatment of spine surgery patients in whom postoperative motor and sensory function are closely monitored. When compared with IM opioids, epidural opioids produce longer-lasting analgesia with smaller doses. A review of the litera-ture reveals that the benefits of administering opioid-only solutions may not outweigh the risks associated with this procedure [83]. Side effects including nausea, vomiting, and pruritus are also commonly seen with this technique. The use of local anesthetic–only solutions also has disadvantages. The dose required for adequate analgesia can produce a motor block, interfering with lower-extremity neurologic examination, and potentially can cause sympa-thectomy-mediated hypotension. The combination of local anesthetic and opioids may provide more advantages than administering either agent alone. Adding opioids to local anesthetic decreases the amount of local anesthetic and opioid necessary to achieve good results, thereby decreasing the incidence of side effects. It has also been documented that this combination improves the quality of dynamic pain relief [84] when compared with opioid-only infusion.

The choice of opioid and local anesthetic varies among different practices. Ropivacaine seems to provide an advantage over bupivacaine with respect to safety index and the selectivity of ropivacaine toward sensory rather than motor blockade, although this may be apparent only at the higher dose range. Different techniques for epidural injection have been studied including single and double catheters, intermittent boluses, patient-controlled epidural analgesia, and continuous infusion of medication. The placement of the epidural catheter intraoperatively can be done by the surgical team under direct vision with relative ease and high success rate. As with parenteral administration, intermittent bolus administration of epidural opioids may result in patients who are more likely to experience pain and unnecessary suffering, whereas patients being treated with epidural PCA experience overall lower pain scores and decreased side effects [85]. The advantages of epidural opioids and the combination of opioids and local anesthetics include low pain scores [86,87], decreased parenteral opioid requirements [88,89], decrease in the incidence of pulmonary morbidity [90], and better patient satisfaction. Other studies report that both patient-controlled epidural analgesia and IV PCA are equally effective [33,89,91], with no difference observed in the epidural groups in time to oral intake of liquids or solids, ambulation, bowel sounds, or length of stay when compared with placebo [91], but a greater incidence of side effects has been reported with the patient-controlled epidural analgesia group [89]. The divergent conclusions can be explained because of the lack of a standardized method of infusion (intermittent bolus versus continuous infusion, versus patient-controlled epidural analgesia with or without baseline infusion) and the different drugs, doses, and combinations used. It is not clear at this time which method is most effective for postoperative analgesia in patients following spine surgery.

Other agents

Alpha-2 agonists have been used for epidural analgesia as adjuncts to opioids, local anesthetic, or the combination of both to potentate their action. They produce minimal respiratory depression when compared with opioids. Clonidine is effective in the treatment of neuropathic pain, especially when administered in the epidural space [92]. This theoretically makes it a good addition to the management of postoperative pain, because patients who still feel neuropathic, referred pain after surgery tend to have higher VAS scores and are more challenging to manage. In a study by Ekatodramis and colleagues [93], a double-catheter approach of bupivacaine, fentanyl, and clonidine infusion was used with good results. Jellish and colleagues [94] concluded that epidural clonidine (150 µg), in addition to subcutaneous bupivacaine at the incision site, improved postoperative pain and hemodynamic stability in patients undergoing lower spine procedures. Epidural doses of clonidine higher than 4 µg/kg have been associated with reduced pain by more than 70% and effects lasting for 4 to 5 hours. Bradycardia, hypotension, and sedation were reported as the most common side effects [95].

Tizanidine and dexmedetomidine have also been studied, but further randomized controlled trials involving spine procedures need to be performed. These agents provide a fast onset of analgesia and may provide a smooth transition between intraoperative anesthesia and epidural infusion of opioids with or without local anesthetics.

Summary

Until recently, perioperative pain management in neurosurgical patients has been inconsistently recognized and inadequately treated. An increased awareness of pain management in general along with advances in understanding of pain modulation and pathophysiology has led to improved practice and perioperative care of patients. The greatest challenge to managing neurosurgical patients is the need to assess neurologic function while providing superior analgesia with minimal side effects. To achieve this goal, a multimodal approach to analgesia using various drugs and techniques is used. In addition to opioids, several classes of drugs are currently available or under investigation for use as adjuvants or alternative therapies. There still remains a need, however, to conduct randomized, controlled trials to determine the best combination of drugs or techniques for treating perioperative pain in this patient population. Improved awareness, assessment, and treatment of pain result in better care and overall patient outcome.

References

[1] Rahimi SY, Vender JR, Macomson SD, et al. Postoperative pain management after craniotomy: evaluation and cost analysis. Neurosurgery 2006;59(4):852–7.

[2] Quiney N, Cooper R, Stoneham M, et al. Pain after craniotomy: a time for reappraisal? Br J Neurosurg 1996;10(3):295–9.

[3] Verchere E, Grenier B, Mesli A, et al. Postoperative pain management after supratentorial craniotomy. J Neurosurg Anesthesiol 2002;14(2):96–101.

[4] De Benedittis G, Lorenzetti A, Migliore M, et al. Postoperative pain in neurosurgery: a pilot study in brain surgery. Neurosurgery 1996;38(3):466–9.

[5] Dunbar PJ, Visco E, Lam AM. Craniotomy procedures are associated with less analgesic requirements than other surgical procedures. Anesth Analg 1999;88:335–40.

[6] Stoneham MD, Walters FJ. Post-operative analgesia for craniotomy patients: current attitudes among neuroanaesthetists. Eur J Anaesthesiol 1995;12(6):571–5.

[7] Roberts GC. Post-craniotomy analgesia: current practices in British neurosurgical centres— a survey of post-craniotomy analgesic practices. Eur J Anaesthesiol 2005;22(5):328–32.

[8] Julius D, Basbaum AI. Molecular mechanisms of nociception. Nature 2001;413:203–10.

[9] Kerr FWL. The structured basis of pain: circulatory and pathway. In: Ng LWY, Bonica JJ, editors. Pain, discomfort and humanitarian care. New York: Elsevier; 1980. p. 49.

[10] Nguyen A, Girard F, Boudreault D, et al. Scalp nerve blocks decrease the severity of pain after craniotomy. Anesth Analg 2001;93(5):1272–6.

[11] Ayoub C, Girard F, Boudreault D, et al. A comparison between scalp nerve block and morphine for transitional analgesia after remifentanil-based anesthesia in neurosurgery. Anesth Analg 2006;103(5):1237–40.

[12] Bala I, Gupta B, Bhardwaj N, et al. Effect of scalp block on postoperative pain relief in craniotomy patients. Anaesth Intensive Care 2006;34(2):224–7.

[13] Pinosky ML, Fishman RL, Reeves ST, et al. The effect of bupivacaine skull block on the hemodynamic response to craniotomy. Anesth Analg 1996;83:1256–61.

[14] Law-Koune JD, Szekely B, Fermanian C, et al. Scalp infiltration with bupivacaine plus epinephrine or plain ropivacaine reduces postoperative pain after supratentorial craniotomy. J Neurosurg Anesthesiol 2005;17(3):139–43.

[15] Biswas BK, Bithal PK. Preincision 0.25% bupivacaine scalp infiltration and postcraniotomy pain: a randomized double-blind, placebo-controlled study. J Neurosurg Anesthesiol 2003; 15(3):234–9.

[16] Stein C. The control of pain in peripheral tissue by opioids. N Engl J Med 1995;332: 1685–90.

[17] Jellish WS. Morphine/ondansetron PCA for postoperative pain, nausea, and vomiting after skull base surgery. Otolaryngol Head Neck Surg 2006;135(2):175–81.

[18] Stoneham MD, Cooper R, Quiney NF, et al. Pain following craniotomy: a preliminary study comparing PCA morphine with intramuscular codeine phosphate. Anaesthesia 1996;51(12): 1176–8.

[19] Svensson CI, Yaksh TL. The spinal phospholipase-cyclooxygenase-prostanoid cascade in nociceptive processing. Annu Rev Pharmacol Toxicol 2002;42:553–83.

[20] Brater DC. Renal effects of cyclooxygenase-2-selective inhibitors. J Pain Symptom Manage 2002;23:S15–20.

[21] Barden J, Edwards J, Moore RA, et al. Single dose oral rofecoxib for postoperative pain. Cochrane Database Syst Rev 2005;(1):CD004604.

[22] Remy C, Marret E, Bonnet F. State of the art of paracetamol in acute pain therapy. Curr Opin Anaesthesiol 2006;19(5):562–5.

[23] Sakaguchi Y, Takahashi S. Dexmedetomidine. Masui 2006;55(7):856–63.

[24] Souter MJ, Rozet I, Ojemann JG, et al. Dexmedetomidine sedation during awake craniotomy for seizure resection: effects on electrocorticography. J Neurosurg Anesthesiol 2007; 19(1):38–44.

[25] Grant SA, Breslin DS, MacLeod DB, et al. Dexmedetomidine infusion for sedation during fiberoptic intubation: a report of three cases. J Clin Anesth 2004;16(2):124–6.

[26] Sato K, Kamii H, Shimizu H, et al. Preoperative sedation with dexmedetomidine in patients with aneurysmal subarachnoid hemorrhage. Masui 2006;55(1):51–4.

[27] Arain SR, Ruehlow RM, Uhrich TD, et al. The efficacy of dexmedetomidine versus morphine for postoperative analgesia after major inpatient surgery. Anesth Analg 2004;98(1):153–8.

[28] Unlugenc H, Gunduz M, Guler T, et al. The effect of pre-anaesthetic administration of intravenous dexmedetomidine on postoperative pain in patients receiving patient-controlled morphine. Eur J Anaesthesiol 2005;22(5):386–91.

[29] Dickenson AH. Spinal cord pharmacology of pain. Br J Anaesth 1995;75:193–200.

[30] Helmy SA. The effect of the preemptive use of the NMDA receptor antagonist dextromethorphan on postoperative analgesic requirements. Anesth Analg 2001;92(3):739–44.

[31] McCartney CJ, Sinha A, Katz J. A qualitative systematic review of the role of N-methyl-D-aspartate receptor antagonists in preventive analgesia. Anesth Analg 2004;98(5): 1385–400.

[32] Bianconi M, Ferraro L, Ricci R, et al. The pharmacokinetics and efficacy of ropivacaine continuous wound installation after spine fusion surgery. Anesth Analg 2004;98:166–72.

[33] Cohen BE, Hartman MB, Wade JT, et al. Postoperative pain control after lumbar spine fusion: patient-controlled analgesia versus continuous epidural analgesia. Spine 1997;22:1892–7.

[34] Klimek M, Ubben J, Ammann J, et al. Pain in neurosurgically treated patients: a prospective observational study. J Neurosurg 2006;104:350–9.

[35] Kalkman CJ, Visser K, Moen J, et al. Preoperative prediction of severe postoperative pain. Pain 2003;105(3):415–23.

[36] Kotzer AM. Factors predicting postoperative pain in children and adolescents following spine fusion. Issues Compr Pediatr Nurs 2000;23:83–102.

[37] Epker J, Block AR. Pre-surgical psychological screening in back pain patients: a review. Clin J Pain 2001;17(3):200–5.

[38] Fessler RG. The development of minimally invasive spine surgery. Neurosurg Clin N Am 2006;17(4):401–9.

[39] Oskouian RJ, Johnson JP. Endoscopic thoracic microdiscectomy. J Neurosurg Spine 2005; 3(6):459–64.

[40] Waddell G. The back pain revolution. 2nd edition. Edinburgh (UK): Churchill Livingstone; 2004.

[41] McMahon S. Wall and Melzack's textbook of pain. 5th edition. Philadelphia: Elsevier, Churchill Livingstone; 2006.

[42] Devereaux MW. Neck and low back pain. Med Clin North Am 2003;87:643–62.

[43] Sumpton JE. Treatment of neuropathic pain with venlafaxine. Ann Pharmacother 2001; 35(5):557–9.

[44] Tremont-Lukats IW. Anticonvulsants for neuropathic pain syndromes: mechanisms of action and place in therapy. Drugs 2000;60(5):1029–52.

[45] Backonja MM. Anticonvulsants (antineuropathics) for neuropathic pain syndromes. Clin J Pain 2000;16(Suppl 2):S67–72.

[46] Jaffe RA, Samuels SI. Anesthesiologist's manual of surgical procedures. 3rd edition. Philadelphia: Lippincott Williams & Wilkins; 2004.

[47] Bernard JM, Surbled M, Lagarde D, et al. Analgesia after surgery of the spine in adults and adolescents. Cah Anesthesiol 1995;43(6):557–64.

[48] Bollish SJ, Collins CL, Kirking DM, et al. Efficacy of patient-controlled versus conventional analgesia for postoperative pain. Clin Pharm 1985;4(1):48–52.

[49] Egbert AM, Parks LH, Short LM, et al. Randomized trial of postoperative patient-controlled analgesia vs intramuscular narcotics in frail elderly men. Arch Intern Med 1990; 150(9):1897–903.

[50] Izquierdo E, Fabregas N, Valero R, et al. Postoperative analgesia in herniated disk surgery: comparative study of diclofenac, lysine acetylsalicylate, and ketorolac. Rev Esp Anesthesiol Reanim 1995;42(8):316–9.

[51] Le Roux PD. Postoperative pain after lumbar disc surgery: a comparison between parenteral ketorolac and narcotics. Acta Neurochir (Wien) 1999;141(3):261–7.

[52] Gwirtz KH, Kim HC, Nagy DJ, et al. Intravenous ketorolac and subarachnoid opioid analgesia in the management of acute postoperative pain. Reg Anesth 1995;20(5):395–401.

[53] Sevarino FB, Sinatra RS, Paige D, et al. The efficacy of intramuscular ketorolac in combination with intravenous PCA morphine for postoperative pain relief. J Clin Anesth 1992; 4(4):285–8.

[54] Turner DM, Warson JS, Wirt TC, et al. The use of ketorolac in lumbar spine surgery: a cost-benefit analysis. J Spinal Disord 1995;8(3):206–12.

[55] O'Keefe RJ, Tiyapatanaputi P, Xie C, et al. COX-2 has a critical role during incorporation of structural bone allografts. Ann N Y Acad Sci 2006;1068:532–42.

[56] Reuben SS. High dose nonsteroidal anti-inflammatory drugs compromise spinal fusion. Can J Anaesth 2005;52(5):506–12.

[57] Wong HK, Tan KJ. Effects of corticosteroids on nerve root recovery after spinal nerve root compression. Clin Orthop Relat Res 2002;(403):248–52.

[58] King JS, Gallant P, Myerson V, et al. The effects of anti-inflammatory agents on the responses and the sensitization of unmyelinated (C) fiber polymodal nociceptors. In: Zotterman Y, editor. Sensory functions of the skin in primates with special reference to man

[Wenner-Gren Center International Symposium Series, vol. 28]. Oxford (UK): Pergamon Press; 1976. p. 441–61.

[59] Aminmansour B, Khalili HA, Ahmadi J, et al. Effect of high-dose intravenous dexamethasone on postlumbar discectomy pain. Spine 2006;31(21):2415–7.

[60] King JS. Dexamethasone: a helpful adjunct in management after lumbar discectomy. Neurosurgery 1984;14:697–700.

[61] Vuilleumier PA, Buclin T, Biollaz J, et al. Comparison of propacetamol and morphine in postoperative analgesia. Schweiz Med Wochenschr 1998;128(7):259–63.

[62] Delbos A, Boccard E. The morphine-sparing effect of propacetamol in orthopedic postoperative pain. J Pain Symptom Manage 1995;10:279–86.

[63] Moore UJ. Effects of peripherally and centrally acting analgesics on somato-sensory evoked potentials. Br J Clin Pharmacol 1995;40(2):111–7.

[64] Piletta P, Porchet HC, Dayer P. Central analgesic effect of acetaminophen but not of aspirin. Clin Pharmacol Ther 1991;49:350–4.

[65] Flower RJ, Vane JR. Inhibition of prostaglandin synthetase in brain explains the anti-pyretic activity of paracetamol. Nature 1972;240:410–1.

[66] Tjolsen A, Lund A, Hole K. Antinociceptive effect of paracetamol in rats is partly dependent on spinal serotoninergic systems. Eur J Pharmacol 1991;193(2):193–201.

[67] Daluiski A. Cyclooxygenase-2 inhibitors in human skeletal fracture healing. Orthopedics 2006;29(3):259–61.

[68] Reuben SS. The effect of cyclooxygenase-2 inhibition on analgesia and spinal fusion. J Bone Joint Surg Am 2005;87(3):536–42.

[69] Ummenhofer WC. Comparative spinal distribution and clearance kinetics of intrathecally administered morphine, fentanyl, alfentanil, and sufentanil. Anesthesiology 2000;92(3): 739–53.

[70] Rigler ML, Drasner K, Krejcie TC, et al. Cauda equine syndrome after spinal anesthesia. Anesth Analg 1991;72:275–81.

[71] Urban MK, Jules-Elysee K, Urquhart B, et al. Reduction in postoperative pain after spinal fusion with instrumentation using intrathecal morphine. Spine 2002;27(5):535–7.

[72] Dalens B, Tanguy A. Intrathecal morphine for spinal fusion in children. Spine 1988;13: 494–8.

[73] Blackman RG, Reynolds J, Shively J. Intrathecal morphine dosage and efficacy in younger patients for control of postoperative pain following spinal fusion. Orthopedics 1991;14: 555–7.

[74] France JC. The use of intrathecal morphine for analgesia after posterolateral lumbar fusion: a prospective, double-blind, randomized study. Spine 1997;22(19):2272–7.

[75] Hesselgard K, Stromblad LG, Romner B, et al. Postoperative continuous intrathecal pain treatment in children after selective dorsal rhizotomy with bupivacaine and two different morphine doses. Paediatr Anaesth 2006;16(4):436–43.

[76] Hesselgard K, Stromblad LG, Reinstrup P. Morphine with or without a local anaesthetic for postoperative intrathecal pain treatment after selective dorsal rhizotomy in children. Paediatr Anaesth 2001;11(1):75–9.

[77] Strebel S, Gurzeler JA, Schneider MC, et al. Small-dose intrathecal clonidine and isobaric bupivacaine for orthopedic surgery: a dose-response study. Anesth Analg 2004;99(4): 1231–8.

[78] Liu SS, Hodgson PS, Moore JM, et al. Dose-response effects of spinal neostigmine added to bupivacaine spinal anesthesia in healthy volunteers. Anesthesiology 1999;90: 710–7.

[79] Sites BD, Beach M, Biggs R, et al. Intrathecal clonidine added to a bupivacaine-morphine spinal anesthetic improves postoperative analgesia for total knee arthroplasty. Anesth Analg 2003;96:1083–8.

[80] Zhu X, Conklin D, Eisenach JC. Cyclooxygenase-1 in the spinal cord plays an important role in postoperative pain. Pain 2003;104:15–23.

[81] Conklin DR, Eisenach JC. Intrathecal ketorolac enhances antinociception from clonidine. Anesth Analg 2003;96:191–4.

[82] Eisenach JC, Curry R, Hood DD, et al. Phase I safety assessment of intrathecal ketorolac. Pain 2002;99:599–604.

[83] Wheatley RG, Schug SA, Watson D. Safety and efficacy of postoperative epidural analgesia. Br J Anaesth 2001;87:47–61.

[84] Dahl JB, Rosenberg J, Hansen BL, et al. Differential analgesic effects of low-dose epidural morphine and morphine-bupivacaine at rest and during mobilization after major abdominal surgery. Anesth Analg 1992;74:362–5.

[85] Rockemann MG. Epidural bolus clonidine/morphine versus epidural patient-controlled bupivacaine/sufentanil: quality of postoperative analgesia and cost-identification analysis. Anesth Analg 1997;85(4):864–9.

[86] Schenk MR, Putzier M, Kugler B, et al. Postoperative analgesia after major spine surgery: patient-controlled epidural analgesia versus patient-controlled intravenous analgesia. Anesth Analg 2006;103(5):1311–7.

[87] Lowry KJ, Tobias J, Kittle D, et al. Postoperative pain control using epidural catheters after anterior spinal fusion for adolescent scoliosis. Spine 2001;26:1290–3.

[88] Amaranth L, Andrish JT, Gurd AR, et al. Efficacy of intermittent epidural morphine following posterior spinal fusion in children and adolescents. Clin Orthop Relat Res 1989;249: 223–6.

[89] Fisher CG, Belanger L, Gofton EG. Prospective randomized clinical trial comparing patient-controlled intravenous analgesia with patient-controlled epidural analgesia after lumbar spinal fusion. Spine 2003;28(8):739–43.

[90] Ballantyne JC, Carr DB, deFerranti S, et al. The comparative effects of postoperative analgesic therapies on pulmonary outcome: cumulative meta-analyses of randomized, controlled trials. Anesth Analg 1998;87(3):598–612.

[91] O'Hara JF. The effect of epidural vs intravenous analgesia for posterior spinal fusion surgery. Paediatr Anaesth 2004;14(12):1009–15.

[92] Eisenach J, Detweiler D, Hood D. Hemodynamics and analgesic actions of epidurally administered clonidine. Anesthesiology 1993;78:277–87.

[93] Ekatodramis G, Min K, Cathrein P, et al. Use of a double epidural catheter provides effective postoperative analgesia after spine deformity surgery. Reg Anesth Pain Med 2002;49:173–7.

[94] Jellish WS, Abodeely A, Fluder EM, et al. The effect of spinal bupivacaine in combination with either epidural clonidine and/or 0.5% bupivacaine administered at the incision site on postoperative outcome in patients undergoing lumbar laminectomy. Anesth Analg 2003; 96(3):874–80.

[95] Rockemann MG, Seeling W. Epidural and intrathecal administration of alpha 2-adrenoceptor agonists for postoperative pain relief. Schmerz 1996;10(2):57–64.

ELSEVIER
SAUNDERS

Anesthesiology Clin
25 (2007) 675–685

ANESTHESIOLOGY
CLINICS

Controversies in Neurosciences Critical Care

J. Ricardo Carhuapoma, MD, Neeraj S. Naval, MD,
Marek A. Mirski, MD, PhD*

*Neurosciences Critical Care Division, Departments of Neurology,
Neurosurgery and Anesthesiology and Critical Care Medicine,
The Johns Hopkins Hospital, 600 North Wolfe Street, Mayer 8-140,
Baltimore, MD 21287, USA*

The subspecialty of neurosciences critical care has matured during the past several decades, with the greatest strides perhaps being the initially controversial integration of a diverse group of health care professionals specifically trained to optimize acute, ICU-level neurologic management. In the past, neurosurgeons by necessity cared for most neuroscience ICU patients with a skill-set in critical care that only their profession had mastered. In particular, the neurosurgical procedure itself, coupled with perioperative derangements that required a discriminating neurologic eye to diagnose and treat, left most other acute care physicians unable to contribute much to this patient care domain. Anesthesiologists and general critical care physicians, as two good examples, were and continue to be extremely competent in respiratory and hemodynamic therapeutics. In the ICU setting, however, these highly trained professionals may lack the necessary neurologic expertise to be pre-emptive, rather than reflexive, in their approach to the prospect of adverse neurologic events. On the contrary, neurologists are commonly trained in the consultant style of in-patient practice, rather than direct patient care. They are capable diagnosticians that support the ICU physician teams, but comprehensive, integrated care delivery in this manner may not be guaranteed.

From this state of neuroscience affairs emerged the concepts and practice of the skilled neurointensivist and self-reliant neurologic ICUs. Indeed, there is strong support in the literature for the finding that the practice of neurosciences critical care has led to improving patient outcomes is an

* Corresponding author.
E-mail address: mmirski@jhmi.edu (M.A. Mirski).

1932-2275/07/$ - see front matter © 2007 Elsevier Inc. All rights reserved.
doi:10.1016/j.anclin.2007.05.006
anesthesiology.theclinics.com

efficient, cost-effective manner to treat such neurologically complex patients [1–4]. In many ways, the visceral physiology embodied by the cardiac, pulmonary, and renal organ systems has dominated general ICU management, with the central nervous system afforded but indirect attention. Outcome measures focused on mortality as a consequence of severe illness, not functional recovery. Thankfully, such is not currently the case, and much credit goes to neurosurgical colleagues who invested themselves into the critical care arena, and to the advent of the subspecialty of neurointensivist. Whether formally trained as anesthesiologists, neurologists, or neurosurgeons, these specialty physicians have elevated the neurologic examination, and the central nervous itself, to their rightful levels of importance. Without sound brain recovery, all else matters little.

In the year 2007, there is much to be pleased about concerning acute and perioperative neurologic disease. Improvements in anesthetic drugs (rapid on–rapid off), surgical techniques (microscopy, image guidance, stereotactic expertise), interventional neuroradiology (embolization, thrombolysis, stents, angioplasty), and acute neurologic care (thrombolysis, hemapharesis, continuous electrical and intracerebral physiologic monitoring) have all moved the clinical science forward. Nonetheless, there are two very common disease states of the neurocritical care environment that continue to plague physicians regarding best course of therapeutic action: spontaneous intracerebral hemorrhage (ICH) and aneurysmal subarachnoid hemorrhage (SAH). The continued high morbidity and mortality of these two illnesses have spurred a multidisciplinary approach to their management.

Management of spontaneous intracerebral hemorrhage

Intracerebral hemorrhage (ICH) is associated with the worst survival and functional outcomes of all varieties of cerebrovascular diseases [5]. The mortality rate associated with this form of stroke has been reported to be as high as 40%. Furthermore, most ICH survivors never regain functional independence [5]. Although guidelines for the management of spontaneous ICH were developed and released by a Special Writing Group of the American Heart Association in 1999 attempting to set the framework for the care of ICH patients [6], the treatment of ICH victims remains less than uniform. Additionally, the highly anticipated results of a large, prospective, randomized trial comparing the two main forms of therapy for this disease, medical and surgical, have recently become available [7].

Clinical studies identifying early predictors of outcomes after ICH have consistently found intraparenchymal blood clot volume to be independently and directly associated with 30-day survival. Tuhrim and coworkers [8] have reported an exponential increase in mortality when intraparenchymal clot volumes exceed 30 cm^3. Conceivably, the reduced survival associated with this volume cutoff derives from early elevations in intracranial pressure, mass effect, or herniation syndromes. Also, the magnitude of the perihematoma edema that develops following ICH has been repeatedly found to be in direct association with the volume of ICH. Perihematoma edema has been correlated with the delayed peak of neurologic deterioration after ICH reported by Zazulia and coworkers [9]. Although several other outcome-modifying clinical variables are well recognized (eg, admission Glasgow Coma Scale, pulse pressure, hydrocephalus) [10], the impact of perihematomal brain edema on the early and late neurologic outcome of ICH patients is less clear. Plausible mechanisms of neurologic deterioration following the development of perihematomal edema are (1) direct mass effect introduced by perihematomal edema compromising regional perfusion and increasing intracranial pressure, and (2) cascade of secondary neuronal dysfunction triggered by blood and degradation products (hemotoxicity) with potential reversibly or irreversibly to alter brain function [9,11]. Unfortunately, directed therapies for ICH-induced brain edema are lacking. It has been only recently (when thrombolytic agents were used locally to lyse intraparenchymal hematoma in animal models of ICH) that an efficient reduction in the volume of perihematomal edema has been reported [12]. Okuda and coworkers [13] have also suggested a positive effect of early hematoma removal on perihematomal edema formation in a heterogeneously treated cohort of ICH patients. Similarly, Mayer and coworkers [14] demonstrated an association between hematoma size and volume of perihematoma edema. Although the relative safety of using local thrombolysis in different clinical paradigms of acute brain injury (SAH, ICH, ischemic stroke) is well documented, experimental data suggesting that parenchymal clot lysis using thrombolytic agents potentiate brain edema formation and induce direct neurotoxicity have raised concern [15–18].

As early as in 1961, the interest in identifying best treatment options for ICH victims was evident when McKissock and coworkers [19] conducted a seminal clinical trial comparing craniotomy for hematoma evacuation versus best medical therapy alone in this patient group, without statistical success. Although methodologic difficulties with this and other early clinical trials make their results difficult to extrapolate to contemporary ICH patients, application of meta-analysis techniques has spurred inclusion and reanalysis of such data. In 2000, Fernandes and coworkers [20] reported on the meta-analysis including all available clinical trials performed since the initial study by McKissock. The authors identified seven trials of enough homogeneity in their design to permit inclusion for statistical testing. Two well-defined periods were used to stratify the trials, before and after available diagnostic CT technology. Meta-analysis of all seven trials showed a trend toward a higher chance of death and dependency following surgery (odds ratio [OR] 1.2; 95% confidence interval [CI], 0.83–1.74). When the analysis was restricted to modern-day, post-CT, and inclusion of only well-constructed and balanced trials, a trend toward reduced death and dependency in the surgical group remained (OR 0.63; 95% CI, 0.35–1.14). In 2006, Teernstra and coworkers [21] reported on their updated meta-analysis of available clinical trials studying therapies for ICH. Two fundamental contributions were made with this renewed effort: the methodologic criteria list was tailored specifically for this form of disease and related treatment interventions; and this meta-analysis was a more contemporary effort that included trials that followed the report from Fernandes and coworkers [20] from 2000, including the most recent randomized clinical trial lead by Mendelow and coworkers [7], the International Surgical Treatment for Intracerebral Hemorrhage (ISTICH) trial. The overall analysis based on these trials (total of 1258 patients) failed to show a statistically significant effect between the two therapies in reducing the odds of death or independency following ICH. Nevertheless, their subgroup analysis of stereotactic surgery showed a statistically significant effect for reducing mortality (OR 0.29; 95% CI, 0.14–0.59) and death and dependency (OR 0.48; 95% CI, 0.24–0.96) compared with nonsurgical intervention.

The long existing controversy about the "best treatment" for ICH patients remains unresolved. Significant progress has been made, however, in understanding the pathophysiologic mechanisms of brain injury triggered by the interaction between brain tissue and blood, such as neuronal inflammation, vasogenic brain edema, and apoptosis, all in direct association with the amount of blood released in brain tissue. Mechanical injury inflicted by the parenchymal clots is, although likely important, only one of the many clinical challenges these patients pose to the neurointensivist. The available clinical information gathered during the last four decades and recent experimental evidence demonstrating neuronal injury following ICH have allowed clinicians to conclude that clot-tissue interaction following ICH should be minimized. Hematoma evacuation by craniotomy as a standard therapy for all ICH patients is not supported by clinical trials, as confirmed by the recent ISTICH study. Nevertheless, these trials have helped identify the following areas of promising clinical research: (1) the study of surgical treatment effects on ICH patients stratified by location (eg, deep versus superficial); and (2) the role of minimally invasive procedures for hematoma evacuation following ICH (eg, stereotactic hematoma aspiration and thrombolysis). These studies are ongoing. Best medical therapy always remains standard.

Management of nontraumatic subarachnoid hemorrhage

Many aspects of care in patients with aneurysmal SAH remain highly controversial and warrant further resolution with hypothesis-driven clinical or translational research [22]. To provide appropriate care, clinicians must understand current theories for optimal treatment of the ruptured aneurysm and the management of vasospasm related to aneurysmal SAH.

To clip or to coil

Surgical clipping is considered the definitive therapy for the ruptured aneurysm and continues to be considered the gold standard. When neuroradiologic endovascular coiling was in the early development stages of clinical practice, the procedure was primarily considered as an alternative to surgery only in patients deemed poor surgical candidates because of medical comorbidities, high Hunt and Hess grade, or anticipated difficulty with surgery [23]. The International Subarachnoid Aneurysm Trial (ISAT), a multicenter, randomized study of endovascular coiling versus surgical clipping conducted in 2143 patients with aneurysmal SAH who were deemed suitable for either therapy, brought to light the fact that endovascular coiling was not merely an alternative to surgical clipping, but in several cases the treatment of choice. Most of the aneurysms treated in this study were anterior circulation aneurysms less than 10 mm in size. At 1 year, endovascular coiling was associated with dependency or death in 23.5% of patients compared with 30.9% in the surgical group, a relative risk reduction of 22.6% ($P < .001$). This benefit was sustained despite the nonprocedural rebleeding risk within 1 year of 40 recurrent SAH (with 22 deaths) in the endovascular group, which was higher than the surgical group [24,25]. An ISAT trial update based on 3258 patient-years of follow-up after the first year for the endovascular group and 3107 patient-years of follow-up for the neurosurgical group, with a mean follow-up of 4 years, showed a sustained benefit of coiling over clipping with cumulative 7-year mortality curves showing more deaths in the surgical group compared with coiling. This was despite the fact that the risk of recurrent SAH was higher in patients randomized to coiling compared with clipping. In addition, a higher risk for seizures and poor cognitive outcomes was observed in the surgical group.

Despite the results of the ISAT trial, the controversy regarding the optimal treatment of the ruptured aneurysm remains. Because very large, wide-necked, and complex multilobulated aneurysms were by and large excluded from ISAT because of consensus opinion at the time that such patients were better surgical candidates, the results of the ISAT trial do not apply to their treatment. Also, with respect to aneurysm location, coiling was considered the superior modality for securing posterior circulation aneurysms, as were patients with middle cerebral artery (MCA) aneurysms considered better surgical candidates. The ISAT trial did not address these aneurysms in sufficient numbers to draw any conclusion regarding the ideal treatment based on those locations. The low rates of randomization of eligible patients and the higher than expected morbidity in the surgically treated group represent some of the other flaws of the study.

Given the definitive nature of surgical clipping of the aneurysm, the definition of the appropriate follow-up duration posttreatment to compare outcomes is especially difficult because it relates to younger patients with a longer life expectancy. In another study [26] that reported clinical (mean, 19.1 months) and angiographic (mean, 11.6 months) data in 83 patients with SAH treated with endovascular coils, good neurologic outcomes were seen in 77% of patients. But of concern, 26% of patients had a dog-ear remnant, 35% had a residual aneurysm neck, and 3% had residual aneurysm filling. Two or more coiling procedures were required in as many as 34% of patients.

Another important issue not addressed in the ISAT trial was the influence of surgical or endovascular treatment on the prevalence of cerebral ischemic complications. Results from various nonrandomized comparisons of the association of surgery and endovascular therapy of ruptured aneurysms on the rate of symptomatic vasospasm were varied, ranging from a slightly higher rate of vasospasm [27,28] among surgically treated patients to a higher rate of cerebral infarction in patients receiving endovascular compared with surgical therapy [29], whereas still other studies showed no significant difference [30–32].

Summarily, the current available data suggest the relative benefit of endovascular coiling over surgical clipping in small (< 10 mm) aneurysms in the anterior circulation (excluding MCA aneurysms). The experience of the neurosurgeon or the neurointerventional expert is likely to play a major role in the outcomes associated with the procedure and further follow-up data from the ISAT trial are awaited to determine if the stability of the coil is time related and if the benefit of coiling is truly sustained. Despite the ISAT trial, the optimal treatment modality for ruptured aneurysms remains controversial.

Management of vasospasm: when and how to treat

Vasospasm of large arteries in the circle of Willis is a significant determinant of cerebral ischemia after SAH and carries a 15% to 20% risk of stroke or death. Four-vessel cerebral digital subtraction angiography is the gold standard for diagnosing vasospasm, but given the inherent risks and the time and resources required for this procedure, alternative diagnostic tools have been proposed [33].

Transcranial Doppler (TCD) is an ultrasound-based monitor that can be readily used at the bedside to measure cerebral blood flow velocities (CBFV), which correlate with vasospasm and could be repeated as needed, enabling trend analysis [34]. There is debate, however, about the correlation between increased TCD flow velocities and angiographic and clinically significant or symptomatic vasospasm. Although mean MCA CBFV greater than 200 cm/s accurately predict angiographic vasospasm, velocities in the 120 to 200 cm/s range have a far lower predictive value [35]. Also of note, TCD is not as reliable in estimating distal MCA vasospasm compared with the more proximal portions of the MCA [36]. The validity of TCD in diagnosing angiographic vasospasm was summarized in a recent systematic review [37]. For the MCA, sensitivity of TCD was 67% and specificity was 99%, with a positive predictive value of 97% and negative predictive value of 78%. The accuracy of TCD was considerably less for detecting spasm in vessels other than the MCA. Hyperemia secondary to hypervolemia can also elevate measured blood flow velocities and create a false impression of worsening vasospasm based on CBFV measured using TCD. The Lindegaard index overcomes this limitation by computing the ratio of absolute CBFV in the insonated vessel and the ipsilateral extracranial carotid artery [38]. An index greater than 3 is strongly predictive of angiographic vasospasm; however, this methodology continues to have its detractors.

The principal therapy for treating delayed cerebral ischemia is hemodynamic augmentation or "triple-H" therapy (hypertension, hypervolemia, and hemodilution). Several uncontrolled studies have substantiated the clinical efficacy of hemodynamic augmentation in ameliorating vasospasm, and based on these studies and subsequent clinical experience with this method, its use in the setting of vasospasm is considered the standard of care [39–41].

The use of triple-H therapy before vasospasm as a prophylactic method, however, is controversial. Lennihan and coworkers [42] randomly assigned 82 aneurysmal SAH patients on the day after aneurysm clipping to receive albumin fluid boluses titrated to normal or high central venous and pulmonary artery diastolic pressures. The higher cardiac filling pressures were not associated with any significant change in cerebral blood flow (as measured by xenon CT) or cerebral blood volume, nor were there any differences in the rate of symptomatic vasospasm, cerebral infarction, or 3-month Glasgow Outcome Scale. In a study of 32 aneurysmal SAH patients randomized to hypertensive-hypervolemic versus normotensive-normovolemic management protocols, Egge and coworkers [43] reported no difference in vasospasm rates, cerebral blood flow as measured by single-photon emission CT, or 1-year Glasgow Outcome Scale, whereas a higher rate of complications (hemorrhage, coagulopathy, congestive heart failure) was noted in the hypertensive-hypervolemic group. In a systematic review, no significant effect of prophylactic triple-H therapy on the rate of symptomatic vasospasm, delayed ischemic neurologic deficit, or death was noted and a Cochrane meta-analysis reached a similar conclusion [44,45].

More recently, alternative approaches to treating vasospasm have emerged. An argument can be made for the use of cardiac output augmentation as opposed to traditional triple-H therapy. In a recent study, xenon CT was used to evaluate cerebral blood flow in 16 patients with symptomatic vasospasm who underwent volume expansion combined with either mean arterial pressure augmentation with phenylephrine or cardiac output augmentation with dobutamine. The increase in mean cerebral blood flow was similar in both groups. In another study, dobutamine was administered in combination with hypervolemic preload enhancement to 23 patients with vasospasm whose neurologic examination failed to improve after preload enhancement alone. The authors noted a 52% increase in cardiac index, and clinical reversal of ischemic symptoms was evident in 18 of the 23 patients [46].

The more recent development in the use of endovascular therapies for patients with cerebral vasospasm including transluminal balloon angioplasty and the intra-arterial delivery of vasodilating compounds brings into question whether these techniques should be considered as possible first-line options for treatment of clinically significant vasospasm, or if their use should be restricted to patients with symptomatic vasospasm that has been refractory to triple-H therapy [47]. Anecdotal evidence of the use of intra-aortic balloon counter pulsation in patients with delayed cerebral ischemia adds yet another option in the management of vasospasm [48–52].

A randomized trial comparing immediate angioplasty or intra-aortic balloon counter pulsation with triple-H therapy is needed to define the ideal management of delayed cerebral ischemia in patients who have developed symptomatic vasospasm.

Summary

Neurocritical care has come of age, and represents a multidisciplinary approach with neurologists, neurosurgeons, radiologists, and trained subspecialty intensivists who collectively and comprehensively manage the most critically ill neuroscience patients. The central figure that has emerged is the neurointensivist, who directly oversees the patient environment in the neuroscience ICU. The improvement in the outcome of such patients has been supported by several studies in the literature. Continued gains in medical treatment of such pathologies as stroke, traumatic head injury, neuro-oncology, and neuromuscular disease seem forthcoming as attentive and knowledgeable critical care is brought to the ICU bedside. Current diagnoses of SAH and ICH continue to spark controversy as major clinical trials are being completed that assess whether medical versus surgical or interventional radiologic intervention offer the patient the best possible treatment outcome.

References

[1] Diringer MN, Edwards DF. Admission to a neurologic/neurosurgical intensive care unit is associated with reduced mortality rate after intracerebral hemorrhage. Crit Care Med 2001;29:635–40.
[2] Mirski MA, Chang CW, Cowan R. Impact of a neuroscience intensive care unit on neurosurgical patient outcomes and cost of care: evidence-based support for an intensivist-directed specialty ICU model of care. J Neurosurg Anesthesiol 2001;13:83–92.
[3] Suarez JL. Outcome in neurocritical care: advances in monitoring and treatment and effect of a specialized neurocritical care team. Crit Care Med 2006;34(Suppl 9):S232–8.
[4] Varelas PN, Eastwood D, Yun HJ, et al. Impact of a neurointensivist on outcomes in patients with head trauma treated in a neurosciences intensive care unit. J Neurosurg 2006;104:713–9.
[5] Dennis MS. Outcome after brain haemorrhage. Cerebrovasc Dis 2003;16(Suppl 1):9–13.
[6] Broderick JP, Adams HP Jr, Barsan W, et al. Guidelines for the management of spontaneous intracerebral hemorrhage: a statement for healthcare professionals from a special writing group of the Stroke Council, American Heart Association. Stroke 1999;30:905–15.

[7] Mendelow AD, Gregson BA, Fernandes HM, et al. Early surgery versus initial conservative treatment in patients with spontaneous supratentorial intracerebral haematomas in the International Surgical Trial in Intracerebral Haemorrhage (STICH): a randomised trial. Lancet 2005;365:387–97.

[8] Tuhrim S, Horowitz DR, Sacher M, et al. Validation and comparison of models predicting survival following intracerebral hemorrhage. Crit Care Med 1995;23:950–4.

[9] Zazulia AR, Diringer MN, Derdeyn CP, et al. Progression of mass effect after intracerebral hemorrhage. Stroke 1999;30:1167–73.

[10] Tuhrim S, Horowitz DR, Sacher M, et al. Volume of ventricular blood is an important determinant of outcome in supratentorial intracerebral hemorrhage. Crit Care Med 1999;27: 617–21.

[11] Xi G, Keep RF, Hoff JT. Mechanisms of brain injury after intracerebral haemorrhage. Lancet Neurol 2006;5:53–63.

[12] Wagner KR, Xi G, Hua Y, et al. Ultra-early clot aspiration after lysis with tissue plasminogen activator in a porcine model of intracerebral hemorrhage: edema reduction and blood-brain barrier protection. J Neurosurg 1999;90:491–8.

[13] Okuda M, Suzuki R, Moriya M, et al. The effect of hematoma removal for reducing the development of brain edema in cases of putaminal hemorrhage. Acta Neurochir (Wien) 2006;96:74–7.

[14] Mayer SA, Brun NC, Begtrup K, et al. Recombinant activated factor VII for acute intracerebral hemorrhage. N Engl J Med 2005;352:777–85.

[15] Figueroa BE, Keep RF, Betz AL, et al. Plasminogen activators potentiate thrombin-induced brain injury. Stroke 1998;29:1202–7.

[16] Lapointe M, Haines S. Fibrinolytic therapy for intraventricular hemorrhage in adults. Cochrane Database Syst Rev 2002:CD003692.

[17] Rohde V, Rohde I, Thiex R, et al. Fibrinolysis therapy achieved with tissue plasminogen activator and aspiration of the liquefied clot after experimental intracerebral hemorrhage: rapid reduction in hematoma volume but intensification of delayed edema formation. J Neurosurg 2002;97:954–62.

[18] Yepes M, Sandkvist M, Moore EG, et al. Tissue-type plasminogen activator induces opening of the blood-brain barrier via the LDL receptor-related protein. J Clin Invest 2003;112: 1533–40.

[19] McKissock W, Richardson A, Taylor J. Primary intracerebral haemorrhage: a controlled trial of surgical and conservative treatment in 180 unselected cases. Lancet 1961;2:221–6.

[20] Fernandes HM, Gregson B, Siddique S, et al. Surgery in intracerebral hemorrhage: the uncertainty continues. Stroke 2000;31:2511–6.

[21] Teernstra OP, Evers SM, Kessels AH. Meta analyses in treatment of spontaneous supratentorial intracerebral haematoma. Acta Neurochir (Wien) 2006;148:521–8.

[22] Naval NS, Stevens RD, Mirski MA, et al. Controversies in the management of aneurysmal subarachnoid hemorrhage. Crit Care Med 2006;34:511–24.

[23] Guglielmi G, Vinuela F, Duckwiler G, et al. Endovascular treatment of posterior circulation aneurysms by electrothrombosis using electrically detachable coils. J Neurosurg 1992;77: 515–24.

[24] Molyneux A, Kerr R, Stratton I, et al. International Subarachnoid Aneurysm Trial (ISAT) of neurosurgical clipping versus endovascular coiling in 2143 patients with ruptured intracranial aneurysms: a randomised trial. Lancet 2002;360:1267–74.

[25] Molyneux AJ, Kerr RS, Yu LM, et al. International subarachnoid aneurysm trial (ISAT) of neurosurgical clipping versus endovascular coiling in 2143 patients with ruptured intracranial aneurysms: a randomised comparison of effects on survival, dependency, seizures, rebleeding, subgroups, and aneurysm occlusion. Lancet 2005;366:809–17.

[26] Friedman JA, Nichols DA, Meyer FB, et al. Guglielmi detachable coil treatment of ruptured saccular cerebral aneurysms: retrospective review of a 10-year single-center experience. AJNR Am J Neuroradiol 2003;24:526–33.

[27] Groden C, Kremer C, Regelsberger J, et al. Comparison of operative and endovascular treatment of anterior circulation aneurysms in patients in poor grades. Neuroradiology 2001;43:778–83.

[28] Rabinstein AA, Pichelmann MA, Friedman JA, et al. Symptomatic vasospasm and outcomes following aneurysmal subarachnoid hemorrhage: a comparison between surgical repair and endovascular coil occlusion. J Neurosurg 2003;98:319–25.

[29] Gruber A, Ungersbock K, Reinprecht A, et al. Evaluation of cerebral vasospasm after early surgical and endovascular treatment of ruptured intracranial aneurysms. Neurosurgery 1998;42:258–67.

[30] Charpentier C, Audibert G, Guillemin F, et al. Multivariate analysis of predictors of cerebral vasospasm occurrence after aneurysmal subarachnoid hemorrhage. Stroke 1999;30:1402–8.

[31] Dehdashti AR, Mermillod B, Rufenacht DA, et al. Does treatment modality of intracranial ruptured aneurysms influence the incidence of cerebral vasospasm and clinical outcome? Cerebrovasc Dis 2004;17:53–60.

[32] Goddard AJ, Raju PP, Gholkar A. Does the method of treatment of acutely ruptured intracranial aneurysms influence the incidence and duration of cerebral vasospasm and clinical outcome? J Neurol Neurosurg Psychiatry 2004;75:868–72.

[33] Cloft HJ, Joseph GJ, Dion JE. Risk of cerebral angiography in patients with subarachnoid hemorrhage, cerebral aneurysm, and arteriovenous malformation: a meta-analysis. Stroke 1999;30:317–20.

[34] Aaslid R, Huber P, Nornes H. Evaluation of cerebrovascular spasm with transcranial Doppler ultrasound. J Neurosurg 1984;60:37–41.

[35] Vora YY, Suarez-Almazor M, Steinke DE, et al. Role of transcranial Doppler monitoring in the diagnosis of cerebral vasospasm after subarachnoid hemorrhage. Neurosurgery 1999;44:1237–47.

[36] Okada Y, Shima T, Nishida M, et al. Comparison of transcranial Doppler investigation of aneurysmal vasospasm with digital subtraction angiographic and clinical findings. Neurosurgery 1999;45:443–9.

[37] Lysakowski C, Walder B, Costanza MC, et al. Transcranial Doppler versus angiography in patients with vasospasm due to a ruptured cerebral aneurysm: a systematic review. Stroke 2001;32:2292–8.

[38] Lindegaard KF, Nornes H, Bakke SJ, et al. Cerebral vasospasm after subarachnoid haemorrhage investigated by means of transcranial Doppler ultrasound. Acta Neurochir Suppl (Wien) 1988;42:81–4.

[39] Awad IA, Carter LP, Spetzler RF, et al. Clinical vasospasm after subarachnoid hemorrhage: response to hypervolemic hemodilution and arterial hypertension. Stroke 1987;18:365–72.

[40] Giannotta SL, McGillicuddy JE, Kindt GW. Diagnosis and treatment of postoperative cerebral vasospasm. Surg Neurol 1977;8:286–90.

[41] Kosnik EJ, Hunt WE. Postoperative hypertension in the management of patients with intracranial arterial aneurysms. J Neurosurg 1976;45:148–54.

[42] Lennihan L, Mayer SA, Fink ME, et al. Effect of hypervolemic therapy on cerebral blood flow after subarachnoid hemorrhage: a randomized controlled trial. Stroke 2000;31:383–91.

[43] Egge A, Waterloo K, Sjoholm H, et al. Prophylactic hyperdynamic postoperative fluid therapy after aneurysmal subarachnoid hemorrhage: a clinical, prospective, randomized, controlled study. Neurosurgery 2001;49:593–605.

[44] Rinkel GJ, Feigin VL, Algra A, et al. Circulatory volume expansion therapy for aneurysmal subarachnoid haemorrhage. Cochrane Database Syst Rev 2004:CD000483.

[45] Treggiari MM, Walder B, Suter PM, et al. Systematic review of the prevention of delayed ischemic neurological deficits with hypertension, hypervolemia, and hemodilution therapy following subarachnoid hemorrhage. J Neurosurg 2003;98:978–84.

[46] Levy ML, Rabb CH, Zelman V, et al. Cardiac performance enhancement from dobutamine in patients refractory to hypervolemic therapy for cerebral vasospasm. J Neurosurg 1993;79:494–9.

[47] Morgan MK, Jonker B, Finfer S, et al. Aggressive management of aneurysmal subarachnoid haemorrhage based on a papaverine angioplasty protocol. J Clin Neurosci 2000;7:305–8.

[48] Apostolides PJ, Greene KA, Zabramski JM, et al. Intra-aortic balloon pump counterpulsation in the management of concomitant cerebral vasospasm and cardiac failure after subarachnoid hemorrhage: technical case report. Neurosurgery 1996;38:1056–9.

[49] Nussbaum ES, Sebring LA, Ganz WF, et al. Intra-aortic balloon counterpulsation augments cerebral blood flow in the patient with cerebral vasospasm: a xenon-enhanced computed tomography study. Neurosurgery 1998;42:206–13.

[50] Montessuit M, Chevalley C, King J, et al. The use of intra-aortic counterpulsation balloon for the treatment of cerebral vasospasm and edema. Surgery 2000;127:230–3.

[51] Rosen CL, Sekhar LN, Duong DH. Use of intra-aortic balloon pump counterpulsation for refractory symptomatic vasospasm. Acta Neurochir (Wien) 2000;142:25–32.

[52] Spann RG, Lang DA, Birch AA, et al. Intra-aortic balloon counterpulsation: augmentation of cerebral blood flow after aneurysmal subarachnoid haemorrhage. Acta Neurochir (Wien) 2001;143:115–23.

ELSEVIER
SAUNDERS

Anesthesiology Clin
25 (2007) 687

ANESTHESIOLOGY
CLINICS

Erratum

In the June 2007 issue of *Anesthesiology Clinics*, Fig. 1 on page 5 in the article "Virtual Reality Simulations" should have been credited to the Electronic Visualization Lab at the University of Illinois at Chicago. We apologize for this oversight. The figure, legend, and proper attribution appear below.

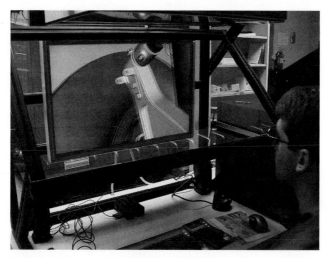

Fig. 1. The ImmersaDesk4 system is suitable for high-fidelity desktop simulations (*Courtesy of* Electronic Visualization Lab, University of Illinois at Chicago).

doi:10.1016/j.anclin.2007.06.004

ELSEVIER
SAUNDERS

Anesthesiology Clin
25 (2007) 689–698

ANESTHESIOLOGY
CLINICS

Index

Note: Page numbers of article titles are in **boldface** type.

1932-2275/07/$ - see front matter © 2007 Elsevier Inc. All rights reserved.
doi:10.1016/S1932-2275(07)00084-5
anesthesiology.theclinics.com

Moving?

Make sure your subscription moves with you!

To notify us of your new address, find your **Clinics Account Number** (located on your mailing label above your name), and contact customer service at:

E-mail: elspcs@elsevier.com

800-654-2452 (subscribers in the U.S. & Canada)
407-345-4000 (subscribers outside of the U.S. & Canada)

Fax number: 407-363-9661

Elsevier Periodicals Customer Service
6277 Sea Harbor Drive
Orlando, FL 32887-4800

*To ensure uninterrupted delivery of your subscription, please notify us at least 4 weeks in advance of move.